Fundamentals of

Person-Centred Healthcare Practice

Fundamentals of
Person-Centred Healthcare Practice

EDITED BY

Brendan McCormack
Queen Margaret University
Edinburgh, UK

Tanya McCance
Ulster University
Northern Ireland, UK

Cathy Bulley
Queen Margaret University
Edinburgh, UK

Donna Brown
Ulster University
Northern Ireland, UK

Ailsa McMillan
Queen Margaret University
Edinburgh, UK

Suzanne Martin
Ulster University
Northern Ireland, UK

WILEY Blackwell

Registered Office(s)
John Wiley & Sons, Inc., 111 River Street, Hoboken, NJ 07030, USA
John Wiley & Sons Ltd, The Atrium, Southern Gate, Chichester, West Sussex, PO19 8SQ, UK

Editorial Office
9600 Garsington Road, Oxford, OX4 2DQ, UK

For details of our global editorial offices, customer services, and more information about Wiley products visit us at www.wiley.com.

Wiley also publishes its books in a variety of electronic formats and by print-on-demand. Some content that appears in standard print versions of this book may not be available in other formats.

Library of Congress Cataloging-in-Publication Data

Names: McCormack, Brendan, editor.
Title: Fundamentals of Person-Centred Healthcare Practice. / [edited by] Brendan McCormack, Tanya McCance, Cathy Bulley, Donna Brown, Ailsa McMillan, Suzanne Martin.
Description: First edition. | Hoboken, NJ : Wiley-Blackwell, 2020. | Includes bibliographical references and index.
Identifiers: LCCN 2020024722 (print) | LCCN 2020024723 (ebook) | ISBN 9781119533085 (paperback) | ISBN 9781119533092 (adobe pdf) | ISBN 9781119533023 (epub)
Subjects: MESH: Patient-Centered Care | Personhood
Classification: LCC R727.3 (print) | LCC R727.3 (ebook) | NLM W 84.7 | DDC 610.69/6–dc23
LC record available at https://lccn.loc.gov/2020024722
LC ebook record available at https://lccn.loc.gov/2020024723

Cover Design: Wiley
Cover Image: © Tim Bird/Getty Images

Set in 9.5/12pt Myriad Pro by SPi Global, Pondicherry, India
Printed and bound by CPI Group (UK) Ltd, Croydon, CR0 4YY

C9781119533085_210824

We dedicate this book to all the persons we have worked with and learned from over the many years of practice, teaching and research. We are indebted to all of you for reminding us to 'always be curious'

Contents

List of contributors

Deborah Baldie
NHS Tayside and Queen Margaret University, Edinburgh, Scotland, UK

David Banks
Queen Margaret University, Edinburgh, Scotland, UK

Owen Barr
Ulster University, Northern Ireland, UK

Derek Barron
Erskine, Bishopton, Scotland, UK

Christine Boomer
Ulster University, Northern Ireland, UK
and
South Eastern Health and Social Care Trust

Donna Brown
Ulster University, Northern Ireland, UK

Robert Brown
Western Health and Social Care Trust, Derry, Northern Ireland, UK

Cathy Bulley
Queen Margaret University, Edinburgh, Scotland, UK

Vivien Coates
Ulster University, Northern Ireland, UK
and
Western Health and Social Care Trust, Londonderry, Northern Ireland, UK

Martina Conway
Health Service Executive, Letterkenny, Republic of Ireland

Neal F. Cook
Ulster University, Northern Ireland, UK

Jean Daly Lynn
Ulster University, Northern Ireland, UK

Jessica Davidson
NHS Lothian and Queen Margaret University, Edinburgh, Scotland, UK

Jan Dewing
Queen Margaret University, Edinburgh, Scotland, UK

Caroline Dickson
Queen Margaret University, Edinburgh, Scotland, UK

Michelle L. Elliot
Queen Margaret University, Edinburgh, Scotland, UK

Ailsa Espie
Queen Margaret University, Edinburgh, Scotland, UK

Caroline Gibson
Queen Margaret University, Edinburgh, Scotland, UK

Patricia Gillen
Southern Health and Social Care Trust
and
Ulster University, Northern Ireland, UK

Jackie Gracey
Ulster University, Northern Ireland, UK

Erna Haraldsdottir
Queen Margaret University, Edinburgh, Scotland, UK
and
St Columba's Hospice, Edinburgh, Scotland, UK

Lindesay Irvine
Queen Margaret University, Edinburgh, Scotland, UK

Dawn Jansch
Queen Margaret University, Edinburgh, Scotland, UK
and
Western General Hospital, Edinburgh Scotland, UK

Ed Jesudason
NHS Lothian, Edinburgh, Scotland, UK

Fiona Kelly
Queen Margaret University, Edinburgh, Scotland, UK

Antonia Lannie
University of Dundee, Dundee, Scotland, UK

Bill Lawson
Queen Margaret University, Edinburgh, Scotland, UK

Lisa Luhanga
Queen Margaret University, Edinburgh, Scotland, UK

Brighide Lynch
Ulster University, Northern Ireland, UK

Jacinta Lynch
Milesian Manor Lifestyle Care Home, Magherafelt, Northern Ireland, UK

Kath MacDonald
Queen Margaret University, Edinburgh, Scotland, UK

Honor MacGregor
NHS Tayside and Queen Margaret University, Edinburgh, Scotland, UK

Fiona Maclean
Queen Margaret University, Edinburgh, Scotland, UK

Suzanne Martin
Ulster University, Northern Ireland, UK

Ruth Magowan
Queen Margaret University, Edinburgh, Scotland, UK

Charlotte McArdle
Department of Health, Belfast, Northern Ireland, UK

Tanya McCance
Ulster University, Northern Ireland, UK

Brendan McCormack
Queen Margaret University, Edinburgh, Scotland, UK

Sonyia McFadden
Ulster University, Northern Ireland, UK

Brian McGowan
Ulster University, Northern Ireland, UK

Lesley McKinlay
Queen Margaret University, Edinburgh, Scotland, UK

Ailsa McMillan
Queen Margaret University, Edinburgh, Scotland, UK

Vidar Melby
Ulster University, Northern Ireland, UK

Kevin Moore
Ulster University, Northern Ireland, UK

Kristina Mountain
Queen Margaret University, Edinburgh, Scotland, UK

Deirdre O'Donnell
Ulster University, Northern Ireland, UK

Lorna Peelo-Kilroe
Health Service Executive, Dublin, Republic of Ireland

Duncan Pentland
Queen Margaret University, Edinburgh, Scotland, UK

Lucia Ramsey
Ulster University, Northern Ireland, UK

Lindsey Regan
University of Central Lancashire, Preston, UK

Helen Riddell
Queen Margaret University, Edinburgh, Scotland, UK

Assumpta Ryan
Ulster University, Northern Ireland, UK

Josianne Scerri
University of Malta and Kingston
and
St George's Medical School, University of London

Margaret Smith
Queen Margaret University, Edinburgh, Scotland, UK

Juliet Spiller
Marie Curie Hospice, Edinburgh, Scotland, UK

Amanda Stears
Queen Margaret University, Edinburgh, Scotland, UK

Fiona Stuart
University of the West of Scotland, Paisley, Scotland, UK

Karl Tizzard-Kleister
Ulster University, Northern Ireland, UK

Angie Titchen
Independent Researcher and Transformative Facilitator
Activist/Eco-Warrior and
Critical-creative Companion

Savina Tropea
Queen Margaret University, Edinburgh, Scotland, UK

Georgios Tsigkas
Queen Margaret University, Edinburgh, Scotland, UK

Lynn Wallace
Queen Margaret University, Edinburgh, Scotland, UK

Catherine Wells
Ulster University, Northern Ireland, UK

Alison Williams
Queen Margaret University, Edinburgh, Scotland, UK
and
Parkinson's UK

Anne Williams
Queen Margaret University, Edinburgh, Scotland, UK

Foreword

The whole of this ground-consolidating, forward-looking book is far greater than the sum of its parts. Exquisitely designed and written, it builds on decades of rigorous research and scholarly inquiry in and on person-centred practice in healthcare in the UK and around the world. Individuals, teams, workplaces and some organisations have aspired to make this practice a reality. However, in recent years, person-centred practice has only become possible for 'moments' due to complex cultural and socio-political contextual reasons that have forced nursing, for example, to go back, almost full circle, to a 21st century version of 20th century task-focussed care. In the UK, these reasons include severe cost-cutting in the National Health Service, resulting in a lack of resources and time to build healthcare systems that support authentic, person-centred practice. Another reason, worldwide at this very moment, is the COVID-19 pandemic.

Writing this foreword, therefore, has been an emotional experience for me because I have been fortunate to play a small and exciting part in a worldwide movement that has enabled health and social care professionals to become person-centred practitioners, leaders, educators, facilitators, life-long-learners, practice developers and researchers. So for me, the 'whole' of this book that goes beyond the sum of its parts, is that it offers hope and a way for recovery towards authentic person-centred practice, at every level of healthcare. The way in this book is a lifelong learning adventure, so the book is crafted for pre-registration students, experienced practitioners, leaders, practice and systems innovators and all those in between. This means that we can dive into parts that are relevant to us as we become more person-centred and progress through our careers.

At the heart of the book is the dynamic Person-Centred Practice Framework, created and fine-tuned by Brendan and Tanya and tested by practitioners nationally and internationally. With an aesthetic minimalism, the theoretical framework reveals the macro context, prerequisites and person-centred processes that come together to create a desired outcome of a healthful culture in which receivers and givers of care flourish.

As if a piece of music, the book weaves the Framework through a four-part structure that enables chapter authors to improvise their unique contribution to the whole. Concepts and constructs of the framework, set out in the first and second sections, flow and harmonise through the third and fourth that are concerned with person-centred practice in different health and social care contexts and facilitating learning and development respectively.

There is an interactive and unifying style of writing and design used by the many authors that lifts the book above being merely a linear textbook to the musical qualities of flow and integration. For example, authors show how the Framework interconnects and fits with the approaches, concepts, models or principles relevant to their professions, roles, service users, students, colleagues, service contexts or learning environments. They also speak directly to us readers as they offer a variety of reflexive, embodied, creative and imaginative activities (alone or with others). They enable us to engage with the whole of ourselves, as we dive into relevant concepts, constructs, dilemmas and challenges of knowing self as a person and active learner and being person-centred within a particular nuanced context. These activities are enriched by web links, clinical vignettes and discussions about what we might have uncovered. Further insights, strategies and practices are offered that we may not have reached ourselves, for instance, on how to reflect upon and re-appraise our practices, help our learning, develop and care for ourselves and create cultures of effectiveness in our workplaces.

So just as a piece of music can jolt us into our bodies and emotions and then being still and silent to go deeper into ourselves to reflect upon what matters to us, this book jolts us to examine issues in relation to our past, current and future practices as well as our ways of active learning, knowing, being and becoming. Thus, it can help us embody or internalise the Framework in our own being and practice.

I finish with a haiku that captures the most important thing for me about this book, at this time in our world's history. I wish you well. You are the future.

Singing the circle round

A call to action
Person-centredness for all
Human flourishing!

Decision-makers!
For moral healthcare systems
This book is a gift

Exemplar for all
Showing how to enculture
Person-centredness

Angie Titchen
July 2020

Acknowledgement

The editors are grateful to Sharon Middlemass for the help and support she provided to us in managing this project. Her attention to detail, unfailing persistence and good humour has enabled the project to be brought to fruition. We are eternally grateful.

Editor Biographies

Brendan McCormack DPhil (Oxon), BSc (Hons) Nursing, FRCN, FEANS, FRCSI, PGCEA, RMN, RGN, FAAN

Professor Brendan McCormack is Head of the Division of Nursing, Occupational Therapy and Art Therapies; Associate Director, Centre for Person-centred Practice Research, Queen Margaret University, Edinburgh, Scotland; and Honorary Nurse Consultant, Erskine Care, Scotland. He also holds adjunct professorial positions at universities in Ireland, Norway, Slovenia, South Africa, Austria, Denmark and Australia. His research has specifically focused on person-centred practice, and over a period of 22 years he has developed models, theories, frameworks and evaluation instruments that have been adopted globally in policy and practice. In addition, he has led the implementation and evaluation of person-centred practices in a variety of clinical settings and in healthcare curricula. Professor McCormack has particular expertise in gerontological nursing and the adoption of person-centred practices with older people.

Tanya McCance DPhil, MSc, BSc (Hons), RGN

Professor Tanya McCance has an international reputation in the development of person-centred practice through the use of participatory research approaches, such as practice development and action research. She has been a registered nurse since 1990 and throughout her career has held several joint posts between higher education institutions and health and social care providers, demonstrating her commitment to the integration of practice, education and research. She has developed a programme of work through engaged scholarship and research that is underpinned by the Person-centred Practice Framework, which is central to the impact of her research. Her most recent work focuses on the identification of a relevant and appropriate set of key performance indicators for nursing and midwifery that are indicative of person-centred care and the development of methods that will demonstrate the unique contribution of nursing to the patient experience. She has been recognised for her research contribution by inclusion in the *Nursing Times* Inspirational Nurse Leaders List (September 2015), was awarded the Nurse of the Year 2017 Outstanding Achievement Award, and was listed as one of 70 influential nurses and midwives in 70 years of the NHS. Tanya's contribution reflects her passion for nursing and her commitment to the development of person-centred practice that will enhance the care experience for patients and their families.

Cathy Bulley PhD, MCSP, SFHEA

Dr Cathy Bulley is a Reader in the School of Health Sciences at Queen Margaret University. She trained in Physiotherapy, and quickly developed a love of research, progressing to PhD studies within Queen Margaret University. Engaging in clinical practice reinforced her love of using research to advocate for people by exploring their experiences of health and healthcare, and Cathy returned to Queen Margaret University.

She is fascinated with the ways in which physiotherapy and other allied health professions enact person-centredness; how different ways of researching interact with person-centred principles; and with the way these concepts mesh with user-centred product design and innovation.

Donna Brown PhD, RN, MA, PGDipHP, PGCert

Donna is currently a Lecturer of Nursing, Postgraduate Tutor for the Institute of Nursing and Health Research and Course Director for the BSc(Hons)/PGDip/MSc Developing Practice in Healthcare Programme, in the School of Nursing, Ulster University. Having qualified as a registered general nurse, Donna has worked across many areas in healthcare and specialised in pain management. She initiated the Acute Pain Service at the Royal Victoria Hospital, Belfast, and was the lead nurse for pain services across the Belfast Health and Social Care Trust. Donna's commitment to developing nursing practice, education and research has been evident throughout her career. She has influenced the development of practice and education programmes both in terms of pain management and facilitating learning in practice.

Donna's work focuses on participatory research approaches, such as action research and practice development, working with teams and individuals to assist them in exploring the culture and context in which they work. She has a particular interest in person-centredness, pain management, knowledge utilisation, critical reflection, facilitation, learning in and from practice and older people.

Ailsa McMillan MSc, PGCert, Prof Ed, RGN

Ailsa McMillan is a senior lecturer in nursing within the Division of Nursing at Queen Margaret University. Her interests include neuroscience, rehabilitation, interdisciplinary practice and leadership while her curiosity is piqued by authenticity and pushing the boundaries of nursing education. Ailsa has been influential in the development of the pre-registration person-centred Masters of Nursing curriculum, engaging in collaborative and creative activities to bring this to fruition.

Suzanne Martin PhD

Suzanne Martin is Professor of Occupational Therapy and Head of School of Health Sciences at Ulster University. She is a Fellow of the College of Occupational Therapists UK and a panel member for the National Institute for Health Research. She is a trainer and contributor to the Cochrane Library and has served on Office Research Ethics Northern Ireland (ORECNI) and the National Institute for Health and Care Excellence (NICE).

Her research focus is on new and emerging technologies within Health and Social Care. Suzanne has successfully led a range of EU and nationally funded research projects to develop new devices and services to support people living with a disability at home.

Introduction

Tanya McCance[1], Brendan McCormack[2], Donna Brown[1], Cathy Bulley[2], Ailsa McMillan[2], and Suzanne Martin[1]

[1] Ulster University, Northern Ireland, UK

[2] Queen Margaret University, Edinburgh, Scotland, UK

Dear reader, welcome to our book on the fundamentals of person-centred practice. We are delighted to work with you through the chapters of this book to enable you to explore the essence of practice and to enhance your understanding of person-centredness within a wide variety of healthcare contexts. You might be a student starting out on your professional journey and excited to learn about your discipline; a newly qualified professional grappling with the realities of practice; an established practitioner or healthcare worker with many years of experience wanting to reaffirm your passion and commitment to trying to make a difference; or a leader aiming to harness a shared vision for your team or organisation that transcends day-to-day professional differences. Whilst we have framed this book in the context of the fundamentals of practice, we believe it has something to offer everyone, regardless of your healthcare discipline or where you might be on your career pathway. But why bother, you might ask, as person-centredness in healthcare has been a focus for many years and is now firmly embedded in the language of healthcare. However, it is our contention that despite a continuous focus on developing healthcare services and practices that place the person at the centre of decision making, the reality and rhetoric of practice are sometimes difficult to dissect!

Let's imagine that someone you love becomes very unwell and has to be admitted to hospital. As a professional, you will have an expectation of the kind of care you want them to experience and what's more, you will instinctively know when their care meets *your* standard. It might not always be clear what members of that healthcare team are doing that makes it a good experience, but it will feel right and you will feel your loved one is in safe hands. Now let's go to a place in your mind where your loved one is getting sicker and no-one seems to know what is happening, nor does there seem any sense of urgency to find out, and, worse still, it gives you a sense that no-one cares.

Understanding what makes the difference between these two scenarios and how you can improve the experience of care for everyone is at the heart of this book. If you want to make a difference to practice that ensures all service users and families have a positive experience of caree, and that you and other staff are also recognised as persons rather than cogs in a wheel, then this book is written for you!

Our desire for all service users and staff to experience person-centredness in their daily contact with healthcare systems may seem like idealism, given that no system is perfect. As a multiprofessional editorial team, we are highly aware that there are challenges in healthcare systems that impact on the development of person-centred workplace cultures. This book is grounded in the realities of practice and our aspiration is to offer a common language that will create a shared understanding of person-centred practice, in the hope that it will generate an impetus for practice change. A shared language is essential if we are to bring about system-wide change. Whilst person-centredness permeates healthcare strategy and policy, the reality is that often stakeholders aren't actually talking about the same thing. We also see this dilemma in the published literature with interchangeable use of terms such as family-centred, patient-centred and relationship-centred, leading to arguments that person-centredness is 'too difficult to define'.

Furthermore, we see this very issue reflected in the campaigns calling for a refocusing on compassion, caring and kindness. Whilst these are important values within healthcare systems, the challenge is how they manifest in our and other people's behaviours and the influence of attitudinal and moral factors. A shared language is the foundation that supports the development of a shared understanding of person-centred practice and the issues that need to be addressed in order to bring about sustainable change. At the level of principle, the understanding of person-centredness is well rehearsed and involves treating people as individuals, respecting their rights as persons, building mutual trust and understanding, and developing therapeutic relationships. Central to this is our explicit focus on all people as persons and the promotion of workplace cultures that promote the well-being of those providing as well as receiving services. This shared understanding, however, needs to be more than an emphasis on the commonly agreed principles that underpin person-centredness. There needs to be an understanding of how these principles can be implemented in practice in order to bring about a positive outcome, that being the development of healthful cultures that enable flourishing for all.

We believe this book offers a unique perspective on person-centredness viewed through the lens of the Person-centred Practice Framework of McCormack and McCance, which is a theoretical model developed from practice, for use in practice. The framework has evolved over two decades of research and development activity and has made a significant contribution globally to the landscape of person-centredness. Not only does it enable the articulation of the dynamic nature of person-centredness, recognising complexity at different levels in healthcare systems, but it offers a common language and a shared understanding of person-centred practice. The Person-centred Practice Framework is used in this book to illuminate the different components that make up person-centredness but, more importantly, how these different components connect to develop a deeper understanding of person-centred practice.

This book is presented in four sections, reflecting different constructs of the Person-centred Practice Framework. The first section focuses on the person in person-centred practice, respecting the centrality of all people as persons. The second section focuses on being person-centred and reflects the person-centred processes. The third section focuses on the many different contexts in which health and social care is delivered, not only recognising the practice context but also the organisational and system issues that can influence practice. The final section brings our focus back to how we equip the workforce to engage effectively in developing this agenda through approaches to learning and development for person-centred practice. Chapters 1–3 form a strong foundation to enhance engagement with the content of subsequent chapters, with Chapter 3 in particular serving as a reference for describing components of the Person-centred Practice Framework. The book, however, is structured in a way that will enable you as the reader to dip in and out as directed by your own learning needs. All the chapters are peppered with activities, encouraging you to reflect on your learning and supporting your development as a person-centred practitioner.

The many contributors to this book have shared their expertise freely and offer a wide range of interesting perspectives on person-centredness. As an editorial team, we are passionate and committed to developing person-centred cultures across health and social care systems, and our wish is that your engagement with the ideas in this book will help you grow as a person and as a healthcare professional. Person-centredness and person-centred practice are not static concepts. Richard Holloway asserted:

> We will go on producing myths, ways of explaining ourselves to ourselves but, like everything else about us, they are in constant transition and we must not fundamentalise any of them.
>
> (Holloway 2001)

It is important that we don't allow person-centredness to become static or fundamentalised. As persons, we are always in a state of becoming and thus, how we engage in person-centred practice also needs to be constantly explored, challenged, questioned and open to change. We hope this book makes an important contribution to that change-making, ensuring that we continue to challenge ourselves and others, as well as coming to know more effective ways of engaging so that all persons receiving healthcare have their personhood reinforced and are able to flourish as persons.

Reference

Holloway, R. (2001). *Doubts and Loves: What Is Left of Christianity*. Edinburgh: Canongate Books.

SECTION 1

The Person in Person-Centred Practice

The first section of this book will guide you through a brief philosophical history of the concepts person, personhood and self. The chapters include a number of activities that we would encourage you to participate in and which will inform your understanding of the concepts. The range of activities are designed to help you to reflect on your self and then to consider the influence you have on others and they on you. We hope you notice and experience the ongoing development of your understanding of your own personhood through critical reflection. This represents some of our beliefs and values that we are never the completed article as there is always capacity to construct new learning and understanding.

The first three chapters in this section of the book introduce you to the key concepts of person-centredness and person-centred practice. These are the foundation chapters that will guide your initial thinking and learning in relation to the different perspectives of what it means to be a person and how person-centredness and person-centred practice may be realised. The focus here is on the continuously evolving nature of person-centred practice. As part of your exploration and learning, you will be introduced to the Person-centred Practice Framework. This framework will be used as a lens to critically examine some of the challenges we face in contemporary healthcare as we try to operationalise person-centredness.

As you work through Chapter 1, you will learn who the person is and consider the importance of personhood and why it is essential to person-centred practice. Chapter 2 builds on notions of being a person and encourages you to explore the concepts and complexities of person-centred practice, paying particular attention to the core values of person-centredness. In Chapter 3, you will be introduced to the Person-centred Practice Framework and guided through its component parts and how it links to the key underpinning theoretical concepts described in Chapters 1 and 2.

Chapter 4 challenges us to explore self. You will be guided to consider different aspects of self and introduced to a variety of different approaches that can be used to know self better. This leads to exploring the concept of human flourishing in Chapter 5. The alignment with person-centred practice emerges as you engage with this chapter and the activities. We encourage you to take time to participate in the activities and reflect afterwards. Some of the activities

Fundamentals of Person-Centred Healthcare Practice, First Edition. Edited by Brendan McCormack, Tanya McCance, Cathy Bulley, Donna Brown, Ailsa McMillan and Suzanne Martin.

can be repeated at various times and we imagine you will become aware of your own development. Chapter 6 will enable you to make links between your practice, the required standards you need to demonstrate for professional practice and how professionalism contributes to person-centred practice. You will also explore the tensions that may exist between the reality of practice and delivering person-centred care. Finally, Chapter 7 examines the future nursing, midwifery and allied health professional in the context of person-centred practice.

1

The person in person-centred practice

Brendan McCormack[1], Tanya McCance[2], and Jan Dewing[1]

[1] *Queen Margaret University, Edinburgh, Scotland, UK*

[2] *Ulster University, Northern Ireland, UK*

Contents

Fundamentals of Person-Centred Healthcare Practice, First Edition. Edited by Brendan McCormack, Tanya McCance, Cathy Bulley, Donna Brown, Ailsa McMillan and Suzanne Martin.

Learning outcomes

- Develop insight into the meaning of 'person' in person-centred practice.
- Distinguish the meaning of 'person' from other concepts such as individual or people.
- Be able to articulate a meaning of personhood and why this meaning is important in person-centred practice.
- Identify and describe the challenges posed for healthcare practitioners when adopting different personhood perspectives

Introduction

Being a person means more than just existing as a human being. There are elements of our make-up as persons that we may struggle to understand or make sense of – the deeper parts of ourselves! In this chapter we will explore some perspectives on what it means to be a person as this is the starting point of person-centredness and person-centred practice.

Who am I?

There is a sense in which the word 'person' is merely the singular version of 'people', yet we are all instinctively aware that it has greater meaning than this – that it represents everything about me as a human being. 'Who am I?' is a question that is probably asked by many of us at various key stages of our lives – as a part of growing up and forming our identity; at a major transition point in our lives (such as reaching a significant birthday) or at a moment of crisis (e.g. the death of a person [or another entity] loved by us). When we reflect on such a question, we sometimes focus on functional aspects of our lives, such as 'my' job, friendships and relationships, ambitions, career prospects, life balance, etc. However, we can also focus on some core aspects of our being, such as the core values, beliefs or attitudes I hold towards particular aspects of my life, i.e. who I REALLY am! To start, we would like to invite you to engage with the following activity.

Activity Who am I as a person?

For 20 minutes, create a collage (this could be either on paper or in digital form) representing your own *self-portrait* based on the following 10 points for creating your portrait. Place your name in the centre of the collage.

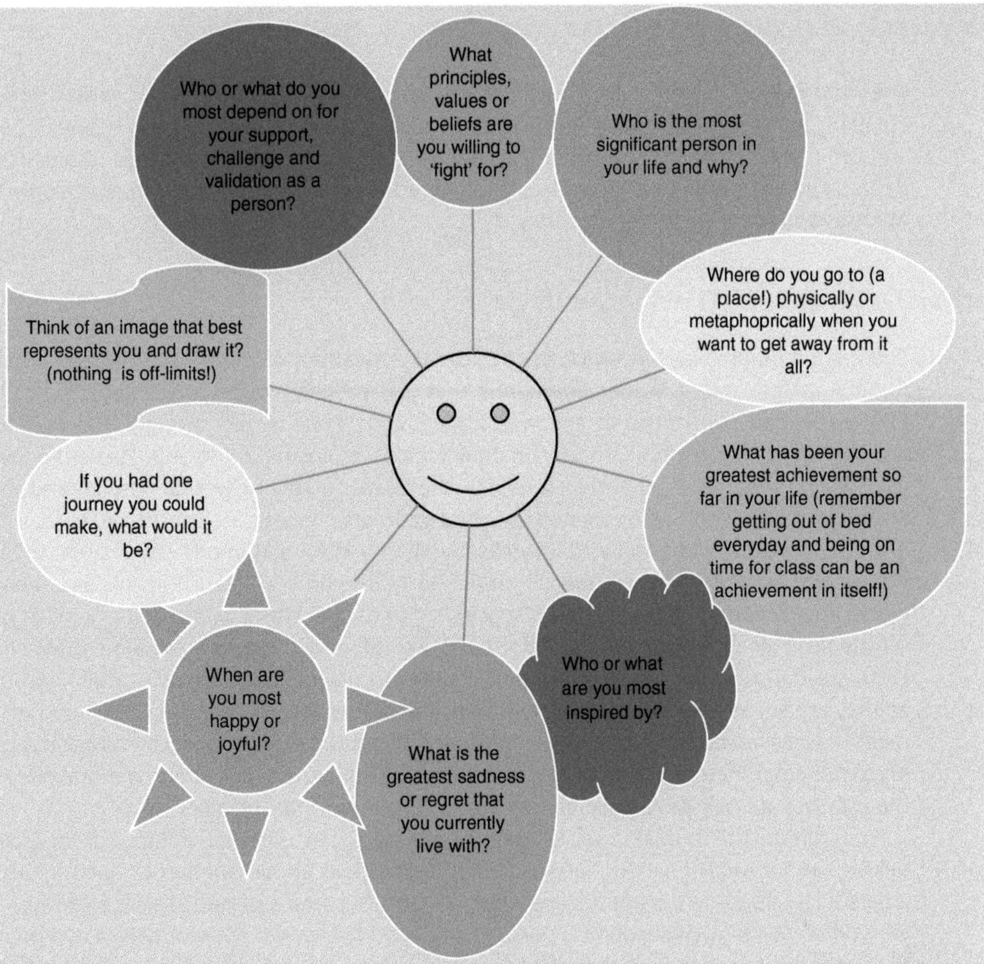
Who or what do you most depend on for your support, challenge and validation as a person?
What principles, values or beliefs are you willing to 'fight' for?
Who is the most significant person in your life and why?
Where do you go to (a place!) physically or metaphoprically when you want to get away from it all?
Think of an image that best represents you and draw it? (nothing is off-limits!)
What has been your greatest achievement so far in your life (remember getting out of bed everyday and being on time for class can be an achievement in itself!)
If you had one journey you could make, what would it be?
Who or what are you most inspired by?
When are you most happy or joyful?
What is the greatest sadness or regret that you currently live with?

Reflect on your answers to these questions. Is there anything that surprises you about your answers? Have you gained new insights about yourself as a person? What do your collective responses tell you about who you are as a person?

Each time we (the chapter authors) do this activity, we are surprised at some of the things that emerge. No two collages are ever the same – there may be some common elements (such as a place of importance) but we are always interested in the things that evolve or transform (a key learning and its influence on us as persons). When we share these with others, the differences reflect changes in us as persons, our different experiences and learning from those, as well as shifts in thinking about our 'being in the world' and what is important over time. All this highlights how we exist in a dynamic state and are constantly evolving as persons.

6 What does it mean to be a person?

The word 'person' has been debated for as long as philosophical thought has existed and there are many perspectives on what it means to be a person. How we distinguish between persons and other species (such as non-human animals and robots) is a key focus for discussion and debate and the differing philosophical stances adopted have influenced the development of theories and frameworks for centuries.

Humans as primary beings

There are multiple ways in which to consider the meaning of 'person' and indeed an animal rights advocate might argue vehemently that it is morally wrong to privilege the rights of human persons over those of animals (Singer 2011). They would strongly believe that it is morally wrong, for example, to test pharmaceuticals or cosmetics on animals before they are used with humans. Their argument would be predicated on the belief that humans and animals are equal and thus should be treated equally. For others, humans are considered to be a higher order species to animals and thus it is reasonable to use animals in this way in order to benefit the greater good of humans. You might like to reflect on your stance in this argument and where your boundaries are regarding speciesism (meaning biases or prejudices against beings on the basis of their species). You might also like to view this short video on speciesism by Professor Peter Singer: www.animalsandsociety.org/human-animal-studies/defining-human-animal-studies-an-asi-video-project/defining-speciesism-with-peter-singer. This kind of argument gets played out in many ways in our daily lives and the fact that such emphasis is placed on preserving different species is not just an ecological argument but also a moral one where the rights of animals have been elevated in importance in recent years.

Even within the 'human species', a 'person' may mean different things, so, for example, debates about abortion are influenced by different ideas about whether or not an embryo is a person; is a foetus a person or when does a foetus become a person? This is a complex issue with different moral philosophical perspectives used to defend different beliefs and practices. We suggest the core issue is that of when a human being becomes a person – is it at the point of fertilisation or is it when the foetus is able to sustain life independent of the womb?

Physical and psychological attributes

For some philosophers (such as Frankfurt 1989), it is not enough to claim that human beings are persons on the basis of a collection of physical and psychological attributes because it is conceptually possible that members of another species could also lay claim to these. If attributes such as sight, taste, smell, sexuality, memory, desires, motives and so forth were to be used as a means of distinguishing persons from non-persons, then we could easily provide a list of other species who would possess similar attributes. For example, the amazing developments in robotics and specifically humanoid robots and androids (i.e. robots or cyborgs made to look like humans on the outside) will find their way more and more into healthcare services in the future. Would it be possible to regard an android worker as a colleague and/or an electronic person? And would we ensure their rights are protected? While advancements are happening, societies and governments will have to find ways of managing or regulating the companies and products (or persons) they produce. In fact, the European Parliament is taking a proactive approach to exploring human-like artificial intelligence, including considering giving rights and responsibilities to robots.

Further, if we argue that personhood is predicated merely on a set of physical and psychological attributes, then what happens to persons who may lose some of these attributes through disease and disability? For instance, a person with dementia may experience deterioration of memory and motivation and loss of physical attributes (e.g. mobility, hand–eye co-ordination, etc.) and so could legitimately, on the basis of this argument, lose the status of person. Even such higher order attributes as 'thought' and decision making fail to distinguish persons from other creatures, as human beings are not alone in having desires and preferences. Members of other species share these attributes with human beings and some species could even be seen to base action on deliberation and even prior thought.

Therefore, distinguishing persons from non-persons on the basis of a hierarchy of attributes is problematic. Some authors, such as Post (2006), argue that a dominant focus in Western cultures on some attributes being more important than others has led to a position whereby cognitive attributes of persons are given greatest importance. We see this played out in all kinds of ways in daily life, in that the ability to connect our thinking with our actions is essential for day-to-day functioning. Thus the loss of these attributes can have significant impact on human beings and their personhood as it can result in reduced ability to engage in daily activities of living, loss of employment, an inability to converse with others, a loss of connection with community, disconnection with friends and family, and increased loneliness and isolation.

So how should we think about 'persons' in ways that help us to not privilege cognition and rationality and in ways that avoid (human-based) hierarchies of attributes? Most philosophers attempt to understand this through a focus on 'personhood' – and it is to this focus that we will turn in the Section 1.4, but first, here's an activity to help you reflect on your reading so far.

Activity

From your perspective, what does it mean to be a person? Does your collage from the previous activity provide you with some insights into those aspects of being a person that you privilege most? Write an approximate 100-word statement that begins with:

I am a person because …

If the activity seems too big, consider today and what it is about you today that makes you a person.

Consider how your statement reflects you as a person. Are you satisfied with your representation of 'you'? Can you identify those parts of your description that are more dominant than others (maybe moral values shaped by your religious beliefs, for example, or beliefs about work and play shaped by your upbringing and childhood experiences)? All of these things are elements of your 'personhood'.

Personhood

Connecting with an innate sense of ourselves as human beings with feelings, emotions, thoughts and desires is an essential component of being a person and de facto having personhood. Leibing (2008) argues that personhood is that inner feeling we have that guides us as a person. It is the sum total of all these feelings, desires, motivations and values – or what Leibing refers to as 'that which really matters' (Leibing 2008, p. 180). This idea of personhood equating with that which really matters to us potentially enables us to rise above discussions of physical attributes and cognition, for example. Instead, it enables a connection with our unique humanness as persons – those inner perspectives that we hold in our body and that influence our being in the world. Leibing uses the term 'interiority' to describe this:

The materialization of certain values in time – and the moral question of what matters to certain people. (Leibing 2008, p. 180)

'What matters to us' is possibly the closest we can get to a neutral understanding of personhood and one that is connected with innate human characteristics. In reading this phrase (what matters to us), you might be reminded of the 'what matters to me' movement that is dominant in healthcare (refer to, for example, the 'What Matters to Me' day in Scotland: www.whatmatterstoyou.scot) which is an attempt by healthcare providers to understand and surface those inner perspectives that we all hold and may not easily articulate.

However, we need to be cautious in viewing this question (what matters to me/you) as the primary consideration, as Leibing argues that in diseases such as Alzheimer's, this interiority may become flattened through disease processes and the medicalisation of the associated symptoms. Accordingly, the response to the 'what matters to you' question may be limited, stunted, stilted or indeed may be voiced by an advocate (family member, friend, partner) and so is an interpretation of the person and who they are.

The reflective person

The work of Christian Smith is also important here (Smith 2003). Smith argues that what distinguishes us as human persons from other non-human persons is that we live within a moral code or framework. This moral code is both inside us (our beliefs, values, desires, motives and feelings) and outside us (societal structures, cultures and processes). Every day, we operate through the lens of this moral code and so control of our actions is not just based on 'interiority principles', as Leibing argues. Like other philosophers such as Frankfurt (1989), Smith suggests that as human persons, we have the unique ability to reflect on our moral behaviour and recalibrate our actions if they misalign with the dominant moral code. We need to be aware, therefore, that our personhood is not just shaped by our internal beliefs, values, desires and feelings but also by our culture, which shapes, forms and reforms us on a continuous basis – thus personhood is not a static fixed concept but something that is continuously evolving and developing.

This is a very important point to reflect on in the context of healthcare practice. So much emphasis is placed on people working in healthcare having the 'right' moral attitude. Indeed, the standards of professional practice for nurses, midwives and associate nurses (NMC 2015) place significant emphasis on the beliefs, values and behaviours of individual nurses. This perspective reinforces and privileges the 'interiority' perspective of Leibing. But what about the culture of the care setting, the team behaviours and practices, the style of management and leadership in operation, the resources available to do the job, and many other elements of organisations that influence our individual effectiveness? To truly be a person-centred accountable person, we also need to operate in cultures that pay attention to these values – more on this in Chapters 3 and 4.

Self and selfhood

In thinking about how we connect with personhood, Sabat (2002) suggests that personhood is connected with different understandings of 'self'. Rejecting the idea of the 'loss of self' that is dominant in dementia discourse and that implies not just a flattening of personhood but its loss, with the consequence of being labelled as a 'non-person', Sabat (2002, p. 27) argues that we have three forms of self – Self 1, Self 2 and Self 3.

Self 1 is 'the self of personal identity' evidenced through our use of personal pronouns: 'I', 'me', 'mine', 'myself', 'ours' (meaning mine and yours). This self relates to our individual and unique view of the world. It expresses how we relate to our being in the world and the words we use to describe this being. It is autobiographical in nature and forms the narrative of our lives. Through Self 1, we tell the stories of our lives, and often how we tell those stories gives some indication of what is important to us. Sabat argues that a loss of words and language (such as happens with people living with dementia) does not mean a loss of self; rather, this Self 1 remains intact but the challenge is how we can enable such persons to voice their stories. Identical diagnosis and apparent severity of dementia, or other conditions, does not mean we can understand all persons in the same way.

Self 2 comprises our physical, mental and emotional attributes past and present – eye colour, height, weight, beliefs, religion, happiness, love, sadness, achievements, hobbies and so forth are all examples of Self 2. Again, these remain relatively intact with the threat of disease and illness. However, Self 2 becomes a problem when others focus on deficits and decline rather than abilities and potentials. Whilst the symptoms of a disease might impact on our physical, mental or emotional attributes, the attributes themselves do not change – what changes is how others engage with this aspect of our self.

Self 3 comprises the different social personas that we construct in different situations in which we live our lives. In different situations and contexts, a person may display very different behaviours – a highly dedicated and professional healthcare person by day and a hard party-goer by night; a focused, targeted and 'hard-nosed' manager versus a loving, sensitive and intimate partner.

Sabat argues that Self 3, the social persona, is most vulnerable when threatened by disease and illness, as it is dependent on a connection with at least one other person in our social world. Whilst this threat is obvious in a person living with dementia, we can also see the potential for loss of Self 3 in all kinds of illness situations where the autobiographical self is not considered; that is, we are concerned with treatment and cure and not with the social construction of that illness and how it threatens our personhood – something central to the argument made for a person-centred approach to practice in many of the chapters in this book. Self 3 fits most closely with Kitwood's ideas on personhood as social status bestowed by others (Dewing 2018).

Of course, these constructions of self can also be challenged and debated as there are a variety of ways in which Self 1–3 can change and/or be altered, and indeed the question needs to be asked, 'are we limited to three kinds of self?'. However, Sabat's ideas demonstrate how interiority (Leibing 2008) links with Smith's (2003) ideas of culture as an important basis for understanding how our behaviours can impact on the personhood of others. Paying attention to Self 1 and 2 is therefore critical for the protection of personhood in situations where a person is vulnerable and in need of care. Sabat's expression of self resonates with Merleau-Ponty's argument about the primacy of a 'perceiving body' in the world (Dewing 2012). Merleau-Ponty argues against any idea of a mind–body split or that we are passive recipients of our history. Instead, he suggests that our knowing is always subjective as we carry through the movement in our bodies, our prehistories that we take up, inherit and transform through our being in the world. Therefore, Self 1 is ever-present, even in the absence of rational thought.

So we could summarise by suggesting that 'persons are persons because of their personhood' and that this is what distinguishes human persons from non-human persons. We are more than our body parts held together by connective tissue – we are interacting persons, guided by whilst also shaping and reshaping our being in the world through our interior and exterior conditions. Yes, persons are complex!

Activity

In our discussion of personhood, a focus on 'values' has been dominant. Consider your core values and what these say about you as a person.

What values did you identify as being important to you? Can you see a connection between your stated values and any of the elements of your collage (self-portrait)? It might be that this is implicit; for example, the place you identified as important might reflect values such as family or relationships. A key learning experience might have influenced your desire to be a healthcare worker. Can you see any connections?

Persons, personhood and person-centred practice

Having some core understandings of persons and personhood is important as you develop your healthcare practice. Knowing who you are as a person, what is important to you, what core values you hold and how these are shaped and developed through different cultures are key considerations as you develop your person-centred practice. As you move through this book and in your day-to-day work, you will read about and hear different ways of understanding how persons and personhood are articulated by you and others, such as person-centred care, family-centred care, woman-centred care, person-centred practice, person-centred culture – to name a few! The ways in which these terms are used reflect different understandings of or engagement with personhood.

Think about 'person-centred care', for example – what does that term say about personhood? Does it reflect a particular set of beliefs and values? We would argue that person-centred care privileges the personhood of the patient/service user over that of the practitioner, i.e. the focus is on ensuring that 'what matters' to the patient is of primary importance. What might the implications of that be for a nurse or physiotherapist, for example? If the nurse or physiotherapist were in a care situation where their values were compromised, does that matter? We would argue that a focus on person-centred culture in healthcare, for example, ensures that the personhood of all persons is equally valued and paid attention to. Drawing on Smith's analysis, different cultural contexts shape how personhood is realised. The Person-centred Practice Framework pays attention to these cultural issues and places something like 'person-centred care' in a broader social context. This focus will be demonstrated in other chapters and in the different ways in which the framework is applied in contrasting contexts.

Conclusion

In this chapter, we have introduced you to the ideas of person and personhood. We have challenged views of persons that privilege cognitive and physical attributes as key characteristics of persons. If you are new to this debate then we realise that this can be challenging to engage with. However, as you consider your own personhood, you will see how you pay attention to other aspects of you as a person and even take these physical and cognitive perspectives for granted – they form the background to your life. As active agents in the world, we constantly evolve, change and grow and through this evolution we influence and are influenced by our interior and exterior qualities, traits and circumstances. Thus being a person is a dynamic state.

Summary

- There are multiple philosophical perspectives to what constitutes a person and personhood.
- Persons are more than their physical and cognitive make-up, but instead constitute a dynamic interrelationship of multiple factors that come together as personhood.
- Personhood is the key characteristic that distinguishes persons from non-persons.
- Values are a key part of our personhood.

References

Dewing, J. (2012). Bringing Merleau-Ponty's inspirations to working with participants. In: *Creative Spaces for Qualitative Researching, Living Research* (eds. J. Higgs, A. Titchen, D. Horsfall and D. Bridges), 65–76. Amsterdam: Sense Publications.

Dewing, J. (2019). On being a person. In: *Dementia Reconsidered*, Revisited (ed. D. Brooker), 17–23. London: Open University Press.

Frankfurt, H.G. (1989). Freedom of the will and the concept of a person. In: *The Inner Citadel: Essays on Individual Autonomy* (ed. J. Christman), 63–76. Oxford: Oxford University Press.

Leibing, A. (2008). Entangled matters – Alzheimer's, interiority, and the 'unflattening' of the world. *Culture, Medicine and Psychiatry* 32 (2): 177–193.

Nursing and Midwifery Council (2015). *The Code: Professional Standards of Practice and Behaviour for Nurses, Midwives and Nursing Associates*. London: Nursing and Midwifery Council.

Post, S. (2006). Respectare: moral respect for the lives of the deeply forgetful. In: *Dementia: Mind, Meaning and the Person* (eds. J.C. Hughes, S.J. Louw and S.R. Sabat), 223–224. Oxford: Oxford University Press.

Sabat, S.R. (2002). Surviving manifestations of selfhood in Alzheimer's disease: a case study. *Dementia* 1 (1): 25–36.

Singer, P. (2011). *Practical Ethics*, 3e. Cambridge: Cambridge University Press.

Smith, C. (2003). *Moral, Believing Animals: Human Personhood and Culture*. Oxford: Oxford University Press.

Further reading

Rogers, C. (2004). *A Therapist's View of Psychotherapy: On Becoming a Person*. London: Constable & Robinson.

Schoenhofer, S.O. (2002). Choosing personhood: intentionality and the theory of nursing as caring. *Holistic Nursing Practice* 16 (4): 36–40.

Singer, P. Ethics, uncertainty and moral progress. www.youtube.com/watch?v=-NMD0g97C64 (18-minute video)

2

What is person-centredness?

Brendan McCormack[1], Tanya McCance[2], and Suzanne Martin[2]

[1]*Queen Margaret University, Edinburgh, Scotland, UK*

[2]*Ulster University, Northern Ireland, UK*

Contents

Fundamentals of Person-Centred Healthcare Practice, First Edition. Edited by Brendan McCormack, Tanya McCance, Cathy Bulley, Donna Brown, Ailsa McMillan and Suzanne Martin.

Learning outcomes

- Understand what person-centred practice is, distinguishing it from other approaches to practice, for example patient-centredness, client-centredness, family-centredness, woman-centredness and child-centredness.
- Identify and describe the different challenges posed for healthcare practitioners when adopting person-centred approaches to practice.
- Understand the importance of the need for the development of person-centred cultures in healthcare organisations.

Introduction

The term 'person-centredness' is increasingly used in healthcare discourse. Reflecting a desire to keep the person in the centre of decision making, a focus on person-centredness challenges traditional ideas of (for example) task-orientated practices, dehumanising of patients through medical labels and system efficiency without considering its impact on persons. In this chapter, we will explore what we mean by person-centredness with a particular focus on person-centred practice. In recognising that there are a variety of terms used in healthcare when considering person-centredness, we will compare and contrast some of these commonly used terms and what they may mean for how person-centredness is operationalised. Being person-centred in everyday practice is challenging and so the need for organisations to adopt a whole-systems approach to person-centred healthcare will be considered.

Activity

Collect a story of a care experience from a relative or friend. Reflect with them the extent to which you consider it to be a person-centred experience. Identify with the relative or friend the key things that led you to think it was or was not person-centred.

In your care story, you may have identified key elements that resonated with aspects of persons and personhood from Chapter 1. The story might include issues that reflect the person's key values and beliefs that are important to them. It might have said something about the kinds of relationships they experienced with different healthcare workers and it may say something about the person-centred processes experienced in the care setting. But you might also be thinking, 'These issues are so basic and ordinary, why are we having to pay such attention to them?' In many respects you are right, of course, but we also know that these fundamental aspects of life, that we value so greatly, often get challenged in different healthcare contexts. This happens because of a variety of complex factors that, taken together, turn the 'ordinariness of the everyday' into the 'extraordinariness of health-care practice'. The Person-centred Practice Framework that we introduce in Chapter 3 picks up on these factors and explores why being person-centred can be so challenging to achieve.

The values of person-centredness

Many of the underpinning values of person-centredness that are dominant in healthcare are not new and, indeed, many can be traced back through the history of healthcare and especially in the context of care and caring, where the core value of 'respect for the person' is paramount (McCance et al. 1997, 1999). Table 2.1 sets out these core values.

Table 2.1 The core values of person-centred practice

Core value	What the value means in practice
Respect for personhood	Holding the person's values central in decision making is essential to a person-centred approach to practice
Being authentic	Being 'real' in our representation of who we are as persons to enable meaningful engagement in relationships
Sharing autonomy	Forming trusted and interconnected relationships between persons for shared, informed decision making
Showing respect for and active engagement with a person's individual abilities, preferences, lifestyles and goals	Balancing all persons' competence and expertise with individual understandings of well-being and potential futures
Demonstrating mutual respect and understanding	Forming positive interactive relationships that create an interdependence and shared energy
Therapeutically caring	Caring as a therapeutic intervention focusing on actions that respond to individual need and that strives for positive outcomes
Committed to healthfulness as process and outcome	Living a positive life and embracing all dimensions of our being

Activity

Consider these core values from the perspective of the work you did for Activity 3 in Chapter 1. Are there similarities between these core values of person-centredness and your personal values? List the similarities and differences. Write a 100-word reflection that captures how you as a person connect with these person-centred values.

In writing your reflection, you might have considered ways in which you respect others as persons and how this respect translates into your ways of being and how you translate those ways of being into your practice. You might have also focused on 'the individual' and the importance of respecting individuality. This is a common focus in twenty-first-century society where respect for the person is often translated into an individualistic perspective where rights, expectations and demands shape our politics, sociocultural norms and behaviours, relationships and societal values. Indeed, some would argue that we have become so dominated by individualism that core values of 'community' have been eroded, leading to a breakdown of society and its supportive interconnected relationships (Everingham 2018).

New and innovative technologies in genetic research, expansion of the genome and the development of treatments that are highly individualised and personalised (e.g. personalised medicine) mean that healthcare professionals have to work in very different ways from those articulated in early writings about care and caring. Such developments have also influenced how healthcare teams are formed, how interdisciplinary practice is understood and operationalised and how knowledge and evidence is used in practice. Thus person-centred practice cannot be understood in simplistic terms of 'caring for a person' or 'providing care to a person' or 'working therapeutically with a person' but instead needs to embrace a variety of individual, personal, contextual and political attributes that shape how we provide healthcare.

You can read more about these issues in the context of the development of person-centredness as health strategy in McCormack et al. (2017) and in the context of research in van Dulman et al. (2017).

Person-centredness and related concepts

We need to challenge individualistic views of persons and person-centredness, especially in healthcare, where shared values, team identity, organisational cultures and norms have a major effect on how we work and how service users experience healthcare. In Chapters 13 and 16, this is discussed in the context of 'human agency' and providing holistic care. We are all 'persons' and so the values of person-centredness need to apply to all of us in any context – this is why person-centredness and person-centred practice are not just about 'patient care' but instead these core values apply to all persons. This is one of the clear distinctions between person-centredness and other similar concepts, such as patient-centredness, client-centredness, woman-centredness and child-centredness. We define some of these associated concepts in Table 2.2.

Table 2.2 Associated concepts

Concept	Definition
Patient-centredness	Patient-centred care seeks to ensure that the needs of individuals requiring care are met with respect and responded to as persons, through respect for their values, preferences, choices and relationships and is inclusive of the individual's family
Client-centredness	Client-centred care originates from the work of Carl Rogers (1961) and his approach to psychotherapy (also called person-centred therapy). By using the term 'client' instead of 'patient', Rogers placed importance on the individual seeking assistance, making autonomous decisions and engaging in self-work to overcome their difficulties. Self-direction is a central principle in client-centred practice and the role of the nurse is that of 'professional guide'
Woman-centredness	Woman-centred care is a term used to describe a holistic philosophy of maternity care that recognises each woman's biopsychosocial, emotional and spiritual needs as defined by her own context
Child-centredness	Child-centred care means placing children and their interests at the centre of practice and recognises children and young people as active participants in their care

Table 2.2 *(Continued)*

Concept	Definition
Family-centredness	Family-centred care is a term used in healthcare services for children and young people. It means that a child in need of care can never be considered as a single individual patient, but that the family is the unit of care as the parents and wider family are central to the child's health and well-being
Relationship-centredness	Relationship-centred care originates from the work of Nolan et al. (2004). It emphasises the promotion of positive relationships in meeting the needs of persons needing care as well as relatives/friends and staff

These associated concepts may have some similarities with person-centredness, as they may share some of the values of personhood, but not all. You may also notice that not all persons are considered equal in some of these perspectives and that they differ according to the emphasis they place on the power relationship, the focus of the relationship and equality of decision making.

Person-centred practice

Dear Oscleans,
I am writing to you to welcome you to our planet. We as a planet of people who care for one another are moving towards becoming more person-centred. I am aware that you are not familiar with the term person-centred, therefore, this letter aims to provide you with an understanding of what it means to be person-centred. Moreover, I hope to provide you with my understanding of person-centredness and how my learning on the topic has changed the way I view my practice. McCormack and McCance (2017, p. 41) have provided a definition of person-centredness:

> person-centredness focuses on the formation and fostering of healthful relationships with service users and others significant to them in their lives, as well as between all care providers. It is underpinned by values of respect for persons (personhood), individual right to self determination, mutual respect and understanding. It is enabled by cultures of empowerment that foster continuous approaches to practice development.

The idea of person-centredness has been formed from the theory of personhood which has been widely described in the literature. Many scholars have presented their views of the theory. One philosopher who has written about what it means to be a person is Immanuel Kant who believed that personhood was the ability for a person to think and act morally and this is what differentiated humans from other species (von Bertalanffy 1968). His philosophy is one which I most associate with. It is what I consider to be the basis of the care that I provide. My view of person-centredness and particularly person-centred practice is that it is focused largely on being with the person and connecting on a human level. I believe that the most person-centred care I provide is when I have been completely authentic with a family. This has included connecting with them on a personal but professional level and remaining transparent throughout my work with them. I encourage the families with whom I have worked to speak freely about their concerns and I have been sympathetically present. I have shared my knowledge with them and worked in partnership to come up with a decision that is suited to their needs.

In addition, I believe that in order to engage authentically with families it is important to recognise our own limitations. A large part of shared decision making with parents and families requires having adequate knowledge/information about a particular illness or treatment. As I am still at the beginning of my career as a specialist community health nurse, I am aware that I do not always have the correct knowledge or information to share with families. Therefore, in order to engage authentically, I inform them of my limitations in knowledge and state that I will seek the correct information in order to support them in making the best decision for their child. This has been generally well received and on reflection it appears that most families appreciate honesty and transparency. So, as I start my career as a newly qualified specialist community health nurse, I will continue to be honest about the extent of my knowledge with families and ensure that I signpost them to the relevant service that will be able to better inform them. Ultimately, my view of person-centred practice has moved on and I have learned that is important to work towards 'person-centred moments' and increasing the frequency of these moments in practice to create a context where person-centred practice can be realised.

I hope this letter better informs you of how I have viewed person-centred practice and how it has shaped the way I will practise in future. I would like to welcome you to our planet and hope that you too can become part of the movement towards person-centred practice.

Yours sincerely,
C Thomson

This letter was written by a student (Caitlin Thomson) who at the time of writing was undertaking education as a specialist community health nurse (also known as a health visitor) at Queen Margaret University, Edinburgh. Caitlin was engaging in an exercise of writing to a fictitious 'alien visitor' known as an Osclean explaining person-centred practice to them.

Activity

Imagine you are 'the Osclean' Caitlin has written to. What would your response be to her regarding your expectation of your care? Does what she says sound interesting? Would you want to be a part of it – why/why not? Are there things missing from Caitlin's description that you would want to be included? Feel free to present your response in any creative way you are drawn to.

As Caitlin recognises in her reflection, consideration of the person and our understanding of personhood in the context of how we relate to each other have a long tradition in philosophy and you have been introduced to some of these perspectives in Chapter 1. In more contemporary theory, the term 'person-centred' is often considered to originate from the work of Carl Rogers and his humanistic psychological and person-centred therapy (Rogers 1961). Rogers' focus was on maximising our potential to fulfil our personal life goals, including our need to be autonomous, social, connected with and respected by others, i.e. to be known as a person.

Drawing on all of these traditions, we can summarise being person-centred as implying the recognition of the broad biological, social, psychological, cultural and spiritual dimensions of each person (i.e. the whole person) in our ways of being and doing as persons.

The core principles of person-centredness can be seen in an array of models and frameworks applied to different health conditions (for example, Parkinson's disease [Buetow et al. 2016]), different client groups – where the most concentrated work has happened with persons living with dementia (see for example Fazio et al. 2018), and different healthcare settings, for example in critical care units (see for example van Mol et al. 2016). In the context of psychiatric medicine, for example, Mezzich et al. (2009) suggest that person-centredness can be seen to be operationalised within four dimensions of practice: (i) care *of* the person (of the totality of the person's health, including its negative and positive aspects), (ii) care *for* the person (promoting the fulfilment of the person's life project), (iii) care *by* the person (with clinicians extending themselves as full human beings with high ethical aspirations) and (iv) care *with* the person (working respectfully, in collaboration and in an empowering manner).

However, we would suggest that these perspectives of person-centredness are myopic and exclusive – what do we mean by that? Earlier we described the core values that underpin person-centredness and we highlighted the importance of these values applying to *all* persons, not just persons using health services. It therefore follows that these values also apply to persons who are directly providing, managing, co-ordinating, funding and planning services. So when we think about person-centred practice, we have to think about it in the context of all persons. It is not enough to just think about person-centred practice in the context of 'doing practice' but we also need to think about it in the context of our 'being' as a person working in healthcare and how we relate to all other persons, and how they relate to us. In addition, we showed in Chapter 1, through an analysis of the work of Leibing (2008) and Smith (2003), that person-centred practice cannot depend solely on the values of individual practitioners and their commitment to working in this way. Smith shows clearly that the prevailing moral values in particular cultures have a significant influence on our ability to work in this way, and so presenting person-centredness from the lens of 'quality of care experienced by service users' is a necessary but insufficient approach to person-centredness. What we need to think about is the continuous development of cultures that can create, nurture, support and reflexively evaluate person-centredness in the everyday experiences of all persons.

Person-centred culture

Imagine a situation where you are not respected at work, because your relationships with other team members feel 'unsafe', the management style is hierarchical and controlling, autonomy is limited and you don't feel you have a 'voice' in decision making. How easy would it be for you to provide person-centred care to service users in that context? We would argue that whilst you might be able to do so intermittently, sustaining your values of person-centredness would be challenging to your personhood and in the end the care you provide would suffer. Evidence of the relationship between the person-centredness of teams in healthcare and quality of care provided to service users is increasing (for example, Albers et al. 2018; ACSQHC 2018; Sinah 2017) and initiatives such as 'Joy in Work' (www.ihi.org/Topics/Joy-In-Work/Pages/default.aspx) have been designed to make explicit the importance of team culture for effective patient care. However, initiatives such as this are not enough to continuously develop healthcare contexts that can sustain excellent person-centred practice.

In Chapter 3 we will introduce the macro healthcare context and this will be further developed in Chapter 17. This is important as we need to consider the qualities of the staff, the specific characteristics of the healthcare setting and the engagement processes we use to develop a person-centred culture – the kind of culture where leaders facilitate meaningful engagement between team members so that they experience the conditions that enable them to provide person-centred care to service users (Cardiff et al. 2018; Lynch et al. 2018). Evidence of the relationship between work environments that lack respect for individual personhood (characterised by staff burnout and staff turnover) and poor outcomes for service users is now well established in the literature (Lyndon 2016; Dyrbye et al. 2017), thus highlighting the need for organisations to commit to the continuous development of person-centred cultures.

Conclusions

In this chapter we have introduced you to some key principles and concepts associated with person-centredness. We have built on Chapter 1, which explored some of the key philosophical principles and especially the idea of personhood. In Chapter 2 we have illustrated why person-centredness in healthcare practice needs to take account of individual personhood in the context of 'all persons'. Person-centred care is just one part of person-centred practice and having a practice context that supports and actively enables these ways of practising is critical to success. Very few healthcare settings are either completely person-centred or not person-centred as it is a much more dynamic process than that. Person-centred practice is continuously being developed and so it is rarely helpful to label individuals, teams or specific workplace settings as being person-centred or not. This dynamic nature of person-centred practice is also influenced by the workplace culture and how the qualities of the workplace help or hinder the continuous being and doing of person-centredness – more about this in Chapter 3 and in many chapters in this book.

Summary

- Person-centred practice is underpinned by core values of respect for personhood, authenticity, shared autonomy, respect, mutuality, therapeutic caring and healthfulness.
- Person-centred practice cannot be understood in simplistic terms of 'caring for a person' or 'providing care to a person' or 'working therapeutically with a person', but instead needs to embrace a variety of individual, personal, contextual and political attributes that shape how we provide healthcare.
- There are several associated concepts that are similar to person-centredness. These associated concepts may have some similarities with person-centredness, as they may share some of the values of personhood, but not all.

- There is significant evidence of the relationship between work environments that lack respect for individual personhood (characterised by staff burnout and staff turnover) and poor outcomes for service users and so having a person-centred culture is critical to practising in a person-centred way.

References

Albers, A., Bonsignore, L., and Webb, M. (2018). A team-based approach to delivering person-centered care at the end of life. *North Carolina Medical Journal* 79 (4): 256–258.

Australian Commission on Safety and Quality in Health Care. (2018). *Review of Key Attributes of High-Performing Person-Centred Healthcare Organisations*. Australian Commission on Safety and Quality in Health Care, Sydney, Australia. www.safetyandquality.gov.au/sites/default/files/migrated/FINAL-REPORT-Attributes-of-person-centred-healthcare-organisations-2018.pdf

von Bertalanffy, L. (1968). *General System Theory: Foundations, Development, Applications*. New York: George Braziller.

Buetow, S., Martinez-Martin, P., Hirsch, M.A., and Okun, M.S. (2016). Beyond patient-centered care: person-centered care for Parkinson's disease. *Parkinson's Disease* 2: 16019.

Cardiff, S., McCormack, B., and McCance, T. (2018). Person-centred leadership: a relational approach to leadership derived through action research. *Journal of Clinical Nursing* 27: 3056–3069.

Dyrbye, L.N., Shanafelt, T.D., Sinsky, C.A., et al. (2017). *Burnout Among Health Care Professionals: A Call to Explore and Address This Underrecognized Threat to Safe, High-Quality Care*. NAM Perspectives. Discussion Paper. National Academy of Medicine, Washington, DC. https://nam.edu/wp-content/uploads/2017/07/Burnout-Among-Health-Care-Professionals-A-Call-to-Explore-and-Address-This-Underrecognized-Threat.pdf

Everingham, C. (2018). *Social Justice and the Politics of Community*. London: Routledge.

Fazio, S., Pace, D., Flinner, J., and Kallmyer, B. (2018). The fundamentals of person-centered care for individuals with dementia. *Gerontologist* 58 (Suppl_1): S10–S19.

Leibing, A. (2008). Entangled matters – Alzheimer's, interiority, and the 'unflattening' of the world. *Culture, Medicine and Psychiatry* 32 (2): 177–193.

Lynch, B.M., McCance, T., and McCormack B, B.D. (2018). The development of the person-centred situational leadership framework: revealing the being of person-centredness in nursing homes. *Journal of Clinical Nursing* 27: 427–440.

Lyndon, A. (2016). *Burnout Among Health Professionals and Its Effect on Patient Safety*. Rockville, MD.: Agency for Healthcare Research and Quality (AHRQ).

McCance, T.V., McKenna, H.P., and Boore, J.R.P. (1997). Caring: dealing with a difficult concept. *International Journal of Nursing Studies* 34: 241–248.

McCance, T.V., McKenna, H.P., and Boore, J.R.P. (1999). Caring: theoretical perspectives of relevance to nursing. *Journal of Advanced Nursing* 30: 1388–1395.

McCormack, B. and McCance, T. (2017). *Person-centred Nursing and Health Care – Theory and Practice*. Oxford: Wiley.

McCormack, B., van Dulmen, S., Eide, H. et al. (2017). Person-centredness in healthcare policy, practice and research. In: *Person-Centred Healthcare Research* (eds. B. McCormack, S. van Dulmen, H. Eide, et al.), 3–18. Oxford: Wiley Blackwell.

Mezzich, J.E., Caracci, G., Fabrega, H., and Kirmayer, L.J. (2009). Cultural formulation guidelines. *Transcultural Psychiatry* 46 (3): 383–405.

Nolan, M., Davies, S., Brown, J. et al. (2004). Beyond 'person-centred' care: a new vision for gerontological nursing. *International Journal of Older People Nursing* (3a): 45–53.

Rogers, C. (1961). *On Becoming a Person*. Boston: Houghton Mifflin.

Sinha, A. (2017). The role of team effectiveness in quality of health care. *Integrative Journal of Global Health*. 1 (1): 1–4.

Smith, C. (2003). *Moral, Believing Animals: Human Personhood and Culture*. Oxford: Oxford University Press.

Van Dulmen, S., McCormack, B., Eide, H. et al. (2017). Future directions for person-centred healthcare research. In: *Person-Centred Healthcare Research* (eds. B. McCormack, S. van Dulmen, H. Eide, et al.), 209–218. Oxford: Wiley Blackwell.

Van Mol, M.M.C., Brackel, M., Kompanje, E.J.O. et al. (2016). Joined forces in person-centered care in the intensive care unit: a case report from the Netherlands. *Journal of Compassionate Health Care* 3: 5.

Further reading

Buetow, S. (2016). *Person-Centred Health Care: Balancing the Welfare of Clinicians and Patients*. London: Routledge.

McCormack, B., Manley, K., and Titchen, A. (eds.) (2013). *Practice Development in Nursing*, vol. 2. Oxford: Wiley-Blackwell.

Sharp, S., Mcallister, M., and Broadbent, M. (2018). The tension between person centred and task focused care in an acute surgical setting: a critical ethnography. *Collegian* 25 (1): 11–17.

3

The Person-centred Practice Framework

Tanya McCance[1] and
Brendan McCormack[2]

[1] Ulster University, Northern Ireland, UK
[2] Queen Margaret University, Edinburgh, Scotland, UK

Contents

Fundamentals of Person-Centred Healthcare Practice, First Edition. Edited by Brendan McCormack, Tanya McCance, Cathy Bulley, Donna Brown, Ailsa McMillan and Suzanne Martin.

Learning outcomes

- Have an awareness of different models and frameworks that are used across the disciplines and how they relate to, and support, the delivery of person-centred practice.
- Acquire a critical understanding of the Person-centred Practice Framework and its component parts.
- Identify and describe the challenges posed for healthcare practitioners in operationalising person-centredness in practice.
- Be able to apply the Person-centred Practice Framework to enhance understanding of professional practice.

Introduction

This chapter will explore the development of models and frameworks to support the delivery of person-centred practice across the professions, taking account of the current evidence base. The Person-centred Practice Framework, the framework of choice for this book, will be introduced and examined to provide a critical understanding of its component parts and how it relates to practice. This will be placed in the context of theory development and will link to key underpinning theoretical concepts described in Chapters 1 and 2. The Person-centred Practice Framework will be used to explore some of the challenges currently faced by healthcare professionals in operationalising person-centredness. The activities provided will illustrate how application of the framework can support learning to enhance professional practice.

What is person-centred practice?

Person-centredness reflects the ideals of humanistic caring in which there is a moral component, and practice has at its basis a therapeutic intent, which is translated through relationships that are built on effective interpersonal processes. Buetow (2016) discusses caring from the perspective of a physician as 'a moral value and an ethical practice defining a connectedness with, and respectful and concerned attention to, concrete needs of others and oneself' (p. 104). This philosophical position has resonance across the caring professions and reflects models for developing person-centred healthcare that fundamentally take account of the humanness of people.

Despite this shared philosophical position, professional groups use a variety of different models and theories to underpin their practice. Within nursing, the use of models has evolved over time, ranging from those based on activities of daily living (Roper et al. 2000) to those that are more relationships centred (Peplau 1997) and many more besides (Fitzpatrick and Whall 2016). The allied health professions have also drawn on a variety of models and theories ranging from the traditional medical model, to biopsychosocial models such as the International Classification of Functioning, Disability and Health (ICF) (WHO 2001) and moving towards the integration of social models for health and well-being.

Social models of health recognise that our health is influenced by a wide range of individual, interpersonal, organisational, social, environmental, political and economic factors. They encourage us to have a deeper understanding of health: 'Health, and what makes people healthy, can only be fully understood by exploring the myriad of interactions and influences that emerge out of the complexities of human experience and the various inter-relationships of the mind, body and society' (Yuill et al. 2010, p. 14). Irrespective of the models or theories that guide practice (and as reflected in Chapter 2), we advocate the importance of the underpinning values of person-centredness, where the core value of 'respect for the person' is paramount.

Person-centredness in practice requires the formation of therapeutic relationships among professionals, patients and others significant to them in their lives. It is generally accepted that the principles underpinning person-centredness as an approach focus on treating people as individuals; respecting their rights as a person; building mutual trust and understanding; and developing positive relationships. Furthermore, these principles reflect a standard of care that practitioners aspire to in their professional practice. The challenge, however, continues to be how these principles are translated into everyday practice to enable multiprofessional teams to deliver this standard of care consistently over time (Mitchell et al. 2015; Wolf et al. 2017; Sharp et al. 2018).

The Person-centred Practice Framework described in this chapter was originally born out of a desire to operationalise person-centredness in a way that would illuminate practice, and provide practitioners with a language that would enable them to name components of person-centredness, and the barriers and enablers that influence its development in the workplace.

Introducing the Person-centred Practice Framework

This book is based around the Person-centred Practice Framework of McCormack and McCance (2017) and is built upon similar values underpinning separate research by both authors.

When they conducted their original research (McCance et al. 1999, 2003; McCormack 2001a,b), McCormack and McCance worked through a humanistic caring lens. McCance made these values explicit in her research on caring, where she identified the key relational focus of care that enabled nurses to connect with other persons and practise effectively. An understanding of human caring was critical to this research and the conceptual and theoretical analysis undertaken by McCance et al. (1999) highlighted the dual nature of caring represented by attitudes/values on the one hand and activities on the other, but with the greatest importance placed on the practitioner–patient relationship. This represents a view of persons embedded in a humanistic tradition reflecting principles including the centrality of human freedom, choice and responsibility; holism whereby persons are interconnected with others and nature; different forms of knowing; and the importance of time and space, and relationships (Watson 1985).

Similarly, McCormack (2001b) focused on the autonomy of persons as a core value. He first problematised autonomy and demonstrated its limitations from behavioural and transcendental perspectives. Then, he identified relational ethics as being critical to demonstrating respect for another person. His research was influenced by humanistic theory that emphasised the centrality of a person's beliefs, values and human desires as core to effective decision making and to 'knowing the person'.

Although she didn't place her research in the same framework as McCormack and McCance, or draw on the same philosophical ideas, Dewing (2012) also adopted a broadly humanistic approach to her research with older persons living with dementia in response to a dominant behaviourist paradigm. Dewing (2012) drew on philosophical ideas about persons and 'being in the world' that challenged the way persons with dementia are viewed as having abnormal, problematic or challenging behaviours. Considering who we are in terms of our bodies and how we use them to be a person, relationships with things or others that matter to us and relationships with time and space/place all offer very different perspectives on what it can mean to be a person. When reading about the Person-centred Practice Framework, it is important to be aware of the dominant philosophical perspectives articulated through the framework as this has shaped its development and may also influence yours!

The development of the Person-centred Practice Framework has spanned over a decade and during that time it has been used in a variety of different ways, across a range of contexts. The framework was developed for use in the intervention stage of a large quasi-experimental research study, which focused on measuring the effectiveness of the implementation of person-centred nursing in a tertiary hospital setting (McCormack et al. 2008). The Person-centred Practice Framework is more than a conceptual model, but has been described as a middle-range theory (McCormack and McCance 2016). In simple terms, this means that the framework is less abstract than a conceptual model as it comprises concepts that are relatively specific, and outlines relationships between the concepts. You will see these relationships within the framework unfold in the remainder of this chapter.

Whilst the framework has its origins in nursing practice and is described in a nursing version of the framework (the Person-centred Nursing Framework), the Person-centred Practice Framework is situated within healthcare systems more broadly. The version of the Person-centred Practice Framework presented in this book is the latest iteration and reflects recent changes made to ensure applicability to a wide range of healthcare workers across multiple contexts. It continues to be tested and refined through an ongoing programme of applied research within a multidisciplinary context (www.cpcpr.org/resources).

The Person-centred Practice Framework comprises four main domains: *prerequisites*, which focus on the attributes of staff; the *practice environment*, which focuses on the context in which healthcare is experienced; the *person-centred processes*, which focus on ways of engaging that are necessary to create connections between persons; and the *outcome*, which is the result of effective person-centred practice. The relationships between the four constructs of the Person-centred Practice Framework are represented pictorially so that, to reach the centre of the framework, the attributes of staff must first be considered, as a prerequisite to managing the practice environment and in order to engage effectively through the person-centred processes. This ordering ultimately leads to the achievement of the outcome – the central component of the framework. It is also important to recognise that there are relationships and overlap between the constructs within each domain.

Finally, the framework sits within the broader *macro context* (the fifth domain), reflecting the factors that are strategic and political in nature that influence the development of person-centred cultures. The macro context will be the focus of Chapter 17.

The Person-centred Practice Framework is presented in Figure 3.1 and the subsequent sections describe the domains of the framework in greater detail.

Prerequisites

The prerequisites (Figure 3.2) focus on the attributes of staff and are considered to be key building blocks in the development of healthcare workers who can deliver effective person-centred care. Attributes include being professionally competent, having developed interpersonal skills, being committed to the job, being able to demonstrate clarity of beliefs and values, and knowing self. There is no hierarchy in relation to these attributes, with all considered of equal importance, but it is the combination of attributes that reflects a person-centred individual who can manage the challenges of a constantly changing context.

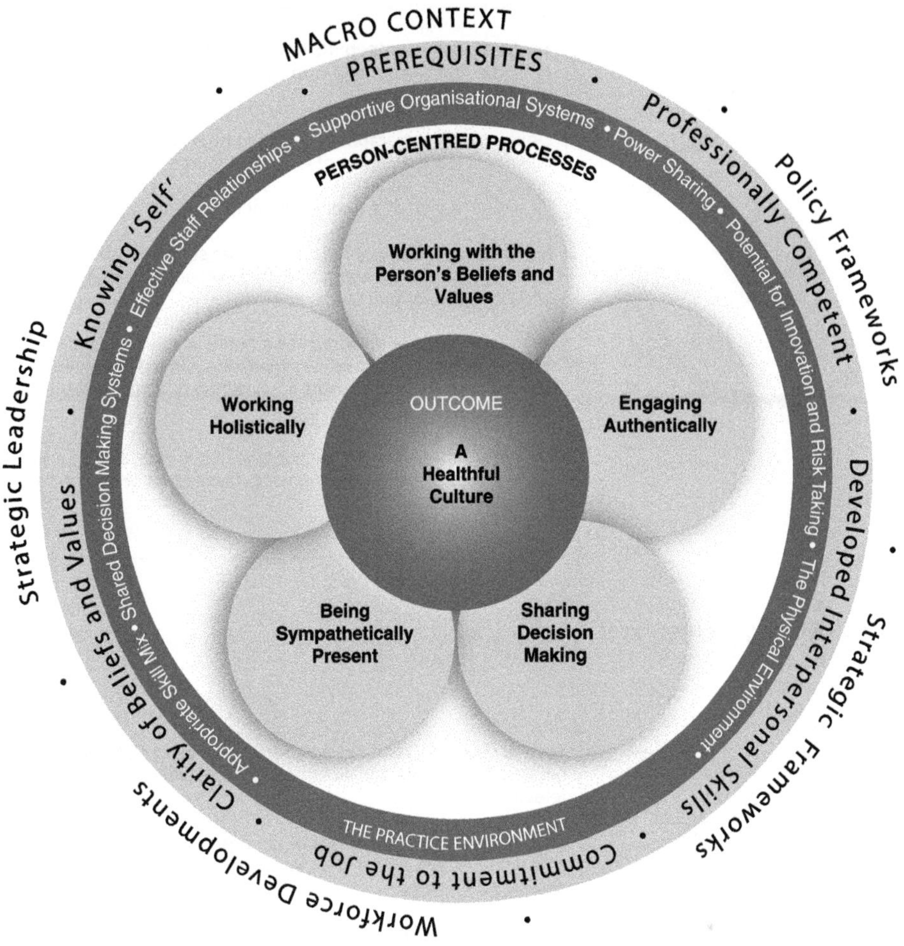

Figure 3.1 Person-centred Practice Framework.

The practice environment

The practice environment reflects the complexity of the context in which healthcare is experienced (Figure 3.3). There is an evidence base in the field of knowledge translation and knowledge utilisation focusing on exploring the meaning of context; identifying the key elements of context and their enabling or hindering qualities (for evidence/knowledge use); and developing approaches to measuring the impact of context on clinical and team effectiveness, including impact on patient outcomes (Rycroft-Malone 2004; Rycroft-Malone et al. 2013). The position taken within the Person-centred Practice Framework is that context is synonymous with the practice environment, and contained within it are multifaceted characteristics and qualities of the environment (people, processes and structures) that impact on the effectiveness of person-centred practice.

To this end, seven characteristics of the care environment are described within the framework: appropriate skill mix; systems that facilitate shared decision making; the sharing of

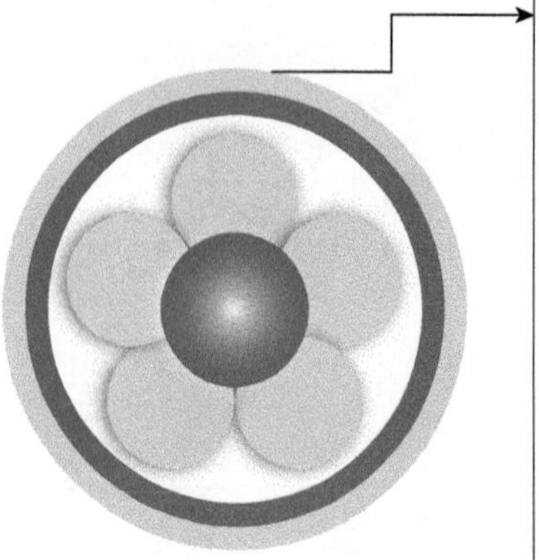

Professionally competent: the knowledge, skills and attitudes of the person to negotiate care options, and effectively provide holistic care

Developed interpersonal skills: the ability of the person to communicate at a variety of levels with others, using effective verbal and non-verbal interactions that show personal concern for their situation and a commitment to finding mutual solutions

Knowing self: the way a person makes sense of his/her knowing, being and becoming through reflection, self-awareness, and engagement with others

Clarity of belief and values: awareness of the impact of beliefs and values on the healthcare experience and the commitment to reconciling beliefs and values in ways that facilitate person-centredness

Commitment to the job: demonstrated commitment of persons through intentional engagement that focuses on achieving the best possible outcomes

Figure 3.2 Defining prerequisites.

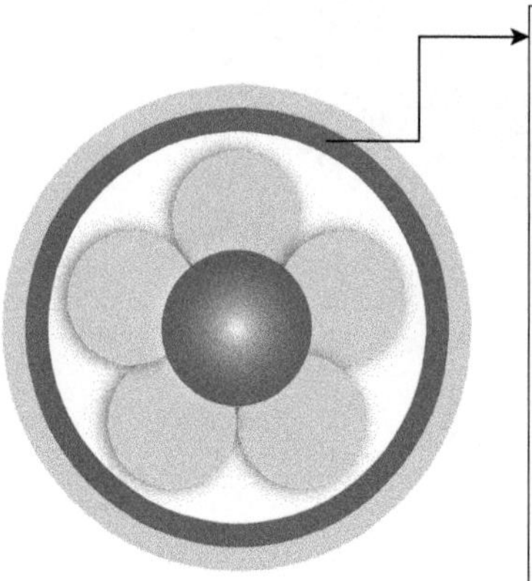

Appropriate skill mix: the number and range of staff with the requisite knowledge and skills needed to provide a quality service relevant to the context

Shared decision-making systems: organisational commitment to collaborative, inclusive and participative ways of engaging within and between teams

Effective staff relationships: interpersonal connections that are productive in the achievement of holistic person-centred care

Power sharing: Non-dominant, non-hierarchical relationships that do not exploit people, but instead are concerned with achieving the best mutually agreed outcomes through agreed values, goals, wishes and desires

Physical environment: healthcare environments that balance aesthetics with function by paying attention to design, dignity, privacy, sanctuary, choice/control, safety, and universal access with the intention of improving patient, family and staff operational performance and outcomes

Supportive organisational systems: organisational systems that promote initiative, creativity, freedom and safety of persons, underpinned by a governance framework that emphasises culture, relationships, values, communication, professional autonomy, and accountability

Potential for innovation and risk taking: the exercising of professional accountability in decision making that reflects a balance between the best available evidence, professional judgement, local information, and patient/family preferences

Figure 3.3 Defining the characteristics of the practice environment.

power; effective staff relationships; organisational systems that are supportive; potential for innovation and risk taking; and the physical environment. Furthermore, we would contend that the constructs that make up the practice environment have a significant impact on the operationalisation of person-centred practice and have the greatest potential to limit or enhance the facilitation of person-centred processes (McCormack et al. 2011).

Person-centred processes

Person-centred processes focus on ways of engaging that are necessary to create connections between persons, which include working with the person's beliefs and values; engaging authentically; being sympathetically present; sharing decision making; and working holistically (Figure 3.4). In the Person-centred Practice Framework the person-centred processes apply to all those involved in healthcare delivery and those in receipt of care. It is important at the outset to acknowledge that the person-centred processes are synergistic and often interwoven in the delivery of healthcare.

Person-centred outcomes

A healthful culture is the outcome expected from the development of effective person-centred practice. A healthful culture is described as one in which decision making is shared, relationships are collaborative, leadership is transformational and innovative practices are supported. The ultimate outcome is to develop a workplace that enables human flourishing. You can read about this in more detail in Chapter 5. This is a key factor in how healthcare is experienced and the extent to which the environment supports and maintains person-centred principles has been shown to be critical to person-centred practice. Use of the term 'healthful' reflects a

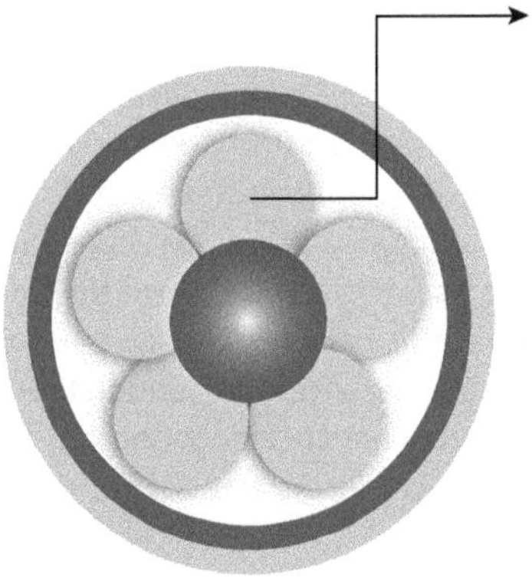

Working with the person's beliefs and values: having a clear picture of the person's values about his/her life and how he/she makes sense of what is happening from their individual perspective, psychosocial context and social role

Sharing decision making: engaging persons in decision making by considering values, experiences, concerns and future aspirations

Engaging authentically: the connectedness between people, determined by knowledge of the person, clarity of beliefs and values, knowledge of self and professional expertise

Being sympathetically present: an engagement that recognises the uniqueness and value of the person, by appropriately responding to cues that maximise coping resources through the recognition of important agendas in their life

Working holistically: ways of connecting that pay attention to the whole person through the integration of physiological, psychological, sociocultural, developmental and spiritual dimensions of persons

Figure 3.4 Defining the person-centred processes.

broader notion of health in line with the work of Seedhouse (1986) that reflects living a positive life, which embraces all dimensions of our being. This is also more relevant from the perspective of staff where a healthful culture is one in which they are supported and enabled to maximise their potential in line with their values. Development of a healthful culture has the potential to create conditions that enable human flourishing for those who give care and those who receive care.

Applying the framework in practice

The Person-centred Practice Framework has been developed over more than a decade, as a means of enhancing understanding of person-centred practice and to provide insights that challenge accepted norms and ways of working. It has been described as a tool that can illuminate practice and provides a language that can operationalise person-centredness at individual, team, organisational and systems levels. The following are some examples of how the framework has been used:

- as a tool for reflection that supports active learning
- to underpin delivery of improvements in practice
- to underpin strategy and policy frameworks
- as a theoretical framework in research
- as a curriculum framework for preregistration and postregistration nursing
- to inform outcome measures and drive instrument development.

Throughout the chapters in this book, there are many activities that will enable you to use the Person-centred Practice Framework to enhance your understanding of person-centredness and how it relates to your practice.

Conclusions

Within this chapter we have introduced the Person-centred Practice Framework as a theoretical model that is multiprofessional in nature and is aimed at operationalising person-centredness across healthcare systems. The Framework takes account of the attributes of staff that are required to manage the practice environment in order to engage in processes that enable the delivery of effective person-centred practice and explains how this can influence the development of healthful cultures. Activities throughout the rest of this book encourage you to apply the Framework in a range of diverse practice situations, to enhance your understanding of professional practice. Chapters 1–3 form a strong foundation to enhance engagement with the remainder of this book. This chapter in particular should serve as a reference for describing components of the Person-centred Practice Framework.

Summary

- The Person-centred Practice Framework was originally born out of a desire to operationalise person-centredness in a way that would illuminate practice.
- The Person-centred Practice Framework is a theoretical framework that is suitable for use across multiple contexts.

- The Person-centred Practice Framework comprises four main domains: *prerequisites*, which focus on the attributes of staff; the *practice environment*, which focuses on the context in which care is delivered; the *person-centred processes*, which focus on delivering care to people through a range of activities; and the *outcome*, which is the result of effective person-centred practice.
- The Person-centred Practice Framework sits within the broader *macro context* (the fifth domain), reflecting factors that are strategic and political in nature that influence the development of person-centred cultures.
- The Person-centred Practice Framework provides a language that enables people to name components of person-centredness and barriers and enablers that influence its development in the workplace.

References

Buetow, S. (2016). *Person-Centred Health Care: Balancing the Welfare of Clinicians and Patients*. London: Routledge.

Dewing, J. (2012). Bringing Merleau-Ponty's inspirations to working with participants. In: *Creative Spaces for Qualitative Researching, Living Research* (eds. J. Higgs, A. Titchen, D. Horsfall and D. Bridges). Amsterdam: Sense Publications.

Fitzpatrick, J.J. and Whall, A.L. (2016). *Conceptual Models of Nursing: Global Perspectives*, 5e, 118–131. Boston, MA: Pearson.

McCance, T.V. (2003). Caring in nursing practice: the development of a conceptual framework. *Research and Theory for Nursing Practice: An International Journal* 17 (2): 101–116.

McCance, T.V., McKenna, H.P., and Boore, J.R.P. (1999). Caring: theoretical perspectives of relevance to nursing. *Journal of Advanced Nursing* 30 (6): 1388–1395.

McCormack, B. (2001a). Autonomy and the relationship between nurses and older people. *Ageing and Society* 21: 417–446.

McCormack, B. (2001b). *Negotiating Partnerships with Older People – A Person-Centred Approach*. Basingstoke: Ashgate.

McCormack, B. and McCance, T. (2016). United Kingdom: the person-centred nursing model. In: *Conceptual Models of Nursing: Global Perspectives*, 5e (eds. J.J. Fitzpatrick and A.L. Whall), 118–131. Boston, MA: Pearson.

McCormack, B. and McCance, T. (2017). *Person-Centred Practice in Nursing and Healthcare: Theory and Practice*. Oxford: Wiley-Blackwell.

McCormack, B., McCance, T., Slater, P. et al. (2008). Person-centred outcomes and cultural change. In: *International Practice Development in Nursing and Healthcare* (eds. K. Manley, B. McCormack and V. Wilson), 189–214. Oxford: Blackwell.

McCormack, B., Dewing, J., and McCance, T. (2011). Developing person-centred care: addressing contextual challenges through practice development. *Online Journal of Issues in Nursing* 16 (2): 3.

Mitchell, E., McCance, T., McCormack, B., and Gribben, B. (2015). Patients' experiences of in-hospital care when nursing staff were engaged in a practice development programme to promote person-centredness: a narrative analysis study. *International Journal of Nursing Studies*. 52: 1454–1462.

Peplau, H. (1997). Peplau's theory of interpersonal relations. *Nursing Science Quarterly* 10 (4): 162–167.

Roper, N., Logan, W., and Tierney, A. (2000). *The Roper-Logan-Tierney Model of Nursing*. London: Churchill Livingstone.

Rycroft-Malone, J. (2004). PARIHS framework – a framework for guiding the implementation of evidence based practice. *Journal of Nursing Care Quality* 19 (4): 297–304.

Rycroft-Malone, J., Seers, K., Chandler, J. et al. (2013). Role of evidence, context, and facilitation in an implementation trial: implications for the development of the PARIHS framework. *Implementation Science* 8 (28) article no. 28.

Seedhouse, D. (1986). *Health: The Foundations for Achievement*. London: Wiley.

Sharp, S., Mcallister, M., and Broadbent, M. (2018). The tension between person-centred and task focused care in acute surgical setting: a crtical ethnography. *Collegian* 25: 11–17.

Watson, J. (1985). *Nursing: Human Science and Human Care – A Theory of Nursing*. New York: National League of Nursing Press.

Wolf, A., Moore, L., Lydahl, D. et al. (2017). The realities of partnership in person-centred care: a qualitative interview study with patients and professionals. *British Medical Journal Open* 7: e016491.

World Health Organization (2001). *International Classification of Functioning, Disability and Health (ICF)*. Geneva: World Health Organization.

Yuill, C., Crinson, I., and Duncan, E. (2010). *Key Concepts in Health Studies. Sage Key Concepts*. London: Sage.

Further reading

Manley, K., Sanders, K., Cardiff, S., and Webster, J. (2011). Effective workplace culture: the attributes, enabling factors and consequences of a new concept. *International Practice Development Journal* 1 (2): 1–29.

McCance, T., Hastings, J., and Dowler, H. (2015). Evaluating the use of key performance indicators to evidence the patient experience. *Journal of Clinical Nursing* 24: 3084–3094.

Slater, P., McCance, T., and McCormack, B. (2017). The development and testing of the person-centred practice inventory – staff (PCPI-S). *International Journal of Quality in Healthcare* 29 (4): 541–547.

4

Knowing self

Donna Brown[1] and Savina Tropea[2]

[1]*Ulster University, Northern Ireland, UK*

[2]*Queen Margaret University, Edinburgh, Scotland, UK*

Contents

Fundamentals of Person-Centred Healthcare Practice, First Edition. Edited by Brendan McCormack, Tanya McCance, Cathy Bulley, Donna Brown, Ailsa McMillan and Suzanne Martin.

Learning outcomes

- Gain some understanding of the different perspectives of self.
- Determine how the choices we make impact upon our professional and personal self and vice versa.
- Refine our personal self-awareness

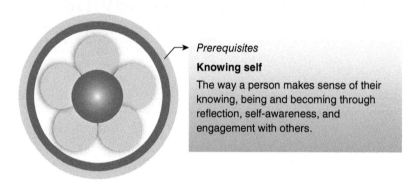

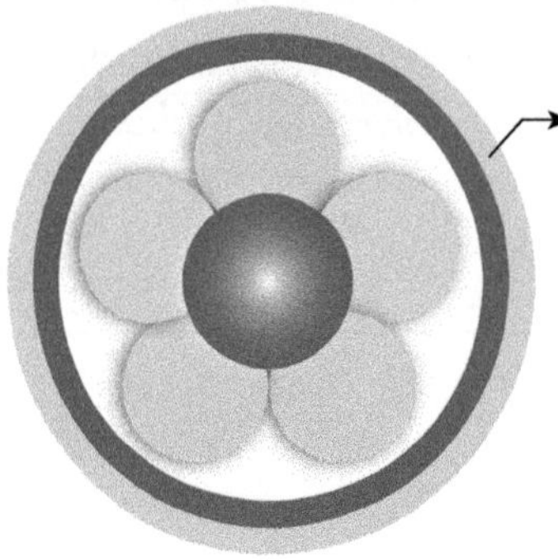

Prerequisites

Knowing self

The way a person makes sense of their knowing, being and becoming through reflection, self-awareness, and engagement with others.

Introduction

This chapter will primarily focus on the prerequisite of knowing self. It will also consider the importance of knowing self in relation to the care environment and to the person-centred processes. We will explore the value of knowing self, as a person, and consider ways in which we can become more aware of self, of how this awareness impacts on working relationships between colleagues and the person using health services.

Understanding and defining self: different perspectives

In the Person-centred Practice Framework, *knowing self* is defined as the way a person makes sense of their knowing, being and becoming through reflection, self-awareness and engagement with others. This definition will guide our thinking as we work through this chapter. Within this perspective, self is not viewed as something fixed. As persons, we are on a constant journey of learning to 'find and re-fine oneself' (Dworkin 1991, p. 32). With the goal of self-development, we engage with lifelong learning and professional growth, through developing self-awareness and engaging in self-reflection.

Before exploring why it is important to know self and what the process of knowing self may look like, we need to develop an understanding of what self is. Throughout history, philosophers, psychologists, sociologists and social psychologists have formulated different definitions and theories of self which have resulted in conflicting perspectives about what self is, its nature and the method of investigation. We have here provided a brief summary of the key perspectives on self to encourage exploration of how these may relate to you and the person-centred perspective. When consulting other texts, you might see slightly different terminology from the one used here.

Experiential perspectives focus on self as an independent and private entity, and on subjective experience. We experience the world and life from a certain point of view, through the lens of our own self. To be a person means to be aware of these experiences (of our thoughts and feelings, for example) and to be aware of being aware. It also means to be able to reflect on our thoughts and actions, to consider different alternatives and the possibility of change. On the other hand, social constructionist perspectives originating from sociology and social sciences view reality and self as socially constructed, as created through the interaction of individuals and groups in the social context. As we grow, social relationships and interactions with others (as well as language and culture) continue to shape who we are and contribute to our ways of thinking and feeling. Furthermore, there are narrative accounts of self, highlighting that selves are agents. Actions take place in time and we can make sense of them when placed within a coherent narrative or life story (temporal and social dimension of self) (Stevens 2002; Zahavi 2014).

There are also realist perspectives of self. These are embraced by various empirical scientists from the areas of psychology, psychiatry and neuroscience, who utilise an experimental approach to the investigation of self, trying to identify measurable variables, to find out the rules that could explain psychological phenomena and the way we behave. As to the biological perspectives of self, these adopt the scientific method to focus on the physiological and genetic processes taking place in the person's body and their influence on behaviour (Stevens 2002; Zahavi 2014).

Some of these perspectives when taken in isolation highlight specific aspects of self, and risk providing a partial and fragmented view. This view clashes with the theory underpinning the Person-centred Practice Framework and the focus on the person as a whole (encompassing the biological, psychological, social, spiritual and environmental dimensions); on personhood (see Chapter 1); and on the five dimensions of being a person (see Chapter 1). The exploration of the possible interrelationships between different perspectives can help us gain interesting insights into the complexity of self. It also inevitably raises questions about the compatibility, or not, of certain points between the different perspectives which are ultimately related to different ways of viewing reality, what is true and what is real (Stevens 2002; Zahavi 2014).

Different aspects of self

Now that we have highlighted the complexities around establishing what constitutes self, we will focus on some of the aspects of self as identified through the literature. The self-concept is the idea we have of ourselves, of who we are in terms of our personal attributes (physical, emotional, social, etc.). It develops as we communicate and interact with others (particularly significant others) during the early stages of our lives, but also as we grow up. It is shaped by the attitudes and reactions others have towards us (Freshwater 2002). Our self-concept does not necessarily align with the way other people see us. According to Rogers (2003, p. 501), the self-concept originates from both the person's direct experiencing (and the values attached to these experiences) and from the 'distorted symbolisation of sensory reactions'. The latter results in the unconscious adoption ('introjection') of values and concepts taken from others (for example, from our parents) as if they were experienced directly. The person can experience freedom from inner tension 'when the concept of the self is at least roughly congruent with all the experiences of the organism', with its genuine reactions and hence starts to feel more his or her real self (Rogers 2003, p. 513).

Activity

Write down 10 words to describe yourself.
Invite a trusted colleague to write down 10 words to describe you.

- Do the words used by your colleague look the same or different from yours?
- Is this what you expected?
- Why do you think the words may look as they do?

This activity might prompt you to think about the way you see yourself and the way others see you. It may also encourage you to explore further different aspects of self, such as the self-concept and the real (or authentic) self and their relevance for person-centred practice.

You are invited to revisit this activity at the end of reading this chapter: have you learned anything new about yourself?

The journey through 'knowing self': tools and approaches

Finding ways to engage in the process of 'knowing self' and improve self-awareness is important for delivering person-centred practice. We need to know self to be authentic and to work collaboratively with others (McCormack and McCance 2017). As you read through this section, you are encouraged to reflect on the examples provided and consider their contribution to the process of 'knowing self' and the role played by yourself and others during the process. The selection of tools and approaches outlined below is not exhaustive. Further ways of knowing self are outlined later in this chapter (reflection and feedback) and in Chapters 1, 5, 12 and 29. This section also requires you to explore what works best for you. For any of these tools and approaches to be able to help during your journey through 'knowing self', they require engagement in critical reflection.

The Johari Window (Luft and Ingham 1955) is a tool normally used within teams or groups (working either one to one or as a group), to help gain more self-awareness about what we know about ourselves and what others know about us. It is divided into four quadrants (windows) that outline potential forms of awareness, behaviours, motivations and feelings in a relationship. The first window represents the behaviours that are openly seen by ourselves and others. The second refers to behaviours, feelings and motivations that you (self) are unaware of (blind spot) but are open for others to see. This highlights inconsistencies between what we say and what we actually do. These behaviours may benefit from feedback from others in order to shrink the blind spot. Quadrant three is a hidden window in which behaviours, motivations and feelings are known to self but are hidden from others (the private self). Finally, the fourth window is an area of aspects unknown to both ourselves and others. As we grow and develop, these 'hidden and unknown' elements of who we are as persons may become known to us – this can be challenging to experience. For more information about this tool see: www.youtube.com/watch?v=KdYo5jn29w4.

Alternatively, journalling is a progressively evolving written record of thoughts, feelings, experiences and learning, designed to increase self-awareness and self-understanding of practice. When developing a journal, we need to consider the medium to use (e.g. paper, computer, phone), how much time to dedicate to writing, if the writing will be private or shared and how structured the journal will be (Dimitroff 2018). Journalling offers an opportunity to be creative. If you are interested in knowing more see: www.americannursetoday.com/journaling-valuable-registered-nurses and https://criticalcreativity.org.

Learning sets offer a structured approach for 6–8 people to meet regularly and learn collectively from one another's experiences. The focus of this approach is on learning (about oneself and others) and on professional development. Participants usually work together for an agreed period of time, taking turns at presenting their issue, in allocated time slots. The 'set' generally has a facilitator who is part of the group but also has responsibility for creating an encouraging, challenging and focused learning environment. To explore this approach further see: https://rapidbi.com/action-learning-sets.

The importance of self-knowledge for developing healthful cultures

The way we see ourselves and the world can influence how we see and relate to other people, and our beliefs and values can affect how we make decisions about healthcare (see Chapters 9 and 12). Thus, developing healthful relationships with the persons we care for and the persons we work with is at the heart of person-centred practice. This requires awareness of self and others.

Health and social care practice can involve situations when difficult topics are approached during conversations between healthcare staff and the person, a significant other, a carer or a colleague. There are situations where the balancing of the risks and enabling choices and preferences may require 'challenging' or 'courageous conversations' (Masterson 2007), not only with the people we care for but with other members of the healthcare team who might have different opinions, values and beliefs (Seedhouse 2009). For these conversations to lead to better outcomes, knowledge and skills are required; for example, knowledge of the research evidence on the topic (see Chapter 32), communication strategies (see Chapter 8), interpersonal skills (see Chapter 10), and awareness of the strong emotions that might arise. To manage these situations and respond effectively, it can be helpful to be aware of those topics and behaviours that might trigger in us strong or negative emotional responses (Masterson 2007, p. 30).

When we feel that our personal self has been attacked (our 'buttons' have been pushed), processes are triggered through the amygdala to protect ourselves by rushing into action (fight-or-flight response) (Goleman 1996; Bruno 2011). To maintain professionalism in these situations, it is important to 'cool down'. Emotional intelligence (see Chapter 10) helps us in this process. By acknowledging and listening to what our feelings are telling us and managing them more effectively to aid our logical thinking, we can regain perspective (through activation of the orbitofrontal cortex) (Goleman 1996; Bruno 2011).

Ways of cooling down include the following.

- Look for alternative ways of explaining a situation (i.e. reframing a discussion).
- Exchange negative thoughts for positive ones (i.e. use of thoughts and phrases that can help to shift the focus to something positive or pleasant).
- Observe thoughts and feelings from a distance (i.e. practice of mindfulness).

Developing self-awareness allows us to know ourselves better, to help make self-regulation possible (to modify our behaviour, choose how to respond to a situation rather than following possible temptations) and to experience greater consistency between the way we behave and our attitudes. To become self-aware, we need to reflect on what we experience when we focus, for example, on our sensations, perceptions, emotions, thoughts, attitudes, preferences and intentions (Morin 2011). Reflection is therefore a central skill in the development of self-awareness.

Using reflection to know self

Reflection and self-awareness are key to knowing self in order to further develop who we are as persons and as professionals. By reflecting on our actions and critically relating to them, we become aware of why we act in certain ways and introduce the potential for learning and change (see Chapter 29). Through reflection, for example, we can work on reconciling the ideal professional self and the actual professional self, the desired practice and the actual practice (Freshwater 2002).

Activity

Reflect on and write down an example of a time in your practice when the care you were providing was not consistent with those desired by the other person. For example, the person did not want to drink the nutrition supplement, try a particular exercise, take medication or vaccinate their baby. What did you do?

This activity may be deeply challenging but has the potential to help you ask yourself difficult questions in order to consider your future behaviours. To develop deep questioning skills, explore the following.

- Did I live out person-centred values?
- Which element(s) of the Person-centred Practice Framework does this map to?
- What organisational pressures obstructed my perception?
- How could my actions have been perceived by others?
- What (if anything) do I need to change to become more person-centred in my practice?
- What is the research evidence on the topic?

Critical reflective practice, whether on an individual level or within groups, is essential to enabling persons who provide healthcare to gain insight into self, the care environment and how these entwine with their practice and the care they deliver (person-centred processes). Reflection encompasses asking challenging questions and being able to live through the discomfort or anxiety of changing deeply held ways of being (Bolton 2014). As heightened anxiety can be counterproductive to learning, it is imperative that we remain mindful of the need to actively contribute to creating spaces in which it is safe to share thoughts and learn from our experiences (see work of Brown and McCormack 2016).

Creating the conditions to know self and others

Looking closely at self requires bravery and living with uncertainty (Bolton 2014). By standing back from the daily grind and assumptions we make and engaging in reflection, we become more aware of the influences that surround us and we are motivated to change (Seedhouse 2017).

As previously highlighted, we can engage in the process of knowing self in a variety of ways. Many of these rely on others to provide us with assistance or feedback so that we can enhance our understanding of our behaviours, actions and reactions through the eyes of others. However, feedback given by the wrong person, at the wrong place or time, in an insensitive way, will add little to our knowledge of self or to creating a healthful culture. Therefore, when considering getting to know and developing self, it is important to consider the following points.

- What feedback do I want and am I ready to hear it?
- Who do I trust and value to assist me?
- Are they the right person?
- Who can support me as a person?
- Is that different from who supports me in a team?
- What do I need to achieve a positive outcome for all?

Activity

Either individually or in a group, reflect on what factors you think are necessary to create the conditions in which to explore knowing self and get to the heart of your practice.

You are encouraged to contemplate things such as time to reflect, quietness, being open, honest, self-confidence, ability to think laterally and non-judgementally about your self and practice. It is easy to be overly critical of our own practice and disappointed in ourselves. It is always good to articulate and work with positive things we have done in practice to affirm values and beliefs and be motivated to acknowledge these to improve our knowledge of self. Perhaps you were thinking of working with others and considered they needed to actively listen, be supportive, generous of self, time and knowledge, approachable, reliable and trustworthy (Heron 1999).

Conclusion

Throughout this chapter we have explored different perspectives of self and possible interrelations between them. As persons, we are constantly involved in a process of being and becoming. Accepting that we are persons, with our strengths and, most importantly, our vulnerabilities, is essential so that any exploration of self is undertaken in a safe environment, through engaging in reflection and gaining feedback. In this way we can become more self-aware and find the motivation to consider the choices we make, as these contribute to making us who we are and who we become (see Chapter 29).

Summary

- Self is not something static.
- To develop self, we need to critically reflect on our practice to gain insight into the deeply enmeshed relationship between self (prerequisites), the care environment and the person-centred processes, and how they connect with one another.
- Using different approaches to knowing self is important in helping us to understand ourselves better and engage in person-centred practice.

References

Bolton, G. (2014). *Reflective Practice. Writing and Professional Development*, 4e. London: Sage.

Brown, D. and McCormack, B. (2016). Exploring psychological safety as a component of facilitation within the promoting action research in health services framework. *Journal of Clinical Nursing* 25: 2912–2293.

Bruno, H.E. (2011). The neurobiology of emotional intelligence. Using our brain to stay cool under pressure. *Young Children* 66 (1): 22–27.

Dimitroff, L.J. (2018). Journaling: a valuable tool for registered nurses. *American Nurse Today* 13: 11.

Dworkin, G. (1991). *The Theory and Practice of Autonomy*. Cambridge: Cambridge University Press.

Freshwater, D. (ed.) (2002). *Therapeutic Nursing: Improving Patient Care Through Self-Awareness and Reflection*. London: Sage Publications.

Goleman, D. (1996). *Emotional Intelligence: Why It Can Matter More than IQ*. London: Bloomsbury Publishing.

Heron, J. (1999). *The Complete Facilitators Handbook*. London: Kogan Page.

Luft, J. and Ingham, H. (1955). *The Johari Window as a Graphic Model of Interpersonal Awareness*. University of California, Los Angeles, Extension Office, Proceedings of the Western Training Laboratory in Group Development.

Masterson, A. (2007). Community matrons: the value of knowing self (part two). *Nursing Older People* 19 (5): 29–31.

McCormack, B. and McCance, T. (eds.) (2017). *Person-Centred Practice in Nursing and Health Care: Theory and Practice*. Chichester: Wiley Blackwell.

Morin, A. (2011). Self-awareness part 1: definition, measures, effects, functions and antecedents. *Social and Personality Psychology Compass* 5 (10): 807–823.

Rogers, C.R. (2003). *Client-Centered Therapy*. London: Constable & Robinson.

Runde, C.E. (2014). Conflict competence in the workplace. *Employment Relations Today* 40 (4): 25–31.

Seedhouse, D. (2009). *Ethics: The Heart of Health Care*. Chichester: Wiley Blackwell.

Seedhouse, D. (2017). *Thoughtful Healthcare: Ethical Awareness and Reflective Practice*. London: Sage Publications.

Stevens, R. (ed.) (2002). *Understanding the Self*. London: Sage Publications.

Zahavi, D. (2014). *Self and Other. Exploring Subjectivity, Empathy, and Shame*. Oxford: Oxford University Press.

5

Flourishing as humans

Brendan McCormack[1], Tanya McCance[2], and Jan Dewing[1]

[1] Queen Margaret University, Edinburgh, Scotland, UK
[2] Ulster University, Northern Ireland, UK

Contents

Fundamentals of Person-Centred Healthcare Practice, First Edition. Edited by Brendan McCormack, Tanya McCance, Cathy Bulley, Donna Brown, Ailsa McMillan and Suzanne Martin.

Learning outcomes

- Understand the meaning of human flourishing.
- Articulate the key attributes of human flourishing and their relationship with person-centredness.
- Consider the conditions necessary for persons to flourish.
- Critically reflect on the attributes of human flourishing and how they connect with persons as spiritual beings.

Introduction

Wakening and entering the day ahead of us is a fundamental part of being alive. How we engage in such a process is dependent on a range of factors that make it either an exciting and joyful start or one that can feel sluggish and listless. Connecting with our immediate environment through observing what is happening or actively connecting with it through physical activity opens up a space for us to consider our being in the world and our day ahead – what some people might see as our spiritual being. This moment of awakening that we each experience every day of our lives can be seen as a micro-context of what we can come to know as 'human flourishing' and the conditions necessary for each of us to flourish in our lives. We would argue that the ultimate manifestation of person-centredness is 'flourishing persons'. In this chapter will encourage you to participate in a reflexive engagement with the idea of human flourishing and what it means for all of us in our lives. We will connect ideas of human flourishing with the 'spiritual self' and our existence as spiritual beings.

Awakening

Water gently lapping over stones
Sunshine rising from the blue horizon
Seabirds swooping in search of morsels of goodness
Morning joggers tracing the outline of the beach
Restaurants waking up from their night-time slumber
The day begins as the world connects

To get us into this reflexive space, we invite you to engage with the following activity.

Activity

Identify a time in your life when you felt you were 'at your best'. What did it feel like? Why was it such a good experience, i.e. what were the key qualities of the experience? What did you do to make it such a good experience (if anything)? Using a creative medium of your choice (drawing, sketching, painting, poetry, prose, photography, etc.), create an image that captures the essence of the experience.

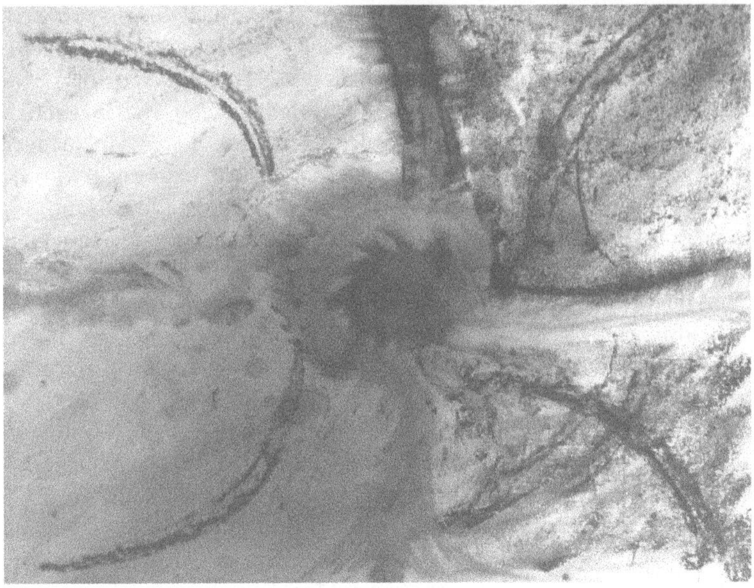

Figure 5.1 'Flourishing in transition'. Source: Brendan McCormack

This image created by one of us (Brendan) expresses his experience of flourishing at a particular stage in his life – a time of significant transition (Figure 5.1). The painting has a central source of energy and four quadrants, each expressing different conditions that enhanced or hindered his flourishing at that point in time. The picture as a whole, however, shows the balance of different energies and all of them working together to create a holistic picture of his experience at that time. Each element has particular meaning for Brendan and came to life as he connected with the flow of creating the image and the intuitive connections arising. The image gives some insight into the dynamic nature of flourishing and its many shapes and energies.

What is human flourishing?

You may not have thought about the term 'human flourishing' prior to reading this chapter, but you might have thought about your spirituality or you as a spiritual person. Spirituality is a broad term with room for many perspectives. Fundamentally, though, spirituality focuses on the deeper aspects of ourselves as persons (our personhood!) and what it means to be alive, happy and connected with the world.

Human flourishing as happiness

The term 'human flourishing' has existed for thousands of years. Originally coined as *eudaimonia* (meaning human flourishing or happiness) by the philosopher Aristotle, the term has existed as a way of expressing all that we know to be human and to live out our personhood. Eudaimonia is an active term meaning we as human beings actively work in pursuit of happiness. Such happiness includes our subjective experiences in pursuit of ends (outcomes or achievements) that are worthy of choosing for human beings.

Eudaimonia is a unifying principle, suggesting that to be happy we have to actively pay attention to such virtues as belonging, harmony, social justice, fairness and equality. Being happy in the world (or to flourish) is not about the pursuit of pleasure, *hedonia* (think about hedonism!), but is the pursuit of a state of well-being by 'concurrently doing what I want to do while at the same time doing what I ought to do'. What Aristotle suggests here is a moral perspective on our being as agents in the world and which should resonate with us as healthcare workers – we are effective as a person when the actions we actually take are the same as those we ought to be taking as a moral agent. To do this requires an understanding of what is required of us as persons (the evidence that informs our practice) whilst at the same time being in a position to want to do the right thing, to enjoy doing it and sometimes to be uplifted by doing it.

So, to flourish means living out the virtues. Virtues are a subset of our character as persons. They are not innate qualities, like eyesight or hearing, but instead are characteristics we acquire and develop through our upbringing, experiences, education, etc. We build them over time and the more we actively work on them, the more attuned we become to how they work for us. The contrary also applies, of course, in that if we don't use them, we lose them and can slide into immoral attitudes and behaviours. If we consider some of the characteristics of persons discussed in Chapter 1, then the possession of virtues could also be seen as a defining characteristic of persons and one that distinguishes us from non-persons. This is because behaving through the lens of the virtues requires us to have 'reason'. That is, we have to reflect on our moral actions and make decisions about our behaviours, practices and actions and if they are morally virtuous or not. Such reflection guides our decisions and ultimately our life as moral agents, i.e. our flourishing. Aristotle identified four primary moral virtues – prudence, justice, temperance and fortitude – but over many years of critique and ongoing development of virtues as a framework for moral action (see for example MacIntyre 1992), the range of possible virtues to include in a virtues-based moral framework has become much more diverse and inclusive.

Human flourishing as psychological wellness

Since the work of Aristotle, human flourishing has grown and developed as a way of capturing our humanness and indeed is the foundation of a branch of psychology called 'positive psychology'. Positive psychologists argue that human flourishing in this context moves beyond the confines of 'happiness' (although this argument is flawed if we view happiness as eudaimonia!) and embraces a wide range of psychological constructs that offer insights into what it means to be happy and to feel well. The origins of such thinking arise from the work of Martin Seligman (2011) who postulated that flourishing arises when we pay attention to and deliberately set out to build and maintain the five components of the PERMA model, designed by him. The five components of the model are:

- **P**ositive emotions
- **E**ngagement
- **R**elationships
- **M**eaning
- **A**ccomplishments.

If we use the PERMA model as a framework for thinking about and reflecting on human flourishing and what that means for us, then we need to consider the following questions.

1. Overall, are our emotions more positive than negative?
2. How engaged are we with the parts of our life that are important to us, such as work or hobbies?

3. Do we have sufficient deep and meaningful relationships to sustain us in our lives?
4. Have we got a sense of purpose in our life, through which we create meaning?
5. Do we apply our talents, gifts and qualities as persons to achieving our goals and then celebrating these achievements (no matter how small)?

PERMA is a useful model for understanding human flourishing and for reflecting on 'where we are at' as spiritual beings. However, living a positive life (just the same as being person-centred as we argued in Chapter 2) is not completely dependent on our own ways of being, actions, relationships and behaviours. The context in which we live our life also plays a key role. So, the success of flourishing is context dependent.

In their paper on engagement in the context of person-centred practice, Dewing and McCormack (2015) argued that for staff to be fully engaged (or to flourish), the conditions necessary for engagement to happen need to be in place. Conditions such as a culture that nurtures positive relationships, consistency between individual goals, desire for achievement and organisational goals, management and leadership styles that invest in people as persons and strategies for learning and development that nurture individual vitality and energy are essential. So, no matter how actively driven we might be towards our own flourishing, it is clear that the cultures in which we work and live have a significant impact on our ability to do so. It is also important not to lose sight of the PERMA attributes plus the essentials of Optimism, Physical Activity, Nutrition, and Sleep. This is now referred to as PERMA+. You might like to see this well-being resource for more details on how PERMA + has been used to shape public health policy for well-being (www.wellbeingandresilience.com/sites/swrc5/media/pdf/permaandcentreoverview.pdf).

Conditions for human flourishing

In recognition that human flourishing is something experienced by persons in context, McCormack and Titchen (2014) developed a set of suggested conditions for human flourishing. These conditions are based on an evolving understanding of human flourishing over 10 years of transformational critical and creative development, research and inquiry. McCormack and Titchen set out this process of evolution of their understanding of human flourishing as something that is intrinsic to persons but is also facilitated through meaningful creative connections with others.

Human flourishing is experienced when people achieve beneficial, positive growth that pushes their boundaries in a range of directions, for example, emotional, social, artistic, metaphysical. And it could be experienced in diverse ways, such as deep fulfilment, radiance, being our real selves and through deep connection with nature, beauty and people. McCormack and Titchen suggest that human flourishing occurs when we move with flow from a point of inner knowing to taking right action effortlessly (Titchen and McCormack 2010). People are helped to flourish (i.e. grow, develop, thrive) during experiences of growth and development that have a focus on well-being for all. Flourishing is supported through contemporary strategies for learning and development, connecting with beauty and nature and blending with ancient, indigenous and spiritual traditions (Titchen et al. 2011, p. 2). As a result of this evolved creative understanding of human flourishing, McCormack and Titchen (Titchen et al. 2011, p. 19) define human flourishing as:

> Human flourishing occurs when we bound and frame naturally co-existing energies, when we embrace the known and yet to be known, when we embody contrasts and when we achieve stillness and harmony. When we flourish we give and receive loving kindness.

Activity

Here are two links to TED talks. The first is a talk by Martin Seligman www.ted.com/talks/martin_seligman_on_the_state_of_psychology?language=en and the second, a talk by Angie Titchen www.youtube.com/watch?v=h0OoeSmA-wA.

Listen to these talks and consider the differences and similarities in how human flourishing is understood and applied. Make notes about these. As a result of listening and reflecting on these talks, we invite you to undertake your own inquiry into your own flourishing. You could do this alone, but you may find that working with others would be more enriching through the reflection itself. We encourage you to start with your own notes you have made from listening to these talks and then think about how these notes compare and contrast with the definitions and descriptions of human flourishing presented in this chapter so far and how you think about your own spiritual existence. Be open to what emerges!

Engaging in this reflective activity may have opened up new insights that you hadn't been aware of before, or it may have revealed new understandings that help you make sense of previous experiences, thoughts and attitudes. In any case, whatever you achieved will help you to expand your consciousness about you as a spiritual person and your flourishing. But as we said earlier, paying attention to the context in which we live and work is important to enriching our capacity for flourishing as persons and the 'conditions for human flourishing' developed by McCormack and Titchen (Titchen et al. 2011) have this explicit purpose in mind. Table 5.1 lists the seven conditions for human flourishing developed by McCormack and Titchen. An explanation of each condition is provided as well as some reflective questions we have developed for you to consider in the context of your work or your life in general. As you read these, you might want to refer back to the work you did for Activity 2 and consider how these conditions resonate with your reflections and new insights and/or if they might be helpful to you in changing particular ways of being that could further enhance your flourishing.

Table 5.1 The conditions for human flourishing

Condition and description	Reflective questions
Bounding and framing Being strong is a characteristic of our humanness that enables us to meet the challenges and opportunities of each day and draw on our inner strengths to achieve what we want to and need to. However, being strong and having strength also place significant responsibilities on us as persons as we strive to meet what may at times seem like unrealistic or unachievable expectations of ourselves and others. Sometimes these responsibilities can seem overwhelming and we need to *bound or frame* our focus so we can make sense of the whole by concentrating on particular parts. Understanding the importance of bounding and framing enables an appreciation of wanting to still the mind and zone out the many distractions that get in the way of us flourishing in life and work. Finding moments of stillness and intentionally focusing only on the issues at hand enables growth, movement and a greater potential to flourish	What do you prioritise in your practice – what is in the foreground and the background of your practice?
	What strategies do you use to create your priorities?
	How do you stay strong?
	What processes do you use to still your mind, create focus and build your strength as a person?

Table 5.1 (*Continued*)

Condition and description	Reflective questions
Co-existence It is the case that in everyday life/practice the context can appear impenetrable, such as navigating through unnecessary hierarchies, being restrained by nonsensical rules, people being resistant to change, and little space for growth and development. However, these challenges are important for us to connect with. Gaffney (2011) identifies 'connectivity' as one of the four elements of flourishing persons. Connectivity implies being attuned to what is happening inside and outside of us. Being attuned to these connections enables us to recognise when disconnections are happening and for us to be able to rise to the challenges associated with such disconnections.	What energy do you use in your daily work/life? (emotional, physical, spiritual, etc.)
	What kinds of energy do you draw upon (these might include inspiration from colleagues, from nature, from art, etc.)?
	How do you stay connected with others to maximise energy and be efficient in your use of energy?
Embracing the known and yet to be known The philosopher John O'Donohue (1997) argues that for persons to be present in the moment, there is a need for us to be rooted in the here and now. 'Being present' is an important element of authentic and compassionate caring and the person who is 'present' has the potential to engage with the other in what O'Donohue has called 'Anam Cara' or soul friend to whom intimate connections can be formed. Through the development of connected relationships, the hidden beauty of each person can be revealed and unfolded. When we move around our workplaces with our eyes, ears, sense of smell, touch and taste wide open, 'hidden gems' emerge. As we rush around at work, our senses are often half shut down. If we do not pay attention we can miss the gems and the beauty around us.	How do you maintain your relationships at work and personally?
	Are you aware of different relationships and how they affect your energy levels?
	What do you do about that?
	What strategies do you use to stay engaged in the moment, i.e. be present?
Living with conflicting energies Gaffney (2011) argues that 'challenge' is a key element of flourishing and that without challenge we would languish in the safety of established habits and norms. Challenges aren't always of our own making, but can arise from unexpected and unanticipated avenues and directions. Every day, we have encounters with others that challenge us and we have a choice in how we react. We may feel irritated and need to work hard to reframe the encounter as an opportunity for loving kindness and connection with the other. This movement and management of feelings draws on our emotional intelligence. Moreover, it also needs us to dance with our spiritual intelligence so that we can give graceful care and focused attention to the person or situation. Being really present for that particular person, persons or situation can also help us to reframe the experience as an opportunity for holding strong to our values and our response to its challenges as a means of enabling our own and others' human flourishing. This is not easy, but it is something we can strive for.	How do you deal with everyday challenges from others?
	What intelligences do you mostly draw upon when you experience challenge?
	Are you aware of your more dominant response to challenge and can you draw on different intelligences to enhance or improve your response?

(Continued)

Table 5.1 (*Continued*)

Condition and description	Reflective questions
Being still Creating different and complementary spaces for different purposes is an important consideration in enabling human flourishing. Creating spaces for quiet reflection and stillness is a real challenge in busy healthcare environments and there is a need for us to pay more attention to the workings of healthcare environments and how they function. We need to be able to clear our minds of the busyness of practice and focus instead on the meanings of our practice and the way these meanings shape our everyday reality. Creating spaces for quiet reflection, critical engagement and meaningful connection with others are essential elements of an environment that enables all persons to flourish.	How do you create stillness in your daily life? Are you aware of the 'mental clutter' that clouds your thinking and a focus on busyness? What strategies do you use to reduce the clutter and busyness?
Embodying contrasts When we are flourishing we bring all aspects of ourselves as we develop our potential. Being attuned to all that is good, beautiful and harmonious brings us closer to recognising the sanctity of person-centred human relationships. It helps us to experience our greater selves, the person we are when we are at our best (as opposed to languishing when we are at our worst). Connecting with what we consider to be 'sacred' is important here. The sacred is not the same as having a religious faith or belief or living a life shaped by doctrines. Whilst some of us may have such a faith, what we are concerned with here is more related to a sense of awe and wonderment at goodness, beauty, harmony, compassion and loving kindness – and with honouring them.	Do you pay attention to issues/ideas/actions that might seem to be insignificant to you or others, but which have the potential for deep learning and development? What strategies do you use in your everyday work and life to create 'wonderment' at the ordinary things of life? Do you appreciate contrasts that exist between you and your co-workers? If so, in what way and how do you make use of these contrasts?
Harmony There is no beginning and no end to flourishing. Each element of our life melds and blends with the whole and with each other element. Another way of looking at this is to see each element as bounding and framing the whole of human flourishing. This realisation and acknowledgement of a continuous and connected journey of flourishing rather than a prescribed structure resonates with the need to respond to the wisdom of our bodies in decision making. No matter how much control we may feel over our lives, many internal and external influences shape us and the conditions that enable us to flourish as persons (or not). This is not to suggest a fatalistic perspective but is instead an understanding and position that recognises the interconnectedness of persons, the environment and the universe. Without an appreciation of these deep connections and an understanding of the need to actively shape our being in the world, then our potential for flourishing may not be realised.	How do you develop your preparedness for a continuous approach to self-growth and development? How do you show loving kindness for yourself and others? What mindful practices do you use to build loving kindness for yourself and others?

A resting place

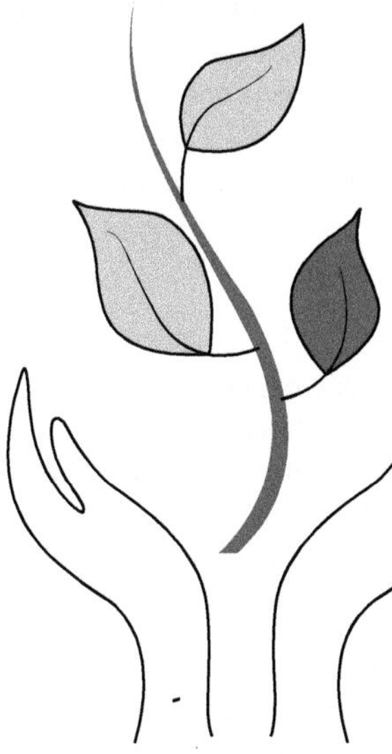

Source: Ilona Krex

You may have experienced engaging with the conditions for human flourishing as both a cognitive, creative and embodied experience. You will have identified how we have focused on using both cognitive and creative approaches to writing and reflecting on our flourishing as persons. There is a growing literature on 'critical creative practices' (cf. Titchen 2013; Titchen and Horsfall 2011; Titchen and McCormack 2008, 2010; Titchen and McMahon 2013) that enables an opening up of our senses and capacity for embodied holistic learning, growth, development and ultimately to transform as persons. Many of these practices are well known and essentially ask us to (re)engage with our innate creative qualities as persons – qualities that expand and extend the horizon of our potentials to flourish, our humanness and capacity as spiritual beings. It is these qualities that surface our moral virtues as persons, bring our personhood to our and others consciousness, create meaning and ultimately build commuinities that are inherently person-centred.

> To be truly happy in this world is a revolutionary act because true happiness depends on a revolution in ourselves. (Salzberg 2002)

Activity

Create an image (poem, painting, etc.) that will act as a 'holder' of your understanding of you as a flourishing person.

Summary

- The term 'human flourishing' has existed for thousands of years, originally coined as *eudaimonia* (meaning human flourishing or happiness) by the philosopher Aristotle.
- Spirituality and human flourishing are inextricably linked and to flourish is an active process of living out the virtues that guide our moral agency.

- Positive psychologists argue that human flourishing embraces a wide range of psychological constructs that offer insights into what it means to be happy and to feel well. The PERMA model is one way of operationalising this approach.
- Considering 'the conditions for human flourishing' enables us to think about the broader landscape of life and how our embodied engagement with all aspects of living provides opportunities for growth, development and transformation.
- Using all our senses in a holistic embodied engagement attunes our senses to the richness of the universe and the riches available to us for our own flourishing and that of others.

References

Dewing, J. and McCormack, B. (2015). A critique of the concept of engagement and its application in person-centred practice. *International Practice Development Journal* 5 article 6.

Gaffney, M. (2011). *Flourishing: How to Achieve a Deeper Sense of Well-Being, Meaning and Purpose – Even When Facing Adversity*. Dublin: Penguin Ireland.

MacIntyre, A. (1992). *After Virtue – A Study in Moral Theory*. London: Duckworth.

McCormack, B. and Titchen, A. (2014). No beginning, no end: an ecology of human flourishing. *International Practice Development Journal* 4 (2): 2.

O'Donohue, J. (1997). *Anam Cara: Spiritual Wisdom from the Celtic World*. London: Bantam Press.

Saltzberg, S. (2002). *Loving-Kindness: The Revolutionary Art of Happiness*. Boston, MA: Shambhala.

Seligman, M. (2011). *Flourish*. New York: Free Press.

Titchen, A. (2013). Writing with flow: publish and flourish through whole-self writing. *International Practice Development Journal* 3 (1): 10.

Titchen, A. and Horsfall, D. (2011). Embodying creative imagination and expression in qualitative research. In: *Creative Spaces for Qualitative Researching: Living Research* (eds. J. Higgs, A. Titchen, D. Horsfall and D. Bridges), 179–190. Rotterdam: Sense.

Titchen, A. and McCormack, B. (2008). A methodological walk in the forest: critical creativity and human flourishing. In: *International Practice Development in Nursing and Healthcare* (eds. K. Manley, B. McCormack and V. Wilson), 59–83. Oxford: Blackwell.

Titchen, A. and McCormack, B. (2010). Dancing with stones: critical creativity as methodology for human flourishing. *Educational Action Research* 18 (4): 531–554.

Titchen, A. and McMahon, A. (2013). Practice development as radical gardening: enabling creativity and innovation. In: *Practice Development in Nursing and Healthcare* (eds. B. McCormack, K. Manley and A. Titchen), 212–232. Oxford: Wiley Blackwell.

Titchen, A., McCormack, B., Wilson, V., and Solman, A. (2011). Human flourishing through body, creative imagination and reflection. *International Practice Development Journal* 1 (1): 1.

Further reading

O'Donohue, J. (2010). *The Four Elements: Reflections on Nature*. London: Transworld Ireland.

McIntosh, P. (2008). Poetics and space: developing a reflective landscape through imagery and human geography. *Reflective Practice* 9 (1): 69–78.

Roth, G. (1990). *Maps to Ecstasy: Teachings of an Urban Shaman*. San Francisco, CA: Mandala.

6

Professionalism and practising professionally

Caroline Gibson[1], Kath MacDonald[1], and Deirdre O'Donnell[2]

[1]Queen Margaret University, Edinburgh, Scotland, UK

[2]Ulster University, Northern Ireland, UK

Contents

Fundamentals of Person-Centred Healthcare Practice, First Edition. Edited by Brendan McCormack, Tanya McCance, Cathy Bulley, Donna Brown, Ailsa McMillan and Suzanne Martin.

Learning outcomes

- Have an understanding of the concept of professionalism in health and social care and its contribution to safe, effective, person-centred practice.
- Be able to apply examples from case-based scenarios to assist you to make professional decisions that are person-centred.
- Be able to critically analyse the tensions between person-centredness, professionalism, and organisational structures.
- Propose professional responses to issues in health and social care that challenge person-centredness.

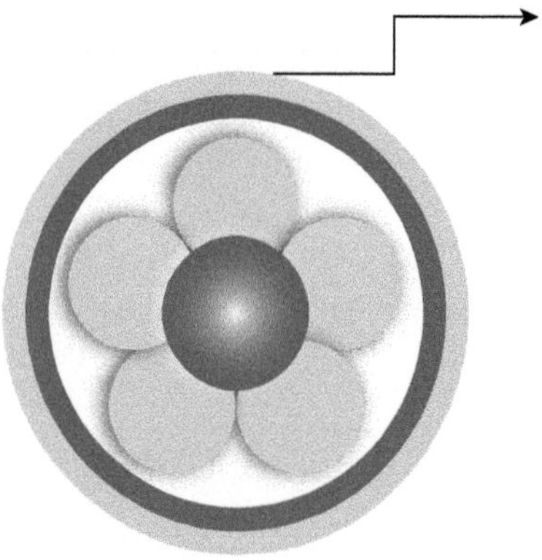

Prerequisites

Professionally competent: the knowledge, skills and attitudes of the person to negotiate care options, and effectively provide holistic care

Knowing self: the way a person makes sense of his/her knowing, being and becoming through reflection, self-awareness, and engagement with others

Clarity of beliefs and values: awareness of the impact of beliefs and values on the healthcare experience and the commitment to reconciling beliefs and values in ways that facilitate person-centredness

Commitment to the job: demonstrated commitment of persons through intentional engagement that focuses on achieving the best possible outcomes

Introduction

This chapter introduces the concept of professionalism and will help you to develop an understanding of what it means to be a healthcare worker. You will have the opportunity to explore the required standards for professional practice and how professionalism contributes to person-centred practice. In the previous chapters you have explored the meaning of person-centredness and been introduced to the Person-centred Practice Framework (PcPF). You have learned about the attributes of staff as prerequisites for person-centredness, the practice environment, the processes that focus on ways of engaging, which are necessary to create connections between persons and how all these considerations influence person-centred outcomes. In this chapter you will have the opportunity to revisit the Person-centred Practice Framework and explore issues about professionalism in health and social care, applied to this model. This will enable you to think about what it means to practise in a professional and person-centred way.

Practising professionally

Traditional models of professionalism promoted professionals as experts in positions of power who practised in a culture that was largely paternalistic (Whitehouse 2015). In the current healthcare climate, people increasingly demand that their voices are heard in a negotiated partnership where decision making is shared (Department of Health 2010). This shift towards person-centred approaches is reflected in global healthcare policy (World Health Organization 2015). The Person-centred Practice Framework supports this position and advocates that health and social care professionals engage authentically, working with people's beliefs and values to place the person at the centre of the care experience. In order to achieve humanistic approaches to care delivery, it is essential that contemporary health and social care professionals can articulate and enact person-centred professional practice (Dalton et al. 2015).

Activity

What is professionalism?

In this first exercise, you are invited to think about a person that you consider to be highly professional.

What is it about that person that you admire?

What does this tell you about the meaning of professionalism?

In your thinking you may have considered the knowledge, skills, attributes and values of a professional. You may have also considered how they present themselves, their behaviour and the way their practice is regulated.

Why is it necessary to define ourselves as professionals? Griffiths and Tengnah (2017, p. 46) suggest that the purpose of professionalism is fourfold: to protect the public; to deter unprofessional or unlawful actions; as a regulatory framework; and to enable learning by other members of the profession. As with many concepts, it is sometimes easier to develop an understanding of what professional practice is by considering behaviour that is unprofessional. Perhaps this may relate to a person's behaviour, for example how they treat you or how they treat other people. It may be in their attitude to others, putting their own needs before those of people in their care, a disregard for professional boundaries or not following policies and procedures. Professional behaviour may also be reflected in how people present themselves, for example timekeeping, their tone of voice, whether they are honest. Furthermore, a healthcare worker's behaviour outside work may also cause concern professionally, such as inappropriate use of social media or disregard for the laws of the country.

Standards for professional practice

Many healthcare-related roles are professionally regulated. This means that each profession is governed by an organisation known as a professional regulator. In understanding the meaning of professionalism, it is important to have an awareness of the role of professional regulators. Some examples are the American Dental Association, Health and Care Professions Council, General Medical Council, Malta Medical Council, Nursing and Midwifery Council, Nursing and Midwifery Board of Australia. The regulator for each professional group generally determines the standards for education and practice for that profession within a country or across a geographical region. On successful completion of a programme of education that is generally approved by a regulator, the names of individuals are added to a professional register. By having your name added to a professional register, you are agreeing to abide by the standards for that profession as set out by your regulator. Each professional regulator provides clear guidance about the required standards of practice, conduct and behaviour for members of the profession. This usually takes the form of a Code of Practice or Good Practice requirements.

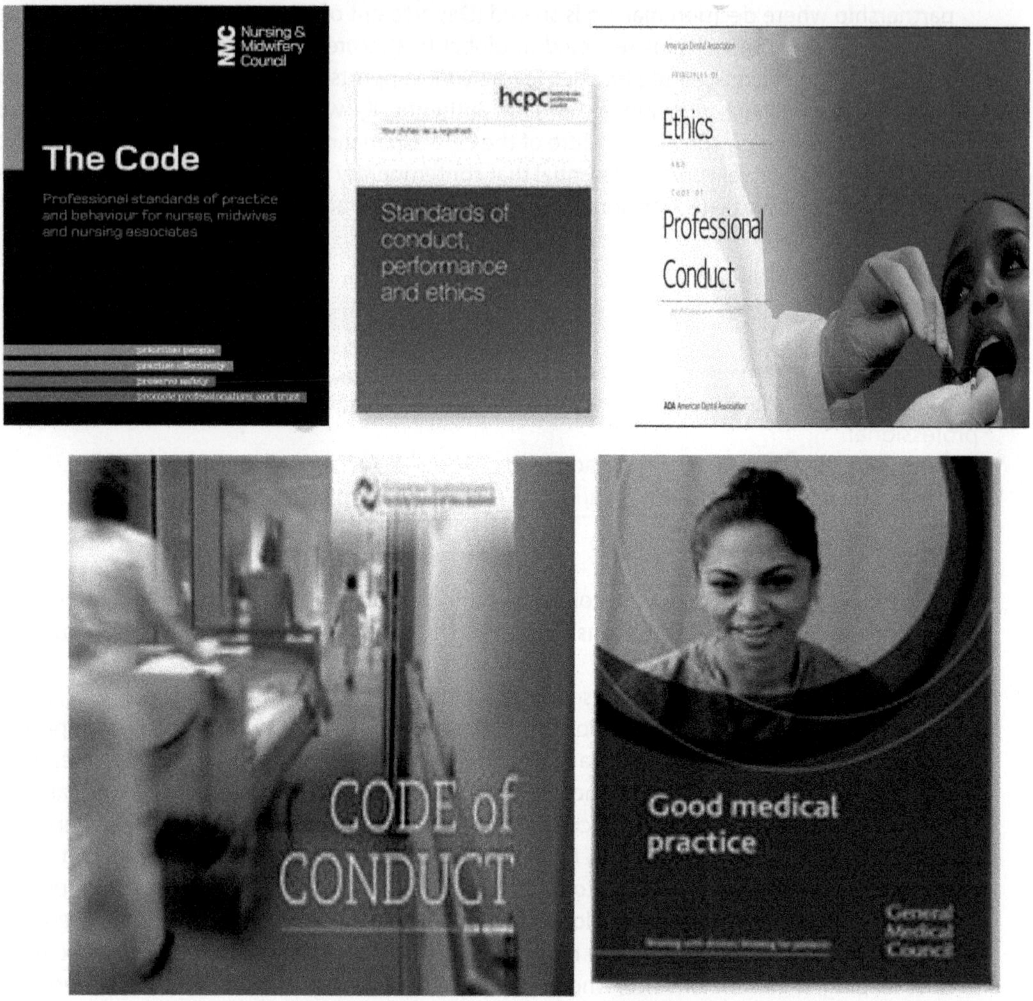

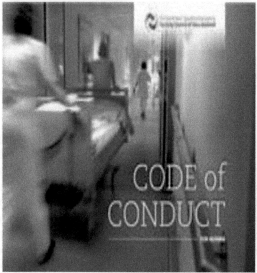

It is important that you are familiar with the requirements for your profession in the jurisdiction where you will be licensed/registered. If you are interested in knowing more about professional standards please see:

- www.nmc.org.uk/standards/standards-for-nurses
- https://ed-areyouprepared.com/wp-content/uploads/2019/01/Nusing-and-Midwifery-Board-Code-Advance-copy-Code-of-conduct-for-nurses-Effective-1-March-2018.pdf
- www.hcpc-uk.org/standards
- www.gmc-uk.org/about/what-we-do-and-why/setting-the-standards-for-doctors
- https://policybase.cma.ca/en/viewer?file=%2fdocuments%2fPolicypdf%2fPD19-03.pdf#phrase=false

Maintaining professional standards

The Code of Practice or requirements for good practice for each profession clarify the standards for education and practice that must be consistently met by all members of that profession. Maintaining standards of professional practice is important because they enable the public to have confidence in the healthcare professionals to whom they entrust their care and that of their families. The public can be satisfied that each registered healthcare professional has met the standards for entry to the register and ongoing requirements in order for their registration to remain live.

Activity

You are invited to consider the professional implications of the behaviour demonstrated by the radiography student in this clinical scenario.

Chan has brought Hu, her 2-year-old toddler, to the emergency department. Chan suspects that Hu has swallowed a small metal key. The key is clearly visible on an X-ray image, which has been viewed by several members of the radiology team. A radiography student takes a picture of the X-ray on his mobile phone and shares it with a friend through social media. The friend posts the photograph to a public social media site and it is viewed by 5000 people.

From your reading of the relevant professional code, what issues does this raise? Do you feel this behaviour is professionally acceptable? Give a rationale for your answer.

Thinking of the Person-centred Practice Framework, consider which component(s) of the prerequisites domain you can draw upon to explore this scenario.

In your discussion, you may have considered professional issues such as dignity, confidentiality and the challenges of using social media. For example, Chan has not given consent for this image to be shared in this way. This may have breached data protection requirements relating to the sharing of information and its justification. In this scenario, there is no apparent permission or justification for sharing the image and the action therefore compromises the privacy and dignity of Chan and the family, which may have serious consequences for the student and the healthcare provider. You may have also considered the Person-centred Practice Framework, specifically the prerequisites domain including clarity of professional beliefs and values such as the need to demonstrate respect for personhood and commitment to the job. The student is not role modelling person-centred behaviour and by sharing this information has breached procedures and shown abuse of his position.

Legal and ethical responsibilities

Our professional codes and standards are underpinned by legal and ethical responsibilities and aligned with values and rights that are fundamental to person-centred practice. These include considerations such as the primacy of the individual, the individual's right to self-determination, social justice and equitable access to healthcare (Levinson et al. 2014). Health and social care regulators also have a role in managing risks to the public, to other healthcare professionals and to individual practitioners themselves, so that only those who are fit to practise are permitted to do so. Regulators depend on registrants, employers, the public and law enforcement bodies to report any concerns that may bring into question a registrant's fitness for professional practice. The following activity encourages you to think about issues of risk.

Activity

John is a second-year student currently undertaking practice learning in a community residential setting for older people. Whilst the registered staff are attending a meeting, Mr Gregor presses the call bell requesting a commode. The safe transfer of Mr Gregor from his bed to commode will require two people to operate the use of a ceiling hoist and there is no-one else around. John has never used this type of equipment and he's frightened of asking for help. Mr Gregor urgently needs to use the toilet. John manages to apply the sling on his own and hoists Mr Gregor onto the commode. Afterwards John asks one of the registered staff to help him return Mr Gregor to bed and comments that Mr Gregor nearly slipped during the earlier transfer.

What professional issues does this raise? Using the Person-centred Practice Framework, what components of the practice environment domain are relevant in this episode of care?

In your discussion, you may have considered professional issues such as competency, accountability and preserving safety. In relation to the care environment domain of the Person-centred Practice Framework, you might have considered appropriate skill mix, shared decision making, power sharing and effective staff relationships. You may have questioned why John did not feel able to ask for help; is this based on his previous experience or current levels of support? Additionally, you may have questioned why John was left alone and why he was prepared to engage in care activities beyond his scope of competency. Consider the potential trauma for Mr Gregor if he had slipped. For John there could also be consequences, both in terms of accountability for his actions and the risk of injury as a result of inappropriate moving and handling. The appropriate professional response would be to prioritise the interests of the client and to seek help. This experience could be used as an opportunity for reflection between John and his practice supervisor, to explore their values and competencies and the culture of the care environment. A possible outcome could be that John attends a moving and handling update, demonstrates safe client transfers and has the confidence to seek help and challenge unsafe practice.

Person-centredness, professionalism and organisational structures

Key learning from a range of international inquiries into high-profile failures in health and social care practices has highlighted the importance of organisational structures and cultures in achieving safe and effective, person-centred practice (Sinclair 2000; Douglas et al. 2001; Francis 2013; Gosport Independent Panel 2018). Recurring issues from such inquiries include failure to raise and challenge concerns, poor performance management, ineffective leadership and inadequate clinical governance systems (Walshe and Shortell 2004). It is therefore essential for healthcare professionals to be vigilant to issues in their own practice, and that of others, which are inconsistent with person-centred values. These may include issues that are explicitly unacceptable. It may, however, include more subtle instances that nonetheless lead you to feel uncomfortable when you believe personhood and dignity have not been respected. The following vignette offers an example of this.

> A clinical manager attends a multidisciplinary bed management meeting in a large NHS teaching hospital. The senior bed manager tells staff that there are 23 patients in the emergency department and only 18 planned discharges.

> Added to this, there are staff shortages on this shift with an additional five staff needed to meet safe staffing levels across the hospital. The bed manager indicates that to increase flow, more patients need to be sent home. One manager reports that:
>
> 'The patient in room 33 will die soon which will free up a bed and we could send another home after 8pm in a taxi when her blood transfusion is finished.' This person lives alone and has been in hospital for a week.

In this vignette, the culture of care appears to prioritise targets over people. This is demonstrated through the use of language that disrespects personhood and dignity. Decisions are being made that affect vulnerable persons, with no acknowledgement of risk management or collaborative working. There is limited opportunity for shared decision making or consideration of the policies and procedures that support safe and effective care delivery. Finally, you may question the manager's position as a leader and role model and the failure of those present to challenge these practices which are at odds with person-centredness.

Such experiences within the practice setting can result in a level of moral distress. This is defined as: 'The painful psychological disequilibrium that results from recognising the ethically appropriate action, yet not taking it. Because of obstacles such as lack of time, supervisory reluctance, an inhibiting medical power structure, institution policy or legal considerations' (Corley 2002, p. 250). For more information on moral distress please see: https://journals.sagepub.com/doi/10.1191/0969733002ne557oa.

Creating person-centred cultures

The Person-centred Practice Framework provides a useful lens for professionals to view, guide and enhance practice. In the previous sections, we discussed prerequisites such as professional competence and developed interpersonal skills. We have also highlighted some of the care processes essential for person-centred practice, such as working with a person's beliefs and values and sharing decision making. The practice environment, such as a ward, community hub, care home or health centre, and the wider organisational structures and leadership that support these environments are also significant in enabling professionals to support human flourishing. In the next section we propose strategies to support professionals to challenge issues that are at odds with their person-centred values and beliefs. These strategies include reflection, self-care and constructive challenge.

Critical reflection is a useful tool for professional learning (Gardner 2014) and can help professionals to discuss, deconstruct and learn from clinical issues. Deep learning is enhanced by a supportive culture and skilled facilitation (Dewing 2008; Mann et al. 2009). Reflective learning can be viewed as occurring at micro, meso, and macro levels. In the above activity, at a micro level John and his supervisor may analyse his actions with Mr Gregor and explore why he felt unable to ask for help. These reflections could be recorded to support continuing professional development and lifelong learning. At the meso level, his supervisor may use this as an opportunity to reflect on expectations of students and the learning culture of the unit. At a macro level, audit results of the learning environment may reveal a high number of critical incidents focusing on safe moving and handling, suggesting that lessons can be learned from this reflection that lead to action at institutional level.

Reflection can also support the development of self-knowledge and such insights might lead to the consideration of strategies to support a professional's own well-being. Some aspects of professional practice, such as long working hours, stressful encounters and placing people's needs ahead of our own, are known to have a detrimental impact on well-being (American Dental Association 2019; Winkel and Morgan 2019), and can result in moral distress and burnout (Hamric 2010). It is important for healthcare professionals to demonstrate self-care and to build resilience to ensure that their fitness for professional practice is not compromised.

In the vignette above we highlighted that staff may experience moral distress regarding discussions about the safety and dignity of people being considered for discharge. Through reflection, practitioners may realise that this is embedded in practice. Challenging values and behaviours that appear to be prioritised within the organisation can create anxiety and contribute to diminished well-being. Strategies that might support well-being could include engaging in clinical supervision to discuss matters and explore how to act. Practice development initiatives, where participants are supported to role play a range of alternative actions in a safe space, may be another means of challenging negative cultures. Additionally, learning mindful practices may support well-being and stress management and help achieve a work/life balance. This is discussed in greater detail in Chapter 15. By engaging in such activities, practitioners may feel empowered to constructively challenge the behaviours and values that were observed at the meeting or speak to another manager to report the concerns that were witnessed.

Conclusion

The realities of current practice require professionals to operate in a challenging and complex system, that is fast paced and dynamic. In order for professionals to lead and influence person-centred practice at micro, meso, and macro levels, they should be positive role models who demonstrate person-centredness in their practice. In this chapter we have used activities to highlight the important role that professionals play in providing safe, effective, person-centred practice. We have considered some of the tensions that arise when upholding professionalism whilst striving to be person-centred and offered some strategies to support professionals in raising concerns or challenging practice that is unprofessional. As a health or social care professional, you will occupy a position of privilege and trust. This position brings with it certain expectations and responsibilities as set out by your regulator. Central to these responsibilities is the need to act at all times with honesty and integrity and to behave in a way that reflects well on the profession and how it is perceived by the public. Being a health or social care professional and acting professionally can also bring a great sense of personal and collegiate pride in knowing that individually and as a profession, you can make a positive difference to the lives of others.

Summary

- Professional standards exist to protect the public and maintain public confidence in the health and social care professions.
- It is important to be familiar with the requirements for professional practice and revalidation as set out by the regulator in the jurisdiction where you practise.
- Reflection and sharing of constructive feedback with others enables health professionals to create accurate perceptions of their practice. This can be used as a basis for developing practice.
- We all have a responsibility for maintaining and promoting acceptable standards. This includes raising concerns without delay when practices are not person-centred.

- Practising professionally involves acting in the best interests of people, being committed to professional development, leading by example and upholding the reputation of the profession to which you belong.

Additional learning activities

We have devised the following learning activities that can be undertaken before, after or during your reading of Chapter 6.

1. *Positioning professionalism within the PcPF*
   Go to the PcPF on page 000 and look at the different domains and make some notes on the following questions.
   - Which components would you associate with professionalism?
   - How do these fit with your earlier thinking of the meaning of professionalism?
   - What other factors not stated in the model link to professionalism?

   Once you have read the chapter go back to your notes. Reflect on any ways in which your thinking has changed or your prior assumptions about professionalism have been changed as a result of your reading.
2. *Standards for professional practice*
   - Identify the relevant documents for your professional group and at least one other.
   - Explore the common elements of professional practice that are included in these documents.
3. *Legal and ethical responsibilities*
   Read the short case study below and make notes on each of the discussion points.

> Jean Jones is a 35-year-old woman who lives alone. She has some learning difficulties and is unable to read and write. She has a key worker who visits three times a week to help with life skills such as budgeting and housekeeping. She has started a relationship with a young man she met at the local community centre. The key worker is concerned about how far this relationship will go and suggests accompanying her to visit the general practitioner to discuss contraception and Jean's sexual health. At the appointment the key worker stresses that Jean is unable to understand the consequences of having unprotected sexual intercourse.

<u>Discussion points</u>

- What professional issues does this case study raise?
- Using the PcPF, explore which of the components of the person-centred processes domain you would apply in considering Jean's needs, preferences, wishes and rights.

<u>Reflective notes</u>

In your discussion you may have considered issues such as capacity to consent, stigma, autonomy and power. As a vulnerable person Jean may lack capacity to consider the consequences of her action, for example an unplanned pregnancy. In addition, the healthcare professionals must also consider whether sex is consensual. This must be balanced with Jean's human rights to engage in an intimate relationship. In relation to the PcPF, you may have highlighted shared decision making, working with the person's beliefs and values and providing holistic care. Jean should not be defined by her disability but as a person with needs, preferences and desires. Professionals may also consider their own responses and assumptions or even prejudices when faced with such ethical dilemmas.

If you are interested in reading further about this issue, see:

- www.bihr.org.uk/learning-disability-autism-and-human-rights
- https://journals.sagepub.com/doi/full/10.1177/1363460715620576
- https://improvement.nhs.uk/improvement-hub/learning-disabilities

References

American Dental Association (2019). *Staying Well in the Dental Profession*. https://success.ada.org/en/wellness/staying-well-in-the-dental-profession

Corley, M.C. (2002). Nurse moral distress: a proposed theory and research agenda. *Nursing Ethics* 9 (6): 636–650.

Dalton, L., Campbell, S.J. and Bull, R. (2015). Preparing graduates for professionalism and person centred practice: developing the patient voice in nurse education. 2nd International Conference: Where's the Patient's Voice in Health Professional Education – 10 Years On? 12–14 November, Vancouver, Canada. http://ecite.utas.edu.au/104840

Department of Health (2010). *Equity and Excellence-Liberating the NHS*. London: HMSO.

Dewing, J. (2008). Becoming and being active learning workplaces: the value of active learning inpractice development. In: *International Practice Development in Nursing and Healthcare* (eds. K. Manley, B. McCormack and V. Wilson), 273–294. Oxford: Blackwell Publishing.

Douglas, N., Robinson, J., and Fahy, K. (2001). *Inquiry into Obstetric and Gynaecological Services at King Edward Memorial Hospital 1990–2000*. Perth: Government of Western Australia.

Francis, R. (2013). The Mid Staffordshire NHS Foundation Trust public inquiry. https://webarchive.nationalarchives.gov.uk/20150407084231/http://www.midstaffspublicinquiry.com/report

Gardner, F. (2014). *Being Critically Reflective. Engaging in Holistic Practice*. London: Red Globe.

Gosport Independent Panel (2018). *Gosport War Memorial Hospital: The Report of the Gosport Independent Panel*. www.gosportpanel.independent.gov.uk/panel-report

Griffiths, R. and Tengnah, C. (2017). *Law and Professional Issues in Nursing*, 4e. London: Learning Matters, Sage.

Hamric, A.B. (2010). Moral distress and nurse-physician relationships. *Journal of the American Medical Association* 12 (1): 6–11.

Levinson, W., Ginsbury, S., Hafferty, F.W., and Lucey, C.R. (2014). *Understanding Medical Professionalism*. New York: McGraw-Hill.

Mann, K., Gordon, J., and MacLeod, A. (2009). Reflection and reflective practice in health professions education: a systematic review. *Advances in Health Sciences Education* 14: 595–621.

Sinclair, C.M. (2000). *The Report of the Manitoba Paediatric Cardiac Surgery Inquest: An Inquiry into Twelve Deaths at the Winnipeg Health Sciences Centre in 1991*. Winnipeg: Provincial Court of Manitoba.

Walshe, K. and Shortell, S. (2004). When things go wrong: how health care organizations deal with major failures. *Health Affairs* 23 (3): 101–111.

Whitehouse, S. (2015). Medical professionalism – what do we mean? In: *Professional and Medical Perspective*. Leeds: Medical Protection Society.

Winkel, A. and Morgan, H. (2019). Collisions at the intersections of competence, wellness and engagement. *Medical Education* 53 (3): 214–216.

World Health Organization (2015). *WHO Global Strategy on People-centred and Integrated Health Services: Interim Report*. https://apps.who.int/iris/bitstream/handle/10665/155002/WHO_HIS_SDS_2015.6_eng.pdf;jsessionid=996BBCD8729F8602908EECA54C38DED8?sequence=1

7

The future nurse, midwifery and allied health professional

Suzanne Martin[1], Charlotte McArdle[2], and Ed Jesudason[3]

[1]Ulster University, Northern Ireland, UK
[2]Department of Health, Belfast, Northern Ireland, UK
[3]NHS Lothian, Edinburgh, Scotland, UK

Contents

Fundamentals of Person-Centred Healthcare Practice, First Edition. Edited by Brendan McCormack, Tanya McCance, Cathy Bulley, Donna Brown, Ailsa McMillan and Suzanne Martin.

Learning outcomes

- Appreciate the link between professionalism and person-centred practice.
- Understand the need for person-centred care to be embedded within professional education (preregistration and postregistration).
- Recognise the need for person-centred principles to be embedded within leadership development.
- Underpin your professional practice with the constructs of person-centredness.
- Be aware of the enablers of professionalism.

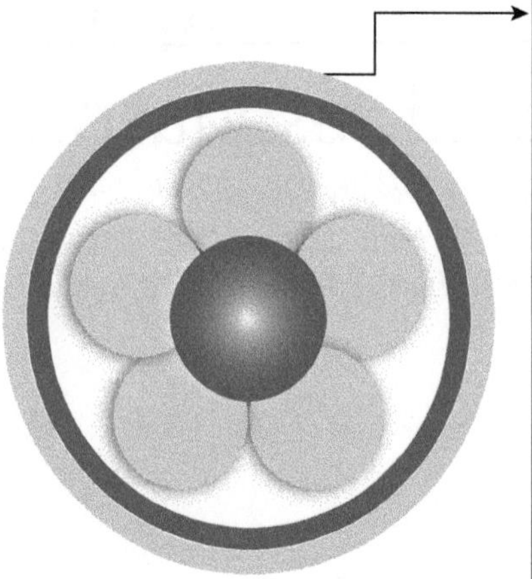

Prerequisites

Professionally competent: the knowledge, skills and attitudes of the person to negotiate care options, and effectively provide holistic care

Developed interpersonal skills: the ability of the person to communicate at a variety of levels with others, using effective verbal and non-verbal interactions that show personal concern for their situation and a commitment to finding mutual solutions

Knowing self: the way a person makes sense of his/her knowing, being and becoming through reflection, self-awareness, and engagement with others

Clarity of beliefs and values: awareness of the impact of beliefs and values on the healthcare experience and the commitment to reconciling beliefs and values in ways that facilitate person-centredness

Commitment to the job: demonstrated commitment of persons through intentional engagement that focuses on achieving the best possible outcomes

Introduction

Electing to study as a nurse, midwife or allied health professional (NMAHP) gives you the opportunity to exit from your university experience with a higher education degree and a professional qualification. Being a person-centred healthcare professional will enable you to develop a unique sense of professionalism as you aspire to be the best role model you can be, working in the interests of those you support. Within the person-centred practice framework, the *prerequisites* focus on the attributes of staff and are the key building blocks in the development of the healthcare professional who can deliver effective person-centred care.

In the United Kingdom, the Nursing and Midwifery Council (NMC) and Health and Care Professions Council (HCPC) are statuted to maintain professional registers for health and social care professionals. They state that the purpose of professionalism is to ensure the consistent provision of safe, effective, person-centred outcomes that support people and their families and carers, to achieve an optimal status of health and well-being (Nursing and Midwifery Council 2015). The HCPC acknowledged the influence personal characteristics have on professionalism and that these continually develop through experiences such as education and work experience (HCPC 2011). The influence of role modelling and contextualising practice should also be considered. This is represented in other constructs of the framework that are discussed in the first section of the book.

Activity

Take some time to note down what it means to you to be professional and what behaviours would be associated with the attributes above. Think about how the prerequisites of the framework might help you achieve this.

Professionalism and person-centredness

Dubree et al. (2017) identified three major elements to help establish and promote a robust and effective way to support professionalism: (i) management, leadership, and peer commitment; (ii) a goal-driven, fair model and process to guide graduated interventions; and (iii) multilevel, system-wide professional training in intervention-related communication skills. However, this alone will not support and promote professionalism. The embodiment of the prerequisites in tandem with positive leadership traits can enable professionals to create positive workplace cultures and therefore sustain professionalism. In addition to this, our professional bodies ensure that person-centred practice is embedded within curricula that you experience in preregistration and postregistration programmes.

As a healthcare worker, you are a leader, working with colleagues at all levels within the health and social care systems to deliver safe and effective services. Contemporary leadership models recognise that leadership can be either formal leadership, gained through specific roles in an organisation, or informal where everyone has the ability to step forward and lead on something which is important to them and their work. A key principle to collective leadership is that everyone has something to contribute and we can all learn from and with each other (West et al. 2014, 2015). Modern healthcare policies have adapted this approach to leadership in an attempt to build cultures shaped through its own staff and that are evidenced through values and behaviours consistent with professional codes of practice and person-centred care.

Collective leaders and person-centred leaders recognise the need and ability to be in the moment with their professional colleagues and those who work in their organisation. Person-centred leaders understand how a person's different traits influence their ability to work effectively and perform duties. Cardiff (2017) outlines this as related connectedness and related individualism with connectedness being achieved through the power of emotional intelligence and inquiry.

Emotional intelligence essentially means that we can recognise and regulate our own emotions and recognise emotions in others. You will see that this is reflected in some of the prerequisites. Goleman identifies five competencies which make up emotional intelligence: motivation, self-awareness, self-regulation, social skills and empathy (Goleman 2011; David 2014). These competencies are necessary to being a collective leader and evident in leadership behaviours which may affect the behaviours of others. This can be best played out when you are feeling under pressure and because emotions are infectious and affect others as well.

Activity

Can you think of a time when your emotion affected another person? Why did that happen? Now can you think of ways in which your behaviour or that of colleague can affect the culture/behaviour in your group or team?

One example of this in action is the collective leadership strategy in Northern Ireland (Department of Health 2017). This is built on four components (Figure 7.1), one of which is compassionate leadership. Compassionate leadership applies to both relationships with colleagues and relationships with people receiving care. It is described as paying attention to staff, really engaging with colleagues, listening to feedback and trying to understand issues through empathy and emotional intelligence before taking action to help a colleague deal with issues they face. This is a similar approach to person-centred leaders being connected and has further synergy with co-production.

Co-production is a person-centred approach which enables partnership working between people with a common goal. Often within healthcare this is to improve the experience and health outcome for the person receiving care.

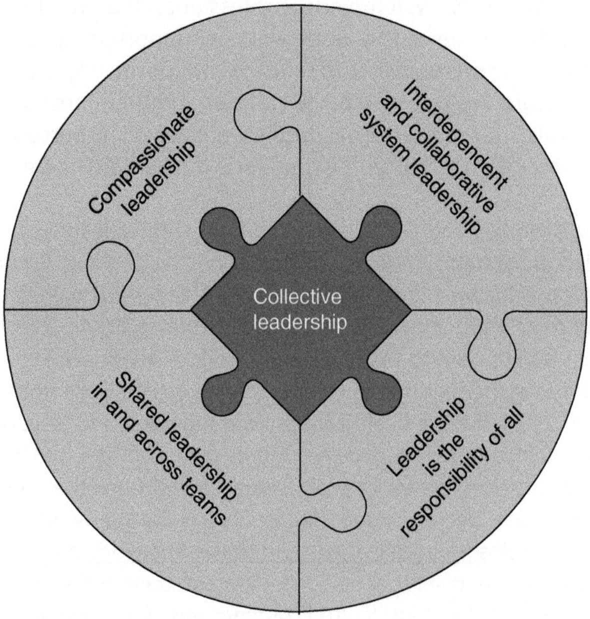

Figure 7.1 Four components of collective leadership.

Co-production and collective leadership can be described as two sides of the same coin. They are both focused on connecting with people and realising opportunity in the health and social care system. Below is a case study illustrating co-production and collective leadership regarding people with lived experience of mental ill-health and health professionals working together for a better outcome. The case study should be read in conjunction with the Department of Health Co-production Guide 2018. It briefly outlines how the 'You in Mind' Mental Health Care Pathway and Recovery College was developed in Northern Ireland.

Step 1 – Build the initial team

This aims to ensure the development of trusting relationships between people who use and people who provide mental health services. Group membership includes those with different roles in health and social care services (e.g. trust director for service, finance, information and clinical expertise). Service users and carers provide their own expertise of lived experience. Staff groups may also be included, for example a professional body or trade union.

When this group was formed, some members had initial anxieties – people with lived experience were worried about professional perspectives being dominant, and some staff had concerns that co-production might undermine professional expertise. This was addressed by developing a collective understanding based on values and vision of recovery-orientated practice. This promoted collective leadership by all working in true partnership with mutual respect, understanding and compassion for each other's point of view.

The co-production and collective leadership approach enables a broader group of people to input to this process without being involved in the actual co-production group through the development of networks led by members of the co-production group.

Step 2 – Identify what we can do

The group identified knowledge gaps whilst respecting each other's expertise, whether their lived experience or in clinical practice. This was vital to develop the recovery college. They used the results of a regional survey of the experiences of people using or caring for someone who uses mental health services. The findings clearly outlined the need for 'good communication', 'shared care', 'timely information' and the importance of respectful and dignified care. This part of the process demonstrates respect for everyone's contribution, ensuring that people are recognised for their input.

Step 3 – Co-create the vision

Having discussed the best way to work together, everyone agreed to be co-productive. This created a culture where the values of hope, control and opportunity became the norm. Working in equal partnership resulted in co-production of a Northern Ireland Mental Health Services Framework that incorporated the 'You in Mind' mental healthcare pathway and the development of recovery colleges.

Step 4 – Co-design the solution

Equal weight was given to people's lived experience and professional expertise. The establishment of an expert by experience writing group ensured the pathway remained practical for everyone involved. The group helped translate clinical evidence into an easily understood practical guide. The vehicle used to facilitate the establishment of recovery colleges was through the Implementing Recovery through Organisational Change Programme (IMROC). The recovery college was designed using a 'hub and spoke' model and programmes are delivered within local communities by both staff and people with lived experience of mental ill health.

Step 5 – Co-delivery

The recovery college is now supported by a network of people with lived experience who are involved in the design and delivery of co-education programmes across Northern Ireland. The collaborative delivery of this work has led to the establishment of peer support worker posts, five recovery college hubs and the appointment of recovery college peer educators in Northern Ireland.

Step 6 – Co-evaluate

Recovery college has made a huge difference to people's lives and is being evaluated using an outcomes-based accountability approach.

Activity

Take some time to consider how you could work more collaboratively with people to develop services. What skills and knowledge will you need to develop to enable you to do this?

Challenges to professionalism

What can you do when things go wrong? Hickson (2007) proposed a model to identify, assess and deal with unprofessional behaviour (Figure 7.2). This model focused on three interventions: informal conversations for a single incident, interventions to raise awareness when a persistent pattern is emerging, and finally moving to uptake disciplinary procedures, if required. Let us keep in mind that the vast majority of your colleagues will work to high professional standards.

Activity

You are in the coffee room with George, one of the physiotherapists. He is complaining to you about one of your colleagues and states that they are unprofessional and 'not good at their job'. You recognise some of what George is saying in the way this person acts but you are concerned about the way George speaks about them and that now everyone in the coffee room can hear. Think about how you can escalate this concern and facilitate conversations that are person-centred.

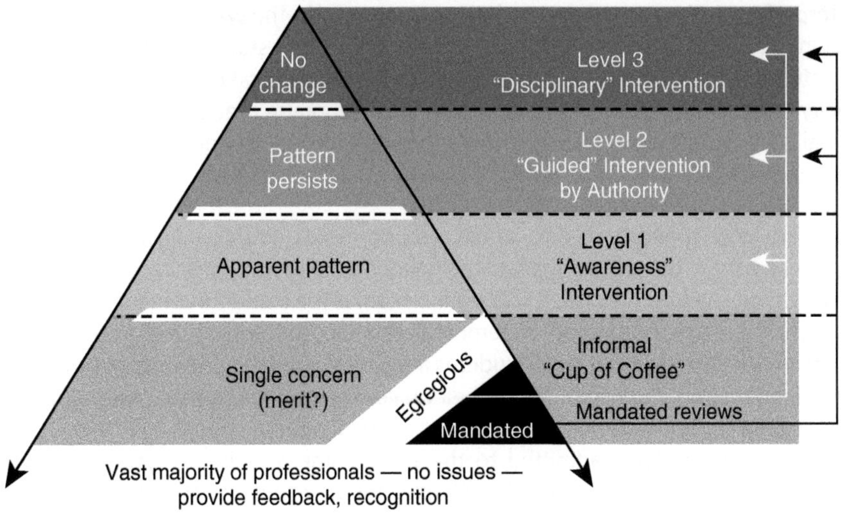

Figure 7.2 Hickson (2007) model to identify, assess and deal with unprofessional behaviour. Source: Adapted from Hickson, G.B. et al. 2007.

Curricula content

Ongoing NMAHP professional development and continuing professional development (CPD) are beneficial to patient care, organisations and each of us as individuals. A strong relationship between education preparation and professionalism is long established (Tanaka et al. 2016). You will be expected to engage in regular CPD (some mandatory) post registration, and may be randomly audited by your professional regulator to ensure compliance with this requirement. The description below is about the motivation and expected outcomes of a Postgraduate Certificate in Education delivered to a mixed cohort of nursing and AHP professionals from practice.

Case study

Learning and teaching takes many forms in clinical/professional practice and is a sizeable portion of any healthcare professional's role. This interprofessional Postgraduate Certificate in Education for healthcare professionals is designed to enable students to facilitate learning and teaching in practice. The course is primarily facilitated through practice learning and supported by university sessions. It prepares the professional to engage in learning and teaching in the workplace with students, colleagues, peers, other professionals and service users.

The course enables practitioners to blend information with experience to help them build new knowledge and develop new skills, which they can use in a variety of ways in their workplace practice. One application of the course has enabled students to develop their skills of supervision in assessment for preregistration students.

Another has enabled students to design and develop education packages to use in practice with their peers (this includes members of their own profession and beyond). These packages have a direct impact on the care provided to people.

The interprofessional nature of the workplace is mirrored in the way in which the PGCEHP has been designed and delivered. We have found that this provides students with an opportunity to create an interprofessional practice education network. Postqualification courses like this also have the capacity to enable practitioners to reflect on and reappraise practice. This includes complex professional issues which either facilitate or compromise the delivery of high-quality care.

Beyond local application, the course also promotes employability. This is a key theme emphasised from the outset that allows students to identify key factors that sustain and enhance their career progression. This stance enables the students to manage their own career development by promoting an incremental and focused approach to the development of professional knowledge and skills. Students are encouraged to participate in personal development planning from the beginning of their university experience, when the value of reflection and personal and professional development are reinforced.

Although the students admitted to the programme are already graduates, the PGCEHP builds on the development of graduate attributes by enabling the students to reflect upon their career and ability through the lens of graduate qualities. This process lends itself well to ongoing professional development and highlights to students how studying this course can be of benefit to them and their future practice.

The NMC and HCPC are explicit in some of the content of programmes that lead to registration. They will participate in the approval and validation of programmes and look for a wide range of stakeholders to be involved in the development, delivery and evaluation of programmes. Your preregistration education establishes your core competencies ensuring your professional approach to service delivery at the point of registration. Each of us then needs to engage in a range of behaviours and activities to maintain this. There are a number of attributes we would expect others to observe in you that would confirm your professionalism.

Activity

Think about the programme you studied or are studying and where you can, notice the constructs of the PcPF. Write down how you have developed as a person as you progressed through the programme. Then take some time to reflect on this in light of the requirements of your registering body.

Within Chapter 12, we further explore the impact of environment on enabling person-centred practice. There is no doubt that the environment is pivotal in supporting professional practice and behaviours. Here are five ways the environment can support this.

- Recognises and encourages leadership.
- Encourages autonomous innovative practice.
- Enables positive interprofessional collaboration.
- Enables practice learning and development.
- Provides appropriate resources.

Activity

For each of the points above, write about two or more things that can support this in the area where you work.

There are many examples from clinical practice where nurses and AHPs work extremely well together, demonstrating high levels of professionalism to deliver outstanding person-centred services. There is no doubt that the drive for interprofessional and multiprofessional working will continue to grow as pressure on acute services, decreased funding and increased community care drive change in how we work. Person-centredness within the workplace is essential to help the professional flourish in these situations. This manifests itself when professionals intentionally develop working relationships based on respect, compassion, kindness, self-determination, trust and understanding (McCormack and McCance 2016).

Our ability to mature and grow professionally is influenced by all the elements of the PcPF. For example, the environment in which we work (Chapter 11), the beliefs and values (Chapter 12) we have and our ability to flourish are all pivotal to our emerging and ever developing and changing professional persona. Flourishing as the natural blending of we ought to do with what we want to do (McCormack and Titchen 2014) is key to the emergence of the future nurse and AHP, and yet the world you will work in is changing dynamically because of the speed of technological change, not only in terms of capability but also availability. You may have a different relationship with specialist knowledge which will be more available electronically to you and your service users. Many people will have looked up material online and constructed a number of options for themselves. They will want your guidance to check they are on the right track and they may want some validation of difficult choices. Professionalism is witnessing a shift from 'telling and doing' to 'listening and advising'. You may be guiding people through choices, and leading them to information and other resources that can help (Chapter 14).

As an emerging professional, post graduation, in order to practise clinically, you will be externally regulated by either the NMC (www.nmc.org.uk/concerns-nurses-midwives/dealing-concerns) or the HCPC (www.hcpc-uk.org/concerns/hearings). Both entities set out professional standards that all registrants must meet not only to become registered but also to retain registration. This is an important part of the monitoring of our professional behaviours in practice.

Conclusion

We know that the purpose of professionalism is to ensure the consistent provision of safe, effective, person-centred outcomes that support people, their families and carers to achieve an optimal status of health and well-being. Preregistration and postregistration education is pivotal in developing the attributes of the professional nurse and AHP of the future, who will work in a very different environment to the one currently existing. In addition, there is a need to understand the evolving needs of people who take a more consumer-based approach to healthcare and have different expectations about how services are designed and delivered. Engaging with all stakeholders and maximising technology will most definitely influence the future workplace and cultures for health and social care professionals.

Summary

- A professionally competent person-centred practitioner has the knowledge, skills and attitudes to negotiate care options and reflectively provide holistic care.
- Nurses and AHPs are independently regulated in terms of professional practice to uphold the safety of the general public.
- There are elements and attributes to professionalism that you can build knowledge and skill in as you gain experience.
- Preregistration and postregistration education is important to the development of professionalism.
- Many elements of the PcPF are relevant to the development of professionalism.

Acknowledgements

We thank Dr Patricia McClure and Dr Brian McGowan who provided the case study on PG education.

References

Cardiff, S. (2017). Person centred nursing leadership. In: *Person Centred Practice in Nursing and Healthcare: Theory and Practice* (eds. B. McCormack and T. McCance), 86–98. Chichester: Wiley Blackwell.

David, L. (2014). *Emotional Intelligence (Goleman).* www.learning-theories.com/emotional-intelligence-goleman.html

Department of Health (2017). *HSC Collective Leadership Strategy. Health and Wellbeing 2026: Delivering Together.* www.health-ni.gov.uk/sites/default/files/publications/health/hsc-collective-leadership-strategy.pdf

Dubree, M., Kapu, A., Terrell, M. et al. (2017). Nurses' essential role in supporting professionalism. *American Nurse Today* 12 (4): 6–8.

Goleman, D. (2011). *The Brain And Emotional Intelligence: New Insights*, 94. Florence, MA: More than Sound.

Hickson, G.B., Pichert, J.W., Webb, L.E., and Gabbe, S.G. (2007). A complementary approach to promoting professionalism: identifying, measuring, and addressing unprofessional behaviors. *Academic Medicine* 82 (11): 1040–1048.

Health and Care Professions Council (2011). *Professionalism in healthcare professions.* www.hcpc-uk.org/resources/reports/2011/professionalism-in-healthcare-professionals/

McCormack, B. and McCance, T. (eds.) (2016). *Person-Centred Practice in Nursing and Health Care: Theory and Practice.* Chichester: Wiley Blackwell.

McCormack, B. and Titchen, A. (2014). No beginning, no end: an ecology of human flourishing. *International Practice Development Journal* 4 (2): article 2.

Nursing and Midwifery Council (2015). *Enabling Professionalism in Nursing and Midwifery Practice.* www.nmc.org.uk/globalassets/sitedocuments/other-publications/enabling-professionalism.pdf

Tanaka, M., Taketomi, K., Yonemitsu, Y., and Kawamoto, R. (2016). Professional behaviours and factors contributing to nursing professionalism among nurse managers. *Journal of Nursing Management* 24 (1): 12–20.

West, M., Armit, L., Eckert, R. et al. (2015). *Leadership and Leadership Development in Health Care: The Evidence Base.* tinyurl.com/KF-west-evidence

West, M., Steward, K., Eckert, R. and Pasmore, B. (2014). *Developing Collective Leadership for Healthcare.* tinyurl.com/KF-west

Further reading

www.nmc.org.uk/standards/guidance/professionalism: take some time to explore three animations available at this link, produced by the Nursing and Midwifery Council, which explain how a framework of enabling professionalism can be used to support professional behaviour.

If you are an allied health professional, please take some time to explore the current tribunal hearings for staff who are challenged in relation to their professionalism at this website: www.hcpts-uk.org

Watch the videos on professionalism produced by the Chief Nursing Officers from Northern Ireland, England, Scotland and Wales located here: www.nmc.org.uk/standards/guidance/professionalism/blogs

Read the Nursing and Midwifery Council's document Enabling Professionalism here: www.nmc.org.uk/standards/guidance/professionalism/read-report

SECTION 2

Being Person-centred

Whilst it is easy in most cases to extol the virtues of person-centredness and person-centred practice, in reality, the translation of these virtues into everyday practice can be challenging. We are all aware of the retort 'that's not very person-centred' when someone does something, says something or expresses a view that might be out of line with established norms. In such instances, person-centredness is used as a 'big stick' with which to punish and blame, reinforcing a mono-dimensional view of person-centredness itself. In reality, no matter how clear we may be about the underpinning values, principles and virtues of person-centredness, living these every day is challenging and all of us will succeed and fail every day!

Therefore in thinking about this book, we agreed that a section that focused on the different dimensions of 'being person-centred' was important. As we have identified in earlier chapters, a lot of the person-centred discourse focuses on the 'doing of person-centredness', something we can turn on and off. This focus on doing may be one reason why we fail every day as much as we succeed. We know that the embodiment of the core values of person-centredness gives us a much greater chance of living out these values and engaging in ways of being that enhance our doing.

Engaging in the nine chapters of this section takes you through key considerations in being person-centred in healthcare practice. We focus on values in Chapter 12 as these form the platform for our being and doing. Sharing decisions is a key component of an effective person-centred relationship and we address shared decision making explicitly in Chapters 9 and 14. Chapter 13 focuses on meaningful engagement, an essential part of decision making and effective relationships. Chapters 10, 15 and 16 focus on how we connect with others with the ultimate goal of providing holistic care. Finally, Chapter 11 locates all of these values, processes and ways of being in the context of the physical environment, which of course has a major influence on our ability to practise effectively.

Fundamentals of Person-Centred Healthcare Practice, First Edition. Edited by Brendan McCormack, Tanya McCance, Cathy Bulley, Donna Brown, Ailsa McMillan and Suzanne Martin.

8

Communicating and relating effectively

Duncan Pentland[1], Helen Riddell[1], and Lindsey Regan[2]

[1]Queen Margaret University, Edinburgh, Scotland, UK
[2]University of Central Lancashire, Preston, UK

Contents

Fundamentals of Person-Centred Healthcare Practice, First Edition. Edited by Brendan McCormack, Tanya McCance, Cathy Bulley, Donna Brown, Ailsa McMillan and Suzanne Martin.

Learning outcomes

- Define communication and its central role in person-centred practice.
- Understand core components of communication.
- Identify strategies that can be used to enhance person-centred communication.
- Examine how to enhance practice and personal professional development by critically engaging with communication.

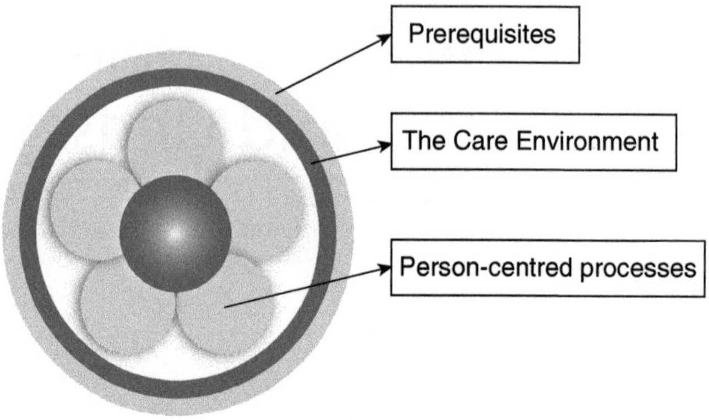

Introduction

The Person-centred Practice Framework identifies communication as a behaviour that contributes to person-centred outcomes. Effective person-centred communication can actively involve a person in their care or therapy and improve their sense of well-being and satisfaction. Many practices in contemporary healthcare require, or can be enhanced by, building relationships with the people involved. Information gathering, assessment, managing physical needs, completing treatment procedures and therapies and giving information are examples most health professionals would recognise as aspects of their practice that require communication with others.

Analysing the theories underpinning interpersonal communication is beyond this chapter's scope; detailed texts are readily available to health professionals. Rather, it considers the core constructs of communication, explores the humanistic principles underpinning person-centred communication and presents strategies that can enhance communication practices and facilitate the development of person-centred practice processes and environments. In this chapter, therefore, we will address the prerequisites, care environment and person-centred processes and constructs of the Person-centred Practice Framework. In so doing, we emphasise the importance of cultivating the positive, mutually trusting, communicative relationships that empower people to take part in decisions about their care, and create person-centred environments and cultures of practice.

Framing communication – definitions and basic concepts

Communication is a multifaceted concept. The OED online (2019) defines it as 'The imparting or exchanging of information by speaking, writing, or using some other medium; The successful conveying or sharing of ideas and feelings and social contact.'

Essentially, communication is the transmission of information between conscious agents, typically people (Robinson 2005). This includes obvious forms, such as talking to a colleague or waving at a friend, but extends to unconscious actions like yawning, subtle body language and behaviours. The importance of communication is hard to overstate. It has long been argued as inseparable from what it is to be human, with some considering all interactions between people to be communication (Watzlawick et al. 1967). Furthermore, communication helps us to understand ourselves and how we relate to others.

Communication has added meaning for person-centred professionals. While the basic idea that communication is about information transfer remains, the nature of what Macke (2014) terms 'the communicative experience' becomes increasingly important. That is, in healthcare, the way in which people communicate, as much as what we communicate, fundamentally affects how people experience practice, both in terms of interactions between persons and professionals, but more widely in how we create (or fail to create) facilitative cultures and environments. Consequently, healthcare professionals must be able to consider communication critically. Central to this is the ability to analyse key components of a situation and their interrelationships, and a basic understanding of communication can help with this.

Communication always has intent

If communication is fundamentally about transferring information, it must occur for a reason. Often, this is about changing someone's understanding of something – an idea, the immediate environment, how they feel. Descriptions of effective communication focus on achieving shared understandings, but this is not an inevitable outcome nor is it invariably positive. Communication, for example, can be intentionally or unintentionally harmful and divisive.

Communication is an interactive process of exchanging content

Language is often the focus when considering communication, but communication content refers to symbols, terms, expressions and artefacts used to encode and share information. Communication processes are the mechanisms by which content is exchanged. Most communicative experiences use aural, visual and kinaesthetic mechanisms. These can happen interpersonally or, for aural and visual mechanisms, remotely using technologies or artefacts to exchange content. Communication is inherently interactive as it is not possible to communicate in the absence of another person. Another important principle is that we cannot not communicate. Non-verbal mechanisms of communication are less amenable to voluntary control than verbal ones.

Communication always occurs in context

The process of communication is affected by the contexts in which communicative experiences occur. Contexts include immediate environments, such as a busy ward where someone might struggle to focus, or a highly charged emotional situation, but also include a person's unique sociocultural history, which affects how they interpret and understand the communication content. Differences in cross-cultural norms can lead to misunderstandings and generational differences and attitudes towards others may be firmly rooted in sociocultural backgrounds.

In summary, critical consideration of communication can be broken down into why (intent), how (process), what (content) and where/when (context).

Fundamental ideas in person-centred communication

As discussed, the complex interactions between intent, process, content and context enable people to participate in the social world. Person-centred communication can be considered as an intentional approach to practice by which strategies and techniques are skilfully applied in ways underpinned by humanistic philosophies. Core to the approach is the development of mutually trusting and healthful relationships that demonstrate respect for persons and uphold their right to self-determinism (McCormack and McCance 2017).

Understanding self and others

Given the mutuality of the helping relationship described above, understanding the 'self', in other words, knowing and accepting who we are and acknowledging our motivations, biases and preferences, can help to improve interpersonal effectiveness. The importance of this in clinical practice cannot be overemphasised, indeed, McCormack and McCance (2017) describe such behaviours as *prerequisites* which are foundational to the development of the person (see Chapter 4 for more information). If people have a sense that their healthcare professional is a competent communicator, with well-developed people skills and self-awareness, they are likely to feel secure. In turn, feeling secure provides a foundation for exploration of the 'self'. From this position, people can identify and articulate what is best for them with the end result of promoting and enabling *person-centred processes*, for example involvement in one's own care and having the feeling of well-being.

It is therefore crucial to grow and learn about our own beliefs and values, biases and prejudices, actions and reactions, emotional responses, desires, likes and dislikes, and, more importantly, to seek to understand the impact of these on practice (see Chapter 30 for further information). Significantly, Luft (1984) emphasised the importance of self-knowledge, arguing that it is the unacknowledged and unknown aspects of our 'self' which often act as barriers to others' potential to grow and flourish. Processes such as conveying empathy through 'sympathetic presencing', being kind and warm, being genuine and trusting self and others are understood to facilitate the process by which others can be known and understood.

Conveying empathy through 'sympathetic presencing'

In reality, one can never *truly* know another's experience. Rather, the healthcare professional, through maintaining an attitude towards others that respects their dignity and uniqueness, is able to offer what McCormack and McCance (2010) refer to as 'sympathetic presencing'.

Similar in function to empathy, sympathetic presencing conveys your willingness to enter the world of another and work with their beliefs and values by suspending your own judgement and being free from the desire to fix the problem/person. It involves you seeking to understand what is known to them, and giving meaning to it in such a way as to ensure the person has a 'felt sense' that you are *with* them. It is inherently healing as it allows strong emotions such as anger, shame and anxiety to be expressed without fear of judgement. For further discussion about sympathetic presencing, please see Chapter 15. Empathy is primarily an attitude, but in the section below we will discuss how it may be enacted through specific strategies.

Being kind and warm

Perceptions of kindness and warmth underpin the process of establishing trusting therapeutic relationships in the opening stages of care, indicating to the other that 'I am with you and for you'. Warmth is conveyed through verbal communication, for example the tone, volume and rate of speech as well as the words used. Verbally 'phatic' communication – the small talk used in everyday life – shows you have an interest in each other's worlds, and helps the other person feel visible and valued. Perhaps most significantly, warmth is conveyed through non-verbal communication, including behaviours such as smiling, appearing interested and attentive, offering eye contact and through the sensitive use of touch. Raphael-Grimm (2014) suggests that positive interactions can occur in very brief encounters, where people share a moment of connectedness.

Activity

Sue is a radiographer in a busy mammography unit. The day's clinic is running late because of some administrative errors accessing case notes. Sue and her colleagues have been rushing to catch up and are aware that the clinic manager has to report on waiting times and screening rates. She calls in her next client, Amy, who has been referred for a screening appointment. Amy has a history of breast cancer in the family and is very anxious that the result of the mammogram will be positive. She does not know what to expect, or how long it will take before she gets her results.

Sue tells her to take her gown off and position herself at the machine, ignoring Amy's attempts at conversation. Sue manoeuvres Amy's breasts into the correct position, leaving Amy balanced uncomfortably on tiptoes whilst she takes the X-ray. When the scan is finished, she tells Amy to put on her gown and go back to the waiting room. Amy leaves the room feeling humiliated and bursts into tears on exiting the waiting room. Reflecting on this scenario, consider what you would do differently during the encounter to make it more person-centred. As you consider the different ways of communicating and the key principles in person-centred communication, what is missing from Sue's practice? What other factors could have contributed to this encounter?

Being genuine

Congruence is the cornerstone of trust in human relationships and is concerned with presenting our authentic self to others. Its presence enables us to build meaningful connections with others transforming what it means to 'be' in the world (McCormack and McCance 2017).

Assuming expert knowledge, using obscure medical jargon and controlling interactions and activities with those in our care introduces an asymmetrical power structure to the caring relationship. In presenting our authentic selves, rather than hiding behind the mystery or superiority of our role, relationships are more egalitarian, allowing us to 'get alongside' rather than dominating others

Trust in self and others

Person-centred communication tends to be non-directional in its orientation. That is to say that communication is used in such a way as to facilitate the person's attainment of their own answers and solutions. Rogers (1961) argued that in a given situation, people can be trusted to 'know' their inner experience and act upon it, and thus intuition is prized over intellect. Guidance from others, therefore, whether solicited or unsolicited, is at best invalid or at worst harmful since it risks disempowering the other. This is welcome news for the learner since the approach enables the person to exercise agency where possible, thus removing the pressure to seek professional-led solutions on their behalf. In the same way that trust (to know and act justly) is afforded to others, it can be helpful to remember that we too can trust in our own ability to *know* what is in our thoughts and to *act* from this place.

Hopefully, the distinction between ordinary communication and person-centred communication is now clear. In delivering person-centred communication, the emphasis is as much on your own growth and development as it is on communicating with others. 'Ways of being' with others that respect their dignity as autonomous people with their own lives, worldviews and emotions have been presented. The following processes are regarded as fundamental to person-centred communication: being kind and warm, being genuine, trusting self and others and conveying empathy. These 'ways of being' form the foundation of a genuinely caring relationship based on egalitarian principles, and imply a moral commitment on behalf of the healthcare professional to their formation and maintenance (Duggan and Thompson 2014).

Activity

From your practice experience, think of an encounter or an episode you experienced or witnessed that left you feeling uncomfortable. If this is not possible, think about an episode that you felt to be excellent practice, or use the vignette above about Sue and Amy to guide your reflections.

In relation to the strategies and practices for person-centred communication, reflect on the following.

- In what ways were you able to present your authentic self? How did you experience the genuineness of others?
- What facilitated or inhibited you (or others) to practise authentically, and what effect did this have?
- In what ways would conveying a sympathetic presence help to build trust and enhance the interaction?

Strategies for putting person-centred communication into action

Noticing

Noticing means focusing your attention on the other person and relies on you being fully present with another. Distractions such as reading computer screens, completing documentation and overtalking can be barriers to the act of noticing. Noting, rather than judging, the other person's mood, emotions, thoughts, attitudes and reactions towards their situation helps facilitate the process of active listening. In the activity above, Sue may have failed to notice Amy's anxiety.

Immediacy

Immediacy involves communicating what is happening in the relationship as it happens in the 'here and now'. It conveys your desire to engage in a relationship and determines the intensity and depth of encounter. It is largely, though not exclusively, negotiated through non-verbal behaviour, including personal distance, smiling, touching and use of eye contact (Hargie 2010). To practise immediacy means to understand how you are perceived by another, to recognise the existence of power dynamics and to demonstrate your appreciation of how this affects the helping relationship. In the vignette, Sue could have enacted person-centred communication by understanding that an imbalance of power exists. Immediacy could have been achieved through simple actions like sitting alongside Amy to explain the procedure and seeking her permission to position Amy during the mammogram.

Asking questions

The judicious use of open questions in assessments or clinical encounters invites the person to respond in the way *they* wish to, as opposed to serving the interests of the healthcare professional. Both open and closed question forms are valid in certain situations but using open questions allows you a glimpse of the other person's 'inner world'. The person can choose to start their response where they wish and from their own perspective. For example, Sue may ask, 'Tell me how you're feeling about your mammogram today' or 'What questions/concerns have you brought with you today?'. A series of closed questions can soon be tiring and interrogatory in tone, and leading questions, such as 'You're ok if I just move your shoulder down slightly, aren't you?', serve to control the responses of the other person. Open questioning shows interest in the other person and leads to further understanding.

Listening and attending

Active listening involves the professional in a process of attending, remembering, responding to and understanding what people are saying. As a skill, it has many therapeutic advantages: making people feel included, respected and valued; providing reassurance, reducing anxiety and setting the appropriate emotional tone for an interaction; assisting decision-making processes (Hargie 2010). Attending, the gentle nods of the head and affirming 'uh-humms' that show we are paying attention, encourages the other to continue speaking. Described in simple terms here, this can require considerable effort, particularly in a busy or noisy environment. This requires some preparation; you will need to empty your head of intrusive thoughts or feelings in order to concentrate, and recognise some of the barriers to your listening well such as 'pretending' to listen, rehearsing your own response whilst the other person is talking, daydreaming, or focusing on some characteristic of the other person. Some people may be harder to listen to by virtue of their personal idiosyncrasies and our own non-verbal communication can serve to encourage or block the speaker.

Responding empathically

Empathic listening enables you to adopt a sympathetic presence and 'hear' what lies behind the words of another. This can include responses to what has and has not been spoken. It requires verbal responses to two messages to show understanding: the facts that are being made explicit (primary empathy) and your hunches about what the person feels about the events/circumstances of the situation (advanced empathy). Empathic reflection, in which the tone/pace/volume of words and gestures used are reflected back verbatim, helps people to gain an insight into their own thoughts and feelings. In all forms, empathy can be regarded as crucial to person-centred communication, having three defining characteristics. First, its purpose is for the listener to understand the other person's 'world from their perspective' in an accepting and non-judgemental way. Second, the listener must be emotionally engaged, and third, the listener should be able to identify closely with the thoughts and feelings of the other person.

Conclusion

So far, our discussion has been confined to ideas about the interpersonal context of the professional/person being cared for in healthcare. However, it is also important to consider other factors that impact communication, in order to develop yourself and your practice. In particular, considering how you *intentionally* use communication is fundamental to improving care processes and creating facilitative environments and cultures that ultimately lead to person-centred outcomes. Healthcare professionals rightly tend to focus on the people for whom they provide care but they should also consider how they communicate with others to create flourishing person-centred cultures (for discussion on this point refer to Chapter 5).

The prerequisites for person-centred practice identify the skills, competencies and values individuals ought to develop to enable them to create and sustain facilitative environments and complete person-centred practice processes. This chapter has discussed core interpersonal skills and strategies to this end, and emphasised the ability to 'know self', demonstrate clarity of beliefs and values and remain professionally competent. Communication plays a key part in social learning processes, transforming professional identity and development. Communication features throughout the person-centred practice framework for good reason; healthcare is inherently interpersonal and no healthcare professional works in isolation. Communicating with people is fundamental to the professional role. However, becoming *person-centred* is to learn how to communicate at each of the levels outlined in the framework, and to do so in ways that allow operationalisation of the key principles of person-centred practice. The theories and strategies outlined in this chapter should help to inform this journey.

Summary

- Effective person-centred communication improves people's experiences of healthcare by promoting autonomy and shared decision making.
- Communication is deemed person-centred when it upholds values and attitudes that are commensurate with respecting human dignity.
- In healthcare, the approach to communication is as important as the skills and strategies used.
- Becoming a person-centred communicator is a developmental process gained through purposeful interaction with self and others.
- The application of person-centred communication extends far beyond clinical practice into areas such as leadership, education and research.

References

Duggan, A. and Thompson, T. (2014). Social interaction contexts processes in healthcare. In: *Interpersonal Communication* (ed. C. Berger), 493. Berlin: De Gruyter.

Hargie, O. (2010). *Skilled Interpersonal Communication: Research, Theory and Practice*, 5e. London: Taylor & Francis Group.

Luft, J. (1984). *Group Process: An Introduction to Group Dynamics*, 3e. New York: McGraw Hill.

Macke, F.J. (2014). *The Experience of Human Communication: Body, Flesh, and Relationship*. Lanham, NJ: Fairleigh Dickinson University Press.

McCormack, B. and McCance, T. (2010). *Person-Centred Nursing: Theory, Models and Methods*. Oxford: Wiley-Blackwell.

McCormack, B. and McCance, T. (2017). *Person-Centred Practice in Nursing: Theory and Practice*, 2e. Chichester: Wiley-Blackwell.

Oxford Dictionaries Online (2019). *Communication*. https://en.oxforddictionaries.com/definition/communication

Raphael-Grimm, T. (2014). *The Art of Communication in Nursing and Health Care: An Interdisciplinary Approach*. New York: Springer.

Robinson, P. (2005). People communicate. In: *E-Communication Skills: A Guide for Primary Care* (eds. L. Simpson, P. Robinson, M. Fletcher and R. Wilson). Oxford: Radcliffe Publishing.

Rogers, C.R. (1961). *On Becoming a Person*. Boston, MA: Houghton Mifflin.

Waltzlawick, P., Bavelas, J.B., and Jackson, D.D. (1967). *Pragmatics of Human Communication: A Study of Interactional Patterns, Paradoxes and Pathologies*. New York: W. Norton and Co.

Further reading

Freshwater, D. (2003). *Counselling Skills for Nurses, Midwives and Health Visitors*. Maidenhead: Open University Press.

Van Servellen, G. (2009). *Communication Skills for the Health Care Professional: Concepts, Practice and Evidence*, 2e. Jones and Bartlett: Sudbury, MA.

9

Systems to support person-centred decision making

Amanda Stears[1] and Dawn Jansch[1,2]

[1] Queen Margaret University, Edinburgh, Scotland, UK

[2] Western General Hospital, Edinburgh, Scotland, UK

Contents

Fundamentals of Person-Centred Healthcare Practice, First Edition. Edited by Brendan McCormack, Tanya McCance, Cathy Bulley, Donna Brown, Ailsa McMillan and Suzanne Martin.

Learning outcomes

- Understand the components of person-centred decision making for the service user, professional and at an organisational level.
- Identify common issues associated with decision making.
- Consider a variety of strategies to enable person-centred decision making.

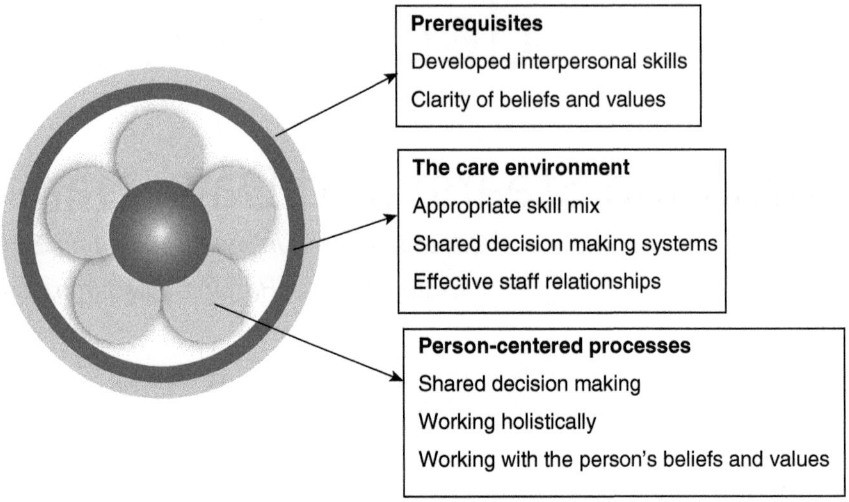

Introduction

This chapter will focus on person-centred decision making which sits within the practice environment domain of the Person-centred Practice Framework (PcPF) that you were introduced to in Chapter 3. The chapter will outline what person-centred decision making is for nursing, midwifery and allied health professionals (NMAHPs). It will discuss the process of decision making both personally and professionally with service users and their family/carers as appropriate and within the wider multidisciplinary team context. At its core, person-centred decision making is facilitation of service user participation by providing information and integrating newly developed perceptions into practice (McCance and McCormack 2017).

What is decision making?

Decision making is something we do every day, impacting on every aspect of our lives, from when we get up in the morning, to what we eat, and what we are going to do each day. Kahneman (2011) describes two systems of decision making: system 1 is our fast system which is to some extent unconscious and instinctive and we use this to make everyday decisions. System 2 is our slow system which is a more conscious thinking process for more complex decisions. When we learn to drive, for example, we would very much use system 2 in the initial stages as we not only learn the mechanics of driving but process the ever-changing environment.

When we become experienced drivers, we switch to fast thinking to react to situations that we may encounter. The process is very much automatic.

In healthcare, it may feel as if decisions are often made on our behalf or we base decisions on advice given to us by professionals such as general practitioners (GP's), nurses and allied health professionals. We can feel that we have had little say in the decision-making process and we can leave with unanswered questions regarding treatment or medication and their expected benefits or potential side effects. This can not only affect adherence to the desired advice or behaviour but can disempower those in our care.

In the 1950s the patient–doctor relationship was hierarchical with the patient as the passive recipient (Szaz and Hollender 1956). In the 1960s there was a recognition of the need to have a relationship that gave the patient autonomy and valued the patient as one who shared in the decision-making process (Arnstein 1969). As healthcare and this concept continued to evolve over the next two decades, Charles and de Maio (1993) proposed that patient involvement in decision making could occur on three levels: consultation, partnership and lay control.

This, however, takes a rather paternalistic view, with the professional having the role of the parent, i.e. they know best, and the service user role limited to being given the information or giving consent for something to happen. Conly (2013) argues that paternalism can be justified where there are self-destructive behaviours such as poor diet or smoking that will impact on the health of the individual. An example of this is the UK government's 'Sugar Tax' or more accurately the Soft Drinks Industry Levy introduced in April 2018. In an attempt to influence the consumption of sugary drinks which are considered detrimental to health when consumed in large quantities, manufacturers must pay the government 24p on drinks containing 8 g of sugar per 100 mL of product. Whether this levy impacts on the rising obesity levels remains to be seen (Thornton 2018).

As shown in Figure 9.1 below Thompson (2007) proposed a continuum of differing levels of service user power correlating to a range of values from exclusion to informed decision making. Shared decision making is not a unilateral process as the healthcare professional, the service user and their families or carers all have differing roles and experiences. The healthcare professional will have expertise and knowledge that they need to share with the service user

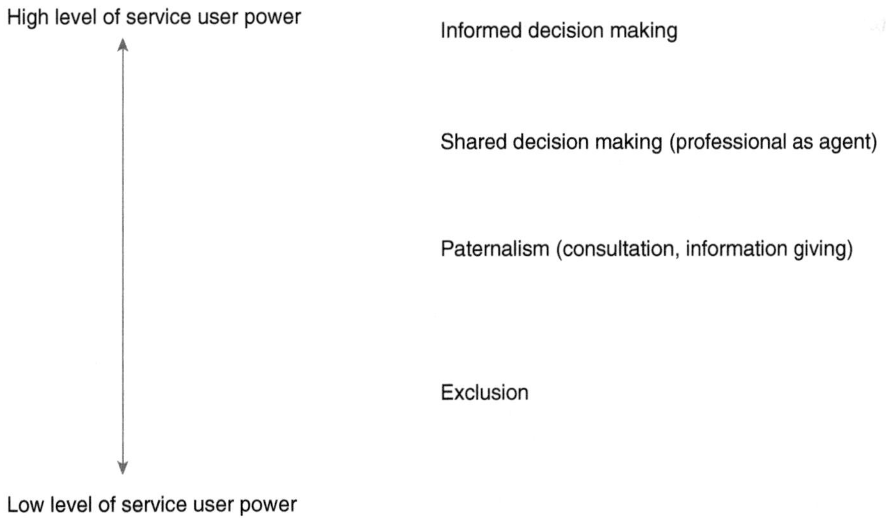

Figure 9.1 Power continuum. Source: Based on Thompson, A.G.H. 2007.

in a way they understand to help inform the decision making. The service user's beliefs and values will come into play as they consider information to make decisions. However, where we have service users who live with long-term (Chapter 26) or life-limiting conditions such as cystic fibrosis or chronic obstructive pulmonary disease (COPD), the service user in many instances is considered the expert in their condition and may know more than the healthcare professional.

Activity

John is an ex-miner who was diagnosed with chronic obstructive pulmonary disease four years ago after a history of declining exercise tolerance and worsening shortness of breath. He is on the maximal drug therapy. He attends for his annual review and reports that he isn't taking his inhaled corticosteroids as he says he doesn't need them, he feels fine. You know that he needs to regularly take all his medication and the corticosteroid in particular as this is what helps with the inflammation, but he is adamant.

Discussion points

- What do you do in this situation?
- Using the continuum proposed by Thompson, where does John currently sit with his views?

It appears here that John has a high level of power, but the choices he is making are detrimental to his health. How do you establish why John doesn't take the medication and how might you explore this with him? Whilst we can recognise and appreciate the continuum that Thompson (2007) identified, it is not what we consider person-centred. This continuum is linear but decision making is not, as healthcare professionals bring a range of personal knowledge, values and experiences to the process. This is further complicated by multidisciplinary team working which can bring its own set of challenges!

Service user perspectives

There are many factors that can influence the perspectives of both service users and health professionals and one of them is social media. This is powerful and offers great potential but as we will discuss, it also has pitfalls! Tennant et al. (2015) report that nearly 90% of older adults have sought information from Facebook and Twitter on health-related issues. Websites such as Mumsnet (www.mumsnet.com) and Gransnet (www.gransnet.com) host forums that offer support and information to a global community on every aspect of child rearing from childbirth to health and parenting to issues of being a long-distance grandparent. This unprecedented rise in social media and the plethora of healthcare information available via the internet can be useful but also misinformed and we need to be mindful of its influence and ensure we guide service users to peer-reviewed resources, discussing where and why that source of information is relevant. It is one thing to seek cancer information online from Cancer Research UK, for example, but quite another to take advice from a social media group which claims that a certain diet or herb can cure all your ills.

The healthcare professional's relationship with the service user is key in helping them feel empowered to improve their health through engaged interactions, fostering self-determination to improve health within healthful relationships. Key to this is creating an environment of mutual respect and understanding, listening to the person's views, interests, priorities and abilities (McCance and McCormack 2017). We need to be mindful of service users such as those with a learning disability or with dementia who may relinquish or delegate decisions to family or carers as this may be a sign of anxiety or a perception of an inability to make informed decisions, as illustrated by Daly et al. (2018) in their work on shared decision making in extended care settings.

Activity

Read the following two interactions.

GP appointment – seven minutes

Harriet is a busy working mother of two small children who are two and four. She has been having some tension headaches and has visited her GP for advice. The GP takes her blood pressure and advises her it is high at 145/90. She is given a prescription for lisinopril and asked to come back to the practice nurse in two weeks' time for review.

Practice nurse appointment – ten minutes

Two weeks later, Harriet attends for a blood pressure review with the practice nurse Sally. Sally asks her how she is feeling and how she has been getting on with the new medication. Harriet says she hasn't taken the medication, she knows she is overweight (BMI 30) and that she should exercise more but she can't see herself at the gym or an exercise class. She says she loves to cook, and enjoys food. She also reports she feels tired as she is also looking after her elderly parents and although she loves them, they can be very demanding as can her two small children.

Discussion points

- What are your thoughts about these interactions?
- What might the person feel after each interaction?
- Are these interactions person-centred?
- What person-centred or communication strategies might you adopt that will facilitate shared decision making?

Person-centred decision making

Person-centred decision making should always respect the service user's experience, values, needs and preferences in the planning, co-ordination and delivery of care. The implementation of a person-centred care model has been shown to contribute to improved outcomes for service users, better use of resources, decreased costs and increased satisfaction with care (Gluyas 2015).

Below (Figure 9.2) is an example of the most common medically focused person-centred model for shared decision making. This model is very unilateral and does not demonstrate the complexities of shared decision making and is a model we must move away from.

Thinking about the model above, the healthcare professional provides the service user with all the best relevant information about their treatment or care plan and the decision is made with a view that the service user has been part of the process. However, this represents a very

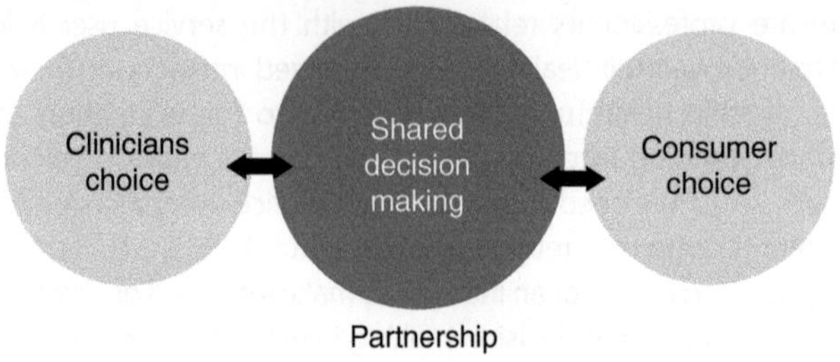

Figure 9.2 A model of shared decision-making. Source: Adapted from The Health Foundation (2019).

simplistic overview of the process. What is disappointing is that it was published in 2019, yet fails to recognise the collaborative nature of shared decision making or the factors that are highlighted in our opening graphic which are the need to work with person-centred processes that are holistic, facilitating shared decision making whilst working with the person's beliefs and values. Added to this are environmental factors, ensuring staff have the appropriate skill mix, can work effectively in the team, whilst developing excellent interpersonal skills with clear shared values and beliefs. These complexities will be explored further in Chapter 15.

From what you have read in previous chapters about the PcPF, there are other factors that should be taken into consideration which may influence the decision-making process. As mentioned earlier, person-centred decision making is a collaborative process where the service user makes a decision about their care that is supported by healthcare professionals.

By interacting and working with service users, we can develop a clearer picture of what their values and beliefs are, understanding what is happening from their perspective physically, psychologically and socially (McCance and McCormack 2017). In doing so we are reinforcing one of the key principles of person-centred care and strengthening relationships. This does not come without its challenges and these are set out with opportunities to overcome them in Chapter 15.

The value of shared decision making

Reflecting on the case in the previous activity, in the second consultation it is clear that the service user has opened up to Sally and disclosed something of who she is, her love of cooking, her fatigue and her health concerns. You know as a health professional that she needs to take the medication. What are the issues that are stopping Harriet taking the medication? How might you discuss these?

Multidisciplinary team

The culture of healthcare is changing, and examples of this are the number of services delivered at times that are outside the standard 9–5 model and using digital technology (Tennant et al. 2015). Whilst Facebook is commonly used by groups of students to share and discuss issues in their education, it is becoming common for groups of staff to use encrypted social media apps as 'virtual huddles'. As societal healthcare challenges continue to emerge, the work of the multidisciplinary team becomes more vital in the co-ordination and integration of care. By coming together and sharing information about a person's wants and needs, their illness and the goals of care in relation to their illness, the management of their care can be improved along with the situational awareness and judgement of the person's situation and ability to make informed clinical decisions (Forte et al. 2018). The team can then incorporate evidence-based practice and the best treatment for that person (Forte et al. 2018). Open communication is key as is organisation and management of resources, including the professionals within the team. They can educate and inform service users and their families/carers whilst providing emotional support and ensuring care can be accessed when required.

Strategies to promote shared decision making

Activity

Sunita is a 29 year old who has recently married. She has lived with type 1 diabetes for the majority of her life. Since being with her husband, she has yearned to become a mother. Sunita feels that she would not be fulfilling her role as a wife if she cannot physically have a child for her husband. She has told the diabetic consultant that she would like to try for a baby. He insists that this would be a bad idea as pregnancy will significantly affect her diabetes control and lead to serious health complications for both Sunita and the foetus and suggests that Sunita should consider adoption instead. The consultant asks if there are any other issues about her diabetes then brings the consultation to an end.

Discussion points

- What are your thoughts about the consultant's response?
- Is this a person-centred or a holistic approach?
- Does it consider Sunita's personal beliefs, values and future aspirations?
- As a healthcare professional, how might you facilitate person-centred decision making?

Therapeutic relationships

A central component of person-centred shared decision making is a therapeutic relationship between the service user and the team of healthcare professionals (Gluyas 2015; McCance and McCormack 2017). Within this relationship, each person acknowledges and respects each other's perception of healthcare. This requires time to listen, understand, and offer support and practical expertise (McCance and McCormack 2017). In the case of Sunita, the consultant imposed his professional position and perceptions of Sunita. Perhaps if he took time to listen, consider and respect Sunita's beliefs and values, he would have gained more understanding of her situation. Using the consultant's expertise and knowledge, together they can explore all other possible options and eventualities and enable a shared decision about what to do about becoming pregnant.

Motivational interviewing

One strategy that can facilitate shared decision making is motivational interviewing (MI). This originated in the early 1980s in the treatment of addiction (Miller and Rollnick 2012). It is a person-centred approach that uses a conversational method to explore a person's health beliefs with the endpoint of facilitating behaviour change. Initiated by the service user, it is being used in a variety of settings from physiotherapy to diabetes care (Christie and Channon 2014). It uses skills such as active listening, reflection, affirmation and summarising to work with the person to positively manage and influence their health. It is often likened to 'dancing and not wrestling' with the person. Thinking about Sunita, do you think the consultant was in harmony with her, in tune with what she wanted, or did he set himself against her so it felt more like a battle of wills? It is outside the scope of this chapter to fully discuss this but more resources are detailed in the Further reading.

Organisational decision making

Whilst the service user should be at the centre of all decisions made in healthcare, it is important to highlight that if a care culture cannot support decision making in a person-centred manner, then it is unlikely that the culture can practise person-centred decision making (Manley et al. 2014). Effective decision making requires an effective team (McCance and McCormack 2017). In an ideal world, all health professionals would collaboratively develop and agree shared purposes and values, that are then 'lived out' in daily practice (McCance and McCormack 2017). The healthcare team should aim to deliver person-centred care to all service users, with the service user involved at each stage. Sadly, this is often not the case. The values that an organisational culture espouses in theory can differ from behaviours displayed in practice.

The PcPF suggests that if the care environment (culture) does not practise and encourage person-centred ways of working, then the potential of the person receiving care may not be realised. Factors that influence or create barriers to this care environment include people, processes and structures. These can include skill mix, systems of decision making, power sharing, staff relationships and organisational support.

Skill mix

Generally, skill mix refers to the expertise and range of staff in the care team that is delivering the care required (McCance and McCormack 2017). This includes the diversity of knowledge, skills and experience that individuals within the team possess (WHO 2000). By developing and maintaining an optimal skill mix in a team, effective collaborative teamwork and high-quality care can be provided (Antunes and Moreira 2013). Investment in all persons in the team in terms of continuing education and professional development is necessary in influencing their professional judgements and ultimately the quality of care.

Systems of decision making

In essence, these are the processes that influence decision making. They include internal factors such as the team's ways of working or external factors and drivers such as policy or finances. For example, in healthcare systems, many decisions about a person's care or treatment will be driven by budget restraints.

Many strategies can be adopted to open up and facilitate discussion and shared decision making. For example, holding regular communicative spaces for all staff to enable team members to reflect, challenge and facilitate discussion about the care environment or care provision more generally. This is more commonly used within education, but reflects qualities that are associated with person-centredness. Communicative spaces and agreed interactions in which thoughtful, mutual listening is encouraged promote understanding and collaborative decision making (Aspfors and Valle 2017).

Similarly, regular 'team huddles' can be implemented to effectively ensure person-centred care. In a busy care environment, huddles are a quick and effective strategy that can provide opportunities for the team to communicate and co-ordinate care. They enable the team to have planned, regular opportunities throughout the working day, to openly communicate relevant issues about care that incorporates the wishes of service users, plan prospective care and prepare for any changes. Huddles give the team space to better understand the person's circumstances, each other's roles and access to resources. They can enhance professional relationships, team communication and work culture (Provost et al. 2015). Ultimately, huddles improve interprofessional working and therefore the care of service users (Yu 2015; Donovan 2018).

Power sharing

Historically, a healthcare team consists of a hierarchy of professions and experience, such as consultant, junior doctor, nurse, occupational therapist, physiotherapist and clinical support worker. This hierarchy generally suggests that knowledge and domination from more senior staff is more powerful when it comes to decision making (McCance and McCormack 2017). In this case, the consultant is the most experienced in the team, so should therefore make all decisions for both the care team and service user. This practice can cause conflict and does not enable person-centred relationships, practices or shared decisionmaking. To promote person-centred decision making in the team, decisions and discussions should be inclusive and non-dominant, encouraging autonomy, mutual respect, equality and shared values, appreciating and valuing what everyone brings to the team.

So what does person-centred decision making look like?

- Has *shared values* which are adopted both individually and collectively (Manley et al. 2011).
- *Shared vision of ways of working* – by having open channels of interaction and communication, staff can actively highlight concerns and then engage in decision making that directly impacts on their workplace culture.
- *Shared learning culture* – creating a workplace culture that supports and develops both individual and group learning needs.
- *Shared governance* – when the workplace culture collectively works together to evaluate, develop and improve practices for their own benefit and to ensure that service users receive the most effective care possible.
- *Effective staff relationships* – which are non-dominant and do not exploit each other. Instead, mutual respect is promoted, paying attention to self and each other and developing positive relationships that ultimately promote productivity and a high standard of care.
- *Creating a culture that promotes high challenge and high support (scaffolding)* – encouraging all team members to provide high-support/high-challenge feedback to each other can increase critical awareness whilst driving for enhanced performance (Wilson and Devereux 2014).

Summary

- Service users are central to the process of decision making.
- Person-centred decision making is a complex process.
- To enable shared decision making, the organisation needs to practise person-centred behaviours and decision making.
- Workplace culture should be non-dominant and inclusive of all regardless of profession and grade.
- Workplace cultures could consider improving communicative practices through the use of 'huddles' or 'communicative spaces'.
- Promotion of person-centred decision making ultimately improves the quality of care provided.

References

Antunes, V. and Moreira, J.P. (2013). Skill mix in healthcare: an international update for the management debate. *International Journal of Healthcare Management* 6 (1): 12–17.

Arnstein, S. (1969). A ladder of citizen participation. *Journal of American Institute of Planners*. 35: 216–224.

Aspfors, J. and Valle, A.M. (2017). Designing communicative spaces – innovative perspectives on teacher education. *Education Inquiry* 8 (1): 1–16.

Charles, C. and DeMaio, S. (1993). Lay participation in health care decision making: a conceptual framework. *Journal of Health Politics, Policy and Law* 18: 887–904.

Christie, D. and Channon, S. (2014). The potential for motivational interviewing to improve outcomes in the management of diabetes and obesity in paediatric and adult populations: a clinical review. *Diabetes, Obesity and Metabolism* 16 (5): 381–387.

Conly, S. (2013). Coercive paternalism in health care: against freedom of choice? *Public Health Ethics* 6 (3): 241–245.

Daly, R.L., Bunn, F., and Goodman, C. (2018). Shared decision making for people living with dementia in extended care: a systematic review. *BMJ Open* 8: 1–11.

Donovan, J. (2018). How our morning 'huddles' improved practice teamworking. *Pulse* www.pulsetoday.co.uk/your-practice/regulation/how-our-morning-huddles-improved-practice-teamworking/20037047.

Eklund, J.H., Holstrom, I.K., Kumlin, T. et al. (2019). "Same same or different?" A review of reviews of person-centred and patient-centred care. *Client Education and Counselling* 102: 3–11.

Forte, D.N., Kawai, F., and Cohen, C. (2018). A bioethical framework to guide the decision-making process in the care of seriously ill patients. *BMS Medical Ethics* 17 (78): 1–8.

Gluyas, H. (2015). Patient-centred care: improving healthcare outcomes. *Nursing Standard* 30 (4): 50.

Kahneman, D. (2011). *Thinking Fast and Slow*. New York: Farrar, Straus and Groux.

Manley, K., Saunders, K., Cardiff, S., and Webster, J. (2011). Effective workplace culture: the attributes, enabling factors and consequences of a new concept. *International Practice Development Journal* 1 (20): 1–29.

Manley, K., O'Keefe, H., Jackson, C. et al. (2014). A shared purpose framework to deliver person-centred, safe and effective care: Organisational transformation using practice development methodology. *International Practice Development Journal* 4 (1).

McCance, T. and McCormack, B. (eds.) (2017). *Person-Centred Practice in Nursing and Health Care: Theory and Practice*. Chichester: Wiley.

Miller, S. and Rollnick, W.R. (2012). *Motivational Interviewing in Health Care*, 3e. London: Guilford Press.

Provost, S.M., Lanham, H.J., Leykum, L.K. et al. (2015). Health care huddles: managing complexity to achieve high reliability. *Health Care Management Review* 40 (1): 2–12.

Szasz, T. and Hollender, M. (1956). A Contribution to the philosophy of medicine: the basic model of the doctor-patient relationship. *Archives of Internal Medicine.* 97: 585–592.

Tennant, B., Stellefson, M., Dodd, V. et al. (2015). eHealth literacy and web.2.0 health information seeking behaviour's among baby boomers and older adults. *Journal of Medical Internet Research* 17 (3): e70.

The Health Foundation (2019). *Shared Decision Making*. London: The Health Foundation.

Thompson, A.G.H. (2007). The meaning of Patient Involvement and participation in health care consultations: taxonomy. *Social Sciences and Medicine.* 64 (6): 1297–1310.

Thornton, J. (2018). *The UK Has Introduced a Sugar Tax, But Will It Work?* London School of Hygiene and Tropical Medicine. www.lshtm.ac.uk/research/research-action/features/uk-sugar-tax-will-it-work.

Wilson, K. and Devereux, L. (2014). Scaffolding theory: high challenge, high support in Academic Language and Learning (ALL) contexts. *Journal of Academic Language and Learning* 8 (3): A91–A100.

World Health Organization (2000). *The World Health Report, 2000 Health Systems: Improving Performance.* Geneva: World Health Organization.

Yu, E. (2015). *Implementing a Daily Team Huddle*. Chicago: American Medical Association.

Further reading

Motivational Interviewing Network of Trainers (MINT): https://motivationalinterviewing.org

10

Connecting with others

Brighide Lynch[1], Derek Barron[2], and Lesley McKinlay[3]

[1] *Ulster University, Northern Ireland, UK*
[2] *Erskine, Bishopton, Scotland, UK*
[3] *Queen Margaret University, Edinburgh, Scotland, UK*

Contents

Fundamentals of Person-Centred Healthcare Practice, First Edition. Edited by Brendan McCormack, Tanya McCance, Cathy Bulley, Donna Brown, Ailsa McMillan and Suzanne Martin.

Learning outcomes

- Be able to analyse person-centred principles and their application in developing relationships with others.
- Have an understanding of the processes used to connect with people and how this contributes to the development of person-centred cultures.
- Development of critical reflection skills in order to explore the concept of emotional intelligence.

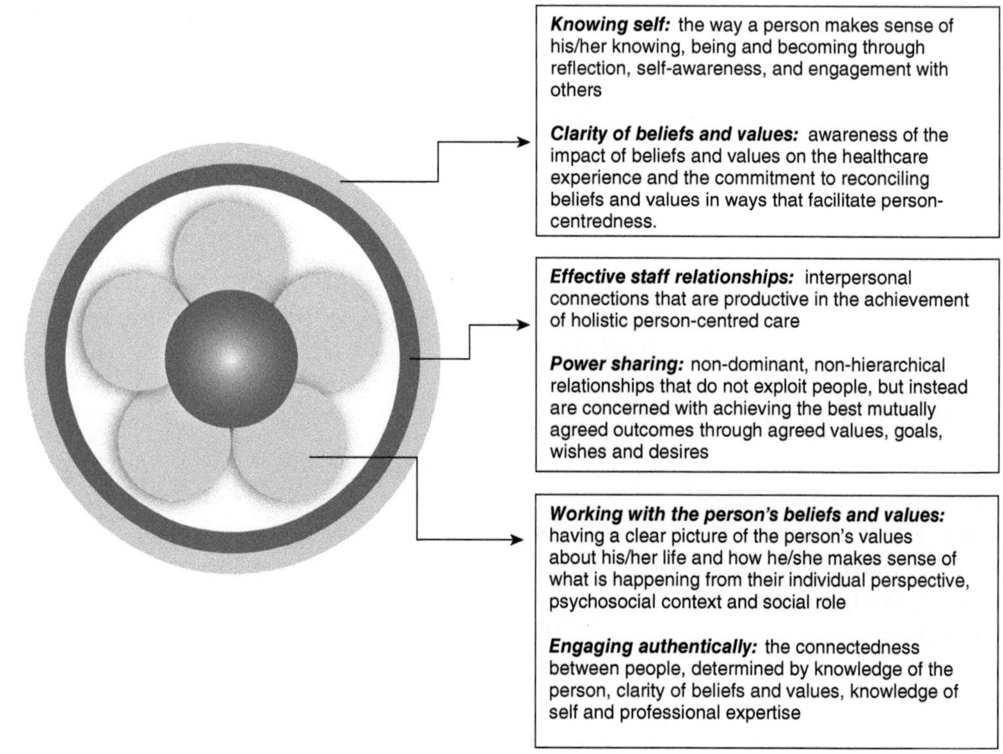

Knowing self: the way a person makes sense of his/her knowing, being and becoming through reflection, self-awareness, and engagement with others
Clarity of beliefs and values: awareness of the impact of beliefs and values on the healthcare experience and the commitment to reconciling beliefs and values in ways that facilitate person-centredness.
Effective staff relationships: interpersonal connections that are productive in the achievement of holistic person-centred care
Power sharing: non-dominant, non-hierarchical relationships that do not exploit people, but instead are concerned with achieving the best mutually agreed outcomes through agreed values, goals, wishes and desires
Working with the person's beliefs and values: having a clear picture of the person's values about his/her life and how he/she makes sense of what is happening from their individual perspective, psychosocial context and social role
Engaging authentically: the connectedness between people, determined by knowledge of the person, clarity of beliefs and values, knowledge of self and professional expertise

Introduction

Person-centred practice is built on the formation of relationships that connect and engage with the other person in a way that is described by McCormack and McCance (2017) as *healthful*. They are relationships that honour the personhood of all persons and therefore include the relationship with self, colleagues, persons being cared for and those significant to them. The development of mutual trust and understanding is fundamental to the formation of healthful relationships with others and can only manifest, and become strengthened, through an increased awareness of one's self from an emotionally intelligent perspective.

Emotional intelligence is about being in touch with, and understanding self, and connects with the prerequisites of *knowing self* and *clarity of beliefs and values* in the Person-centred Practice Framework. Having clarity about one's beliefs and values is fundamental to the development of positive relationships with colleagues and working together effectively. *Power sharing* and *effective staff relationships* are essential characteristics for a supportive context that enables person-centred practice to take place.

Whilst all five person-centred processes can be said to capture the essence of healthful relationships, this section of the chapter will focus on *working with the person's beliefs and values and engaging authentically*, in the context of the relationship with the person and their family. Both processes highlight the importance of the partnership aspect in relationships and are fundamental to the three remaining processes in the Person-centred Practice Framework.

Relationship with self: emotional intelligence

McCance et al. (2011) describe person-centredness as a multidimensional concept, i.e. not a single thing, it is complex and yet simple, it is the essence of our humanity, the basis of our interactions as people. When we begin to unpick the concept, we find that there are multiple layers. The relationship with self, explored in detail in Chapter 4, is the foundation from which other relationships are built. As the foundation, there is a great emphasis on the healthcare worker's relationship with himself or herself, underpinned by a need for them to practise self-compassion and of knowing/understanding himself or herself from an emotionally intelligent perspective. Gilbert et al. (2011) noted that self-compassion is important in mental and emotional well-being, in that it links the qualities of soothing and calming both inwardly and outwards to others. In order to be consistently there for others using a person-centred approach, the healthcare worker not only has a responsibility, but also a duty to care for themselves. Practising self-care is important in being authentic, not only intrapersonally (i.e. within you as a person) but also interpersonally (i.e. with persons you are caring for and colleagues).

Activity

Neff offers a free introductory test of self-compassion (https://self-compassion.org/test-how-self-compassionate-you-are) – you may wish to take a few moments away from the chapter to take this test, remembering that tests such as this are broadly indicative and not absolutely fact.

Take time to reflect on the indicative outcomes of the test.

- Did you learn anything new?
- Will the outcome of the test encourage you to do anything differently?

For your own well-being and efficacy as a person, you need to understand yourself. Emotional intelligence is about understanding self and the impact you have on others. Importantly, it is also the impact they have on you as a person and as a team member. Salovey and Mayer (1990, p. 189), define emotional intelligence as 'the ability to monitor one's own and other's feelings, to discriminate among them and to use this information to guide one's thinking and actions'. Previously, in Chapter 4, we focused on the person's ability to monitor and understand their own feelings in order to care for themselves. Figure 10.1 helps us to explore this 'knowing

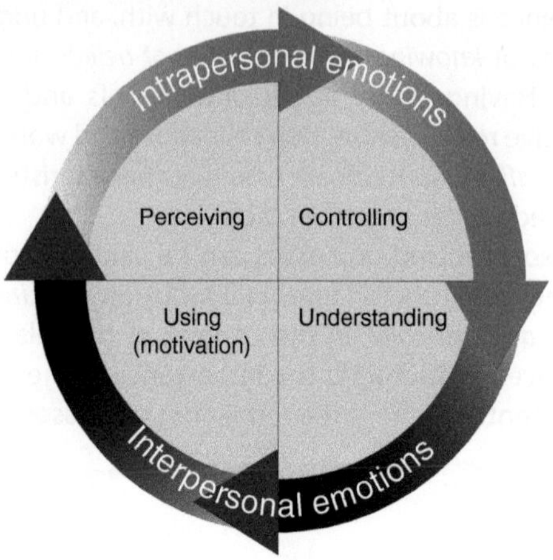

Figure 10.1 Interdependence in relation to emotional intelligence. Source: Barron and Hurley (2012).

self'. Emotions are a key component in guiding our thinking and actions. However, to positively control our actions, feelings need to be understood. Emotions can, when uncontrolled, have a negative impact on our actions. Understanding why you are feeling specific emotions can help shape your response to them.

Reflection

Barron and Hurley (2012) used the diagram in Figure 10.1 in relation to emotional intelligence to demonstrate interdependence and the link between knowing and understanding yourself and the impact you have on others and they have on you.

In understanding the intrapersonal quadrants, the person needs to be aware of their own strengths and weakness from an emotional viewpoint. The skill of reflection is important in enhancing the person's self-awareness. The perceiving and controlling of their emotional response is key in their personal development as well as their effectiveness as a healthcare worker. Cummings et al. (2005) considered that the emotionally intelligent healthcare team member/leader was more supportive and motivating to their colleagues/followers as their approach was most closely linked to both transformational and servant leadership styles. Alimo-Metcalfe and Alban-Metcalfe (2012) noted that the transformational leader showed genuine concern for their colleagues/teams through understanding both themselves and their followers. The lower 'interpersonal' quadrants consider how we interact with others. In the understanding arena, empathy is its core, which is the ability to 'feel' or sense the emotions of others as if you were experiencing those emotions, without losing the 'as if' quality.

Using that understanding to guide our actions with the person, it is important to understand their impact on us as healthcare workers. The motivating quadrant relates to how we are able to use the emotions we sense (in others) to create the emotional setting whereby the other person feels motivated around a course of action or behaviour. For example, through positive influence the person is empowered to take action, rather than it being something given to them.

Relationship with colleagues

When Nolan et al. (2004) introduced the concept of relationship-centred care, they presented it as an exclusive approach that goes beyond person-centredness. These authors suggest that person-centredness concentrates on the relationship between the nurse and the person being cared for, and question the degree to which person-centredness can promote a mutual harmonised and balanced relationship with all parties involved. The authors argue that 'relationship-centred care' is a more suitable term (Nolan et al., 2004, p. 47). In order to provide clarity and enhanced understanding about the difference between relationship-centred care and person-centredness, it is important to point out that conceptually, relationships are a crucial part of the philosophy of personhood. The 'person' includes everyone connected with the care experience and when we pay attention to the significance of meaningful relationships, we enable person-centredness to be realised (McCormack et al. 2012). One can therefore conclude that similarities exist between person-centredness and relationship-centred care and their conceptual underpinnings are complementary.

Our beliefs and values are fundamental to the development of positive relationships with colleagues and working together effectively. They influence our attitudes and often our behaviours and therefore drive the kind of care each member of the healthcare team gives to persons being cared for and those significant to them in their lives. Beliefs and values are interrelated and are buried deep in each person, and in the workplace culture of the practice environment where healthcare teams work. Basic assumptions involve tacit beliefs that team members hold unconsciously about themselves, their relationships and the nature of the organisation in which they work (Schein 1992). A match between what we say we value and believe and what we do in practice is one of the characteristics of effective individuals, teams and organisations. When there is a gap between the theoretical values and the values really being put into action, both individually and collectively, it is extremely unlikely that a person-centred workplace culture will become real in any significant way.

The everyday relationships and interactions that take place between people working in a care setting and the way people act and react within these complex relationships all combine to shape the culture of that workplace. The simplest definition of workplace culture is offered by Drennan (1992): 'The way things are done around here'. Findings from several healthcare scandals, such as the public inquiry led by Robert Francis QC (Francis 2013), highlight the huge influence 'the way things are done around here' has on the delivery of care. One of the major themes identified in the Francis Report on the Mid Staffordshire Trust was the significant lack of power sharing between management at board level and staff at ward level. The values and belief system of the hierarchy in the organisation centred on financial targets and efficiency. These values cascaded down the organisation to the frontline staff, leaving them with feelings of powerlessness as they observed the achievement of financial targets being rewarded and taking greater priority than the delivery of safe, fundamental care to patients.

The issue of power sharing is closely linked to effective staff relationships and decision making. As can be learnt from the Francis Report, when decisions are made high up in the organisation and not shared, these hierarchical relationships can either facilitate or impede person-centredness. A healthcare team may feel they cannot influence such decisions and so they accept the increased monitoring of tasks related to efficiency as 'the way things are done'. This can cause feelings of powerlessness as the team are unable to practise according to their espoused values. In order for a team to be effective in their relationships and in working together to develop a person-centred culture, they need collective commitment to closing the gap between their espoused values and those values that are demonstrated in behaviours observed in practice. Each person in the team needs to be given the opportunity to make their own values clear, to both themselves and others. A values clarification exercise is a practice development tool (McCormack et al. 2013) used to help teams clarify their personal beliefs and values so they can make explicit their vision of what they collectively want to create and how they relate with each other in order to create it.

Relationships with the person and their family

Activity

This poem is a person's professional account of a personal experience. As you read the poem, what do you hear, feel and see? Capture your response in a short paragraph.

Why do we need to build relationships with the people we care for? What does this 'relationship' involve? How do you go about building relationships in your day-to-day practice learning experience? Try to relate these questions to your work with people on a day-to-day basis. Use words or drawings to depict your thoughts.

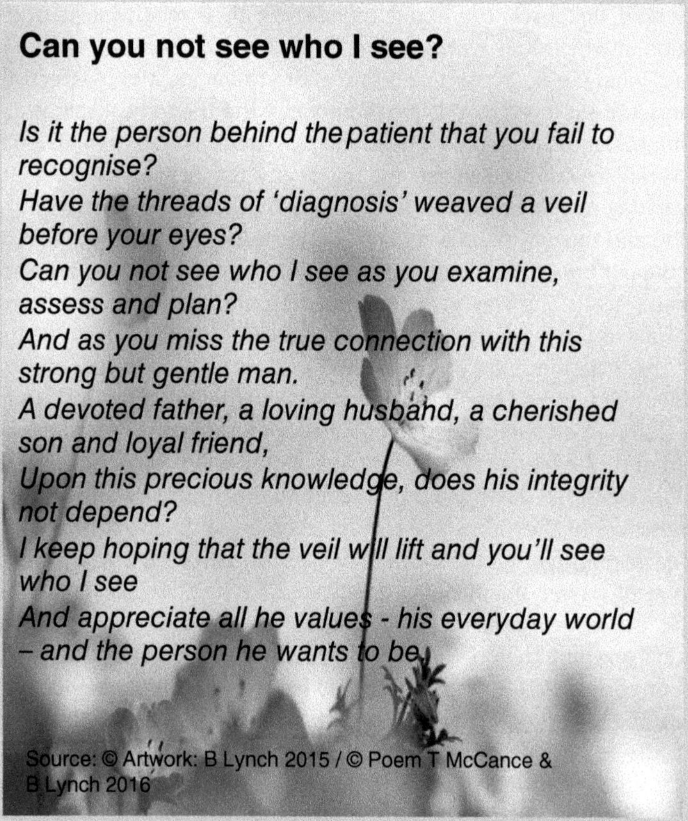
Can you not see who I see?

Is it the person behind the patient that you fail to recognise?
Have the threads of 'diagnosis' weaved a veil before your eyes?
Can you not see who I see as you examine, assess and plan?
And as you miss the true connection with this strong but gentle man.
A devoted father, a loving husband, a cherished son and loyal friend,
Upon this precious knowledge, does his integrity not depend?
I keep hoping that the veil will lift and you'll see who I see
And appreciate all he values - his everyday world – and the person he wants to be.

Source: © Artwork: B Lynch 2015 / © Poem T McCance & B Lynch 2016

One of the key principles of person-centred care is 'being in relation' (McCormack and McCance 2017). Crucially, the healthcare professional must build a relationship with the person in their care and get to know the individual so care can be tailored to their needs. A healthcare worker's role is based on a relationship being formed with an individual who is receiving care which involves recognition, respect and trust (Kitwood 2019). Therapeutic relationships are not a new concept and the building of a relationship between the carer and the person being cared for is a fundamental part of healthcare delivery. In fact, it is such a taken-for-granted fundamental aspect that the detail and the way in which the relationship is formed may not be given the importance or considered in the detail that it deserves. The relationship between the healthcare worker and the person receiving care is crucial to the outcome of a healthful culture.

Back in the 1950s, Peplau wrote that nursing encompasses more than just physical care and it has become of great importance for nurses to focus on additional aspects of a person and 'their world' such as psychological, social and spiritual considerations (Peplau 1952). This involves engaging authentically and is closely related to our relationship with self. If we have the emotional intelligence to know ourselves before we can relate to and form relationships with others, then we can help to lessen the fear, anxiety and distress that a person may be experiencing when facing ill health or a diagnosis/experience that may be difficult.

Engaging authentically with a person and their significant others can move the focus from the physiological response to illness to a more holistic approach, which may have positive health outcomes. Trust can be built through verbal and non-verbal means, such as giving a person time to have a conversation, having a positive and caring attitude, respecting the person and their family and demonstrating mutual respect. The term 'authentic' means being truthful, honest and genuine, which creates a basis for openness and trust between the healthcare worker and the person, as long as they are open to forming a relationship. Taking the time to consider how we are relating to the person and their significant others is an important aspect in ensuring we are engaging authentically. Being mindful of the need to display these attributes will help this become reality in the many interactions that a healthcare worker has with many different people in various settings.

It is essential that we not only have awareness of our own values and beliefs, but we also consider the person's values and beliefs, which helps us appreciate them as a person and what will make their care experience a positive one. Communication is often named as one of the key components that makes a positive or negative impact on a person's experience of healthcare and should be a focus for all healthcare workers. In order to build a relationship with a person and their significant others, the healthcare professional must master the 'art' of good communication. Exploring important aspects of the life history of a patient is part of getting to know the individual and building the relationship. This can give the professional an awareness of how to tailor care delivery to the person's needs and align care to their wishes, values and beliefs.

Activity

If we relate back to the poem 'Can you not see who I see?' the poem portrays a lack of understanding of the person as an individual with a unique life history.

- How could you change that scenario and help build a relationship with this person and those significant to him?
- Reflect on a situation in practice learning in which you feel that good relationships have not been built and how this might be rectified.

Building a relationship between the healthcare professional and a service user/carer/family member may be easier if time can be spent on communicating and getting to know people as opposed to carrying out tasks. Our ultimate aim as healthcare workers is to provide high-quality, safe, effective and person-centred care to the people we work with. Evaluating outcomes for the people we care for is the focus of much work that aims to determine the quality of healthcare delivery and satisfaction with the care people are receiving. The relationships formed between those delivering care and the person being cared for are crucial in determining the person's care experience and the degree to which person-centred outcomes have been achieved. We must have an increased awareness of our ability to build relationships in our professional capacity and ensure we are using person-centred processes to enhance the care to the person and their family. Evidence suggests that improving the person's care experience also has a positive effect on clinical effectiveness and safety (Doyle et al. 2013).

Conclusion

The evidence suggests that relationships that honour the personhood of all persons contribute to an improvement in the care experience of service users and those significant to them. It is therefore essential that this area of healthcare provision is given greater attention. Individuals who have the potential to improve their self-awareness from an emotionally intelligent perspective, and their relationships with colleagues and the people in their care, should consider ways in which they can work on the important aspects of relational connections discussed in this chapter to enhance person-centred practice.

Summary

- Person-centred relationships are those that honour the personhood of all persons.
- Knowing and understanding one's self from an emotionally intelligent perspective underpins all relationships.
- A match between our espoused values and beliefs and our day-to-day practice is a main characteristic of an effective person-centred workplace culture.
- The relationships that are formed between the healthcare worker and the person being cared for are crucial in determining the person's care experience.

References

Alimo-Metcalfe, B. and Alban-Metcalfe, J. (2012). Leadership: time for a new direction? *Leadership* 1 (1): 51–71.

Barron, D. and Hurley, J. (2012). Emotional intelligence and leadership. In: *Emotional Intelligence in Health and Social Care: A Guide for Improving Human Relationships* (eds. J. Hurley and P. Linsley), 75–88. London: Radcliffe Publishing.

Cummings, G., Hayduk, L., and Estabrooks, C. (2005). Mitigating the impact of hospital restructuring on nurses: the responsibility of emotionally intelligent leadership. *Nursing Research* 54: 2–12.

Doyle, C., Lennox, L., and Bell, D. (2013). A systematic review of evidence on the links between patient experience and clinical safety and effectiveness. *BMJ Open* https://bmjopen.bmj.com/content/3/1/e001570.

Drennan, D. (1992). *Transforming Company Culture*. London: McGraw-Hill.

Francis, R. (2013). *Report of the Mid Staffordshire NHS Foundation Trust Public Inquiry: Executive Summary*. London: Stationery Office, Department of Health.

Gilbert, P., McEwan, K., Matos, M., and Rivis, A. (2011). Fears of compassion: development of three self-report measures. *Psychology and Psychotherapy: Theory, Research and Practice* 84: 239–255.
Kitwood, T. (2019). *Dementia Reconsidered, Revisited: The Person Still Comes First*, 2e. London: Open University Press.
McCance, T., McCormack, B., and Dewing, J. (2011). An exploration of person-centredness in practice. *Online Journal of Issues in Nursing* 16 (2), Manuscript 1.
McCormack, B. and McCance, T.V. (2017). *Person-Centred Practice in Nursing and Healthcare: Theory and Practice*. Oxford: Wiley-Blackwell.
McCormack, B., Roberts, T., Meyer, J. et al. (2012). Appreciating the 'person' in long-term care. *International Journal of Older People Nursing* 7: 284–294.
McCormack, B., Manley, K., and Titchen, A. (2013). *Practice Development in Nursing and Healthcare*, 2e, 1–17. Oxford: Blackwell.
Nolan, M., Davies, S., Brown, J. et al. (2004). Beyond 'person-centred' care: a new vision for gerontological nursing. *International Journal of Older People Nursing* 13 (3a): 45–53.
Peplau, H.E. (1952). *Interpersonal Relations in Nursing*. New York: Putnam.
Salovey, P. and Mayer, J.D. (1990). Emotional intelligence. *Imagination, Cognition and Personality* 9: 185–211.
Schein, E.H. (1992). *Organizational Culture and Leadership*, 2e. San Francisco, CA: Jossey-Bass.

Further reading

Pederson, J.S., Brereton, J., and Newbould, E.N. (2013). *The Puzzle of Changing Relationships*. London: The Health Foundation.
Suter, E., Arndt, L., Arthur, N. et al. (2009). Role understanding and effective communication as core competencies for collaborative practice. *Journal of Interprofessional Care* 23 (1): 41–51.

11

The physical environment

Suzanne Martin[1], Assumpta Ryan[1], and Fiona Maclean[2]

[1] Ulster University, Northern Ireland, UK
[2] Queen Margaret University, Edinburgh, Scotland, UK

Contents

Fundamentals of Person-Centred Healthcare Practice, First Edition. Edited by Brendan McCormack, Tanya McCance, Cathy Bulley, Donna Brown, Ailsa McMillan and Suzanne Martin.

Learning outcomes

- To understand the importance of the physical environment for person-centred practice.
- To identify the challenges of delivering person-centred care when the physical environment is not conducive to person-centred practice.
- To explore the construct of the physical environment beyond the built environment including ideas of social connections and the impact on healthfulness.

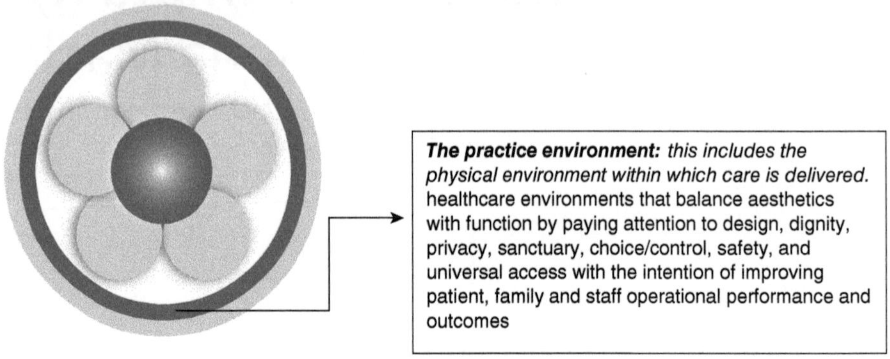

The practice environment: *this includes the physical environment within which care is delivered.* healthcare environments that balance aesthetics with function by paying attention to design, dignity, privacy, sanctuary, choice/control, safety, and universal access with the intention of improving patient, family and staff operational performance and outcomes

Introduction

On entering a healthcare facility, our initial impressions are often influenced by the design, layout, cleanliness, accessibility, and décor of the physical space. In reality, however, we quickly move beyond the concrete interpretation of what we see, hear, smell and touch to establishing perceptions and emotional reactions based on our observations and experiences within the physical space. A study by Lawson and Phiri (2003) found that service users not only said they preferred the appearance of newly built and refurbished healthcare environments, they also felt the clinical staff provided better interactions and services in the new surroundings. There is a growing body of evidence that suggests the physical environment of any healthcare setting (e.g. hospital, health centre or care home) has a significant impact on the well-being of patients, families and staff. This highlights the need to create a psychologically supportive environment that helps people cope with the stress that accompanies ill health (Salonen et al. 2013).

The physical care environment can be described as the visible and measurable environment including the design, lighting, size, decoration and furnishing of a space. It is important for healthcare staff to be mindful of the physical environment as this could have a positive effect on the health and well-being of all service users by enabling a more person-centred approach to care. It has been found that stress levels can be reduced if service users are easily able to navigate their way around a healthcare facility. Despite this, poor design and signposting means that many services users still experience difficulties in finding out where they need to go, adding to an already stressful situation.

Activity

Before you read this chapter, take a few minutes to jot down (i) what you understand by the term 'physical environment' and (ii) how you think the physical environment can enable or hinder the provision of person-centred care.

Salonen et al. (2013) conducted a comprehensive review of the physical factors of the environment that influence health and well-being in healthcare facilities. The review highlighted the following key aspects of the physical environment that have beneficial effects for all user groups.

Ward layout and room type

Several studies have reported the impact of the layout of a healthcare setting on the well-being of service users and staff (Ampt et al. 2008; Nordin and Elf 2019). It is widely accepted that environmental features, such as the placement of doorways, handrails and toilets, flooring type, and the design and location of hazards like furniture can contribute to patient falls and associated injuries. Hendrich (2003) found that most falls occurred when people attempted to get out of bed unassisted or unobserved. In their study, when patients moved from a centralised unit with semiprivate rooms to decentralised units with single-patient rooms that included a family zone, the number of falls was reduced by two-thirds. Creating space that can accommodate family members (who can help or call for aid) in the patient's room, along with better visibility from the nurses' station represent promising design interventions while also promoting a more person-centred approach to care. Decentralised nursing stations have been shown to reduce the amount of walking undertaken by nursing staff and thus increase patient contact time (Ampt et al. 2008). However, nurses working in decentralised units can feel isolated from their colleagues, lose their sense of team connection and have fewer social interactions compared with nurses working in centralised nursing stations. It can be difficult to achieve a balance between the needs of two diverse groups in one space as we try to work in a person-centred way.

There is strong evidence to suggest that single-occupancy rooms have positive healthcare outcomes such as reduced infection rates (Ulrich et al. 2008), improved sleep (Joseph and Ulrich 2007), decreased stress (Ampt et al. 2008), reduced medication errors (Mahmood et al. 2011), improved staff–patient communication (Ampt et al. 2008) and increased family involvement (Ulrich et al. 2008). There are also unintended consequences of single rooms, including the lack of social/emotional support from a roommate, decreased visibility of patients by staff and less staff interaction (Ampt et al. 2008). However, in most cases, the benefits outlined above tend to outweigh these disadvantages.

Acoustic environment (noise reduction)

Noise is one of the features of a healthcare environment that patients complain about most frequently (Ulrich et al. 2008; Salonen et al. 2013). The World Health Organization's guideline for continuous background noise in hospital patient rooms is 35 decibels (dB). Although technological innovations such as sound-absorbing ceilings can minimise noise levels, healthcare staff must also be mindful of other factors that contribute to noise levels.

Salonen et al. (2013) reported that among patients, lower noise levels improved sleep, reduced the use of pain medications, decreased stress, improved communication between patients and families, reduced errors, decreased heart and respiratory rates, reduced confusion and shortened recovery time and hospital stays. Although there has been limited research on the effects of noise on healthcare staff, noise is recognised as a distraction and stressor for staff. Among staff, reduced noise levels in healthcare settings have been associated with reduced stress, reduced fatigue, increased satisfaction, increased effectiveness, increased productivity (Joseph 2007; Ulrich et al. 2008) and improved communication and decreased medical errors (Joseph and Ulrich 2007; Mahmood et al. 2011).

Lighting (natural daylight and artificial light)

Sufficient and controllable lighting is beneficial for both patients and staff (Ulrich et al. 2008; Salonen et al. 2013). Although natural daylight is generally preferred over artificial lighting, artificial lighting is still necessary in healthcare settings. Among patients, daylight has a positive effect on vitamin D metabolism, improves sleep, reduces the use of pain medications, improves mood, reduces agitation and increases patient satisfaction (Ampt et al. 2008; Ulrich et al. 2008).

Among staff, daylight has been associated with reduced stress, improved performance and reduced errors (Cohen and Smetzer 2009). However, it is important to note that in counselling rooms, people feel more comfortable talking, and they talk for longer, with dim lighting as opposed to bright lighting (Ulrich et al. 2008). Improved lighting also reduces falls and allows the older person to function more independently, a key element of person-centred practice in care home settings.

Views, exposure and access to nature

Factoring in elements of nature in a healthcare setting can be an effective way of promoting person-centred care and maximising health outcomes. Research has shown that a connection with nature brings about healing benefits for patients, families and staff (Curtis et al. 2007; Ulrich et al. 2008). Among patients, window views of nature have been associated with reduced levels of stress, anxiety, delirium, depression and pain (Ulrich et al. 2008) and a reduction in blood pressure and sleep disturbances (Ampt et al. 2008). Views of nature have also been associated with faster recovery, emotional well-being and satisfaction with nursing care (Ulrich et al. 2008). Ulrich et al. have advocated the provision of pleasant views from windows. Figure 11.1 shows a children's hospital building.

For staff, views of nature have been shown to reduce stress, improve performance and increase job satisfaction (Ulrich et al. 2008). Scientific evidence strongly suggests that gardens, which provide calming and pleasant views of nature, are effective in fostering access to social support and privacy while also promoting restoration among stressed patients, families and staff (Joye 2007). For people living with dementia, access to secure outdoor environments has been reported to reduce agitation and aggressive behaviour (Curtis et al. 2007). Where views of nature are not possible, artwork depicting natural environments can help to lower stress and anxiety levels for patients, visitors and staff. Fleming et al. (2016) explored the relationship between the quality of the built environment and quality of life of people living with dementia in residential care. Qualitative interviews with 275 residents in 35 facilities confirmed that the quality of the built environment was significantly associated with the quality of life of the resident.

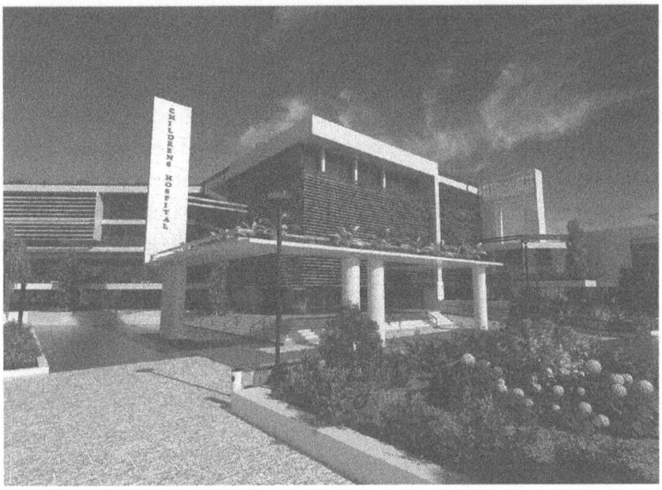

Figure 11.1 Children's hospital building. Source: Soran Shangapour/Shutterstock.com

Consequently, understanding the physical environment from a person-centred perspective does not only include elements of the built design of healthcare facilities, as the research on providing views, exposure and access to nature indicates. In addition, a person-centred view of the physical environment could also embrace a broader perspective to include 'where we live *and* where we go' (Yuen 2019). This is influenced by the emphasis placed on understanding a person's healthfulness, described in person-centred literature as the 'totality of health as lived by the person, reflected through the quality of their relationships and social engagement' (McCormack 2012). In terms of person-centred practice, creating the existence of a healthful culture to sustain and influence positive health and well-being means understanding the quality of a person's relationships with others, including the extent of their social network, and how this is valued and defined by the person. In older people, this is especially important as social isolation and loneliness have been shown to be associated, for example, with poorer cognitive function (Shankar et al. 2013), amongst other factors.

As such, understanding 'where we go', as part of the physical environment, is an important consideration as this can influence the opportunities which exist for people to experience social interaction with others. For example, the presence of public spaces as part of the physical environment is emphasised by Kantartzis and Molineux (2017) who describe the role and value of public squares, local shops, going for a coffee with friends and neighbours, buying a newspaper, to support daily encounters with others. These examples of everyday activities that people do as individuals, in families and as part of our communities, to occupy time and bring meaning and purpose to life are described as collective occupations. These collective occupations, set within the physical environment, offer the opportunity for people to experience social interaction, described as 'a need to go out, to be out, to join the social world' (Kantartzis and Molineux 2017, p. 171).

Acknowledging this need to socially connect with others is especially important in older people, due to the life course transitions often uniquely experienced in later life, such as changing health status and retirement, that can lead to social isolation and loneliness (Hallgren 2010). In older age, where a circle of friends can diminish through bereavement or ill health, the opportunity to connect socially with others may be less available or visible yet all the more important. Seeking to understand the existence of alternative opportunities to experience social connection with others, set within the physical environment, can contribute positively to a person's healthfulness. For example, as part of an occupational therapy internship programme, members of the Scottish Dementia Working Group (SDWG), who live with dementia, were asked to photograph occupations identified as being of importance to them (Maclean and Hunter, 2019). An example given was that of visiting the barber or hair salon to experience a haircut. Revisiting the same hair salon or barber, situated as part of a person's community may, beyond maintaining appearance, support the opportunity to connect with others, through conversations with staff and customers, and in so doing help to retain a sense of identity and provide purpose to the day.

These types of everyday services, situated in people's communities as part of the physical environment, can offer an important source of social connection for older people generally, including people who live with dementia. Consequently, to deliver person-centred healthcare there is a responsibility to understand a person's physical environment in terms of the layout and design of existing care facilities, and also the places where a person may wish to travel, to sustain social connectedness with others. Understanding the physical environment encompasses more than built physical spaces. It includes the extent to which we can value and enjoy our relationships with others, to socially connect, set within the built environment. Consequently, adopting this wider understanding of the physical environment is an important determinant in how we can create, foster and grow healthfulness aligned to the Person-centred Practice Framework.

Activity

- Using a camera, iPhone, etc., photograph occupations (activities) situated in your own physical environment that are important to help you sustain social connection with others. Note in what way(s) your chosen occupation(s) promote social connectedness with others.
- As you travel to the places where you go to connect with friends, family and/or others, what are some of the barriers and enablers of your physical environment that allow you to do this independently?

Having completed the learning activity above, take a few minutes to reflect on your responses. Did you identify enablers and barriers within the physical environment that were not linked to the concrete nature of the space? The relationship between a person, how they function (behave, perform) and the environment is long established. Law et al. (1996) reported published work on this stemming from 1919! How we behave within space is not a linear activity. It is a dynamic, ever changing complex relationship woven into the fabric of our lives (see Chapter 1). This is influenced by many factors, some of which you are exploring within this book. It is not like cause and effect. Each of us is constantly changing and shifting in our physical, mental and emotional well-being and our social connectedness.

As highlighted above, the environment is much broader than the physical space. It is the contexts and situations all around us that significantly influence how we behave, feel and perform. Think for example how in certain places, with specific individuals, you behave in particular ways. Researchers often refer to environmental fit or congruence and that this fit is perceived uniquely by each of us with triggers within the space evoking an emotion and behaviour. It is suggested that work environments are designed to structurally reinforce positive affect and successful performance, because it is in these environments that people are most likely to experience high levels of person–environment fit. Creating an empowering working environment will support thriving at work. In this instance, we are thinking about how we support the emergence and sustained presences of the PCF within the physical space.

Activity

What types of things could a manager do within the work space to help the Person-centred Practice Framework be felt?

(Answers: well-designed job descriptions, ensure resources are available to support CPD and routine training of staff, reward good behaviours, be mindful of the environment design)

History has shown us that, in many instances, services for society's most vulnerable groups do fail. Often there are warning signs in the environment that we as healthcare professionals should pick up on (Francis 2013). Let us explore how you as a student can help deliver a better environment for the people we serve.

How can a better environment be provided to service users?

The physical environment encompasses more than our built physical spaces. It includes the extent to which we can value and enjoy our relationships with others, to socially connect and, as such, is an important determinant in building healthfulness.

As we work towards developing person-centred practice, increasingly our responsibility is to understand that the care environment extends beyond the traditional mechanisms of service delivery which seek to influence health and well-being. The care environment reaches out into our communities, to value social connection, and in so doing can help to establish and build a person's healthfulness. In understanding the person's physical environment, we begin to understand the facilitators and barriers to the existence of healthfulness (Person-centred Practice Framework: Care Environment).

To develop this, we need to capture what a 'healthful' culture as part of our physical environment might look and feel like from a service user's perspective, as opposed to the perspective the healthcare practitioner may hold. Involvement in care is needed to understand and capture quality relationships identified by the person as being of importance to them (Person-centred Practice Framework: Involvement in Care).

This becomes increasingly important as we age, as the mechanisms of support that can hold us up may be less obvious. Indeed, in later life, when our circle of friends can diminish through bereavement or ill health, and as loneliness can often increase, the opportunity to connect socially with others may be far less available or visible, yet all the more important. Often these mechanisms can exist but in forms that are less recognised or valued. For example, as part of a small photo-voice project we recently undertook, we asked people living with dementia which occupations (activities) as part of their community or environment were important to them. Visiting the hairdresser and having a haircut was noted in several instances (Person-centred Practice Framework: Feeling of Well-Being). It may be that, beyond looking good, visiting the hairdresser can offer the opportunity to experience the sense of positive touch, often limited or lost as we age, and an opportunity to connect socially with others, to continue to 'belong' as part of our communities, and to provide routine and structure to the day (Person-centred Practice Framework: Feeling of Well-Being).

Conclusion

This chapter has considered more broadly a definition of what the physical environment is to people, with a specific focus on the care environment. It offers the perspective that to promote person-centred practice, understanding the physical environment must consider the quality of a person's social relationships, as well as the facilitators and barriers to social connection. In so doing, it challenges person-centred practitioners to offer holistic care, which values and privileges the importance of our social relationships with others, and the ways through which this can sustain and maintain our health and well-being.

Summary

- Environment includes the physical space but also other dimensions such as cultural and social interactions that impact on behaviours.
- The physical environment should have a positive effect on the health and wel-lbeing of all service users by enabling a more person-centred approach to care.
- Understanding the physical environment encompasses more than built physical spaces. It includes the extent to which we can value and enjoy our relationships with others, to socially connect, set within the built environment.

References

Ampt, A., Harris, P., and Maxwell, M. (2008). *The Health Impacts of the Design of Hospital Facilities on Patient Recovery and Wellbeing, and Staff Wellbeing: A Review of the Literature*, 92. Liverpool, NSW: Centre for Primary Health Care and Equity.

Cohen, M.R. and Smetzer, J.L. (2009). ISMP Medication Error Report Analysis. *Hospital Pharmacy* 44: 1062–1065.

Curtis, S., Gesler, W., Fabian, K. et al. (2007). Therapeutic landscapes in hospital design: a qualitative assessment by staff and service users of the design of a new mental health inpatient unit. *Environment and Planning C: Government and Policy* 25 (4): 591–610.

Fleming, R., Goodenough, B., Low, L.F. et al. (2016). The relationship between the quality of the built environment and the quality of life of people with dementia in residential care. *Dementia* 15 (4): 663–680.

Francis, R. (2013). *Report of the Mid Staffordshire NHS Foundation Trust Public Inquiry*. https://assets.publishing.service.gov.uk/government/uploads/system/uploads/attachment_data/file/279124/0947.pdf

Hallgren, A. (2010). Alcohol consumption and harm among elderly Europeans: falling between the cracks. *European Journal of Public Health* 20: 616–618.

Hendrich, A. (2003). *Optimizing Physical Space for Improved Outcomes: Satisfaction and the Bottom Line. Proceedings of Minicourse*. Atlanta, GA: Institute for Healthcare Improvement and the Center for Healthcare Design.

Joseph, A. and Ulrich, R. (2007). *Sound Control for Improved Outcomes in Healthcare Settings*, 17. Concord,CA: Center for Health Design www.healthdesign.org/sites/default/files/Sound%20Control.pdf.

Joye, Y. (2007). Architectural lessons from environmental psychology: the case of biophilic architecture. *Review of General Psychology* 11 (4): 305–328.

Kantartzis, S. and Molineux, M. (2017). Collective occupation in public spaces and the construction of the social fabric. *Canadian Journal of Occupational Therapy* 84 (3): 168–177.

Law, M., Cooper, B., Strong, S. et al. (1996). The person-environment-occupation model: a transactive approach to occupational performance. *Canadian Journal of Occupational Therapy* 63 (1): 9–23.

Lawson, B. and Phiri, M. (2003). *The Architectural Healthcare Environment and Its Effects on Patient Health Outcomes: A Report on an NHS Estates Funded Research Project. Stationery Office*. London.

Maclean, F. and Hunter, E. (2019). *Occupation Matters to Me*. Edinburgh: Alzheimer Scotland.

Mahmood, A., Chaudhury, H., and Valente, M. (2011). Nurses' perceptions of how physical environment affects medication errors in acute care settings. *Applied Nursing Research* 24 (4): 229–237.

McCormack, B. (2012). *The Person-centre Practice Research International Community of Practice*. www.fons.org/library/journal.aspx

Nordin, S. and Elf, M. (2019). The importance of the physical environment to support individualised care. In: *Individualized Care* (eds. R. Suhonen, M. Stolt and E. Papastavrou). Cham.: Springer.

Salonen, H., Lahtinen, M., Lappalainen, S. et al. (2013). Physical characteristics of the indoor environment that affect health and wellbeing in healthcare facilities: a review. *Intelligent Buildings International* 5 (1): 3–25.

Shankar, A., Hamer, M., McMunn, A. et al. (2013). Social isolation and loneliness: relationships with cognitive function during 4 years of follow-up in the English longitudinal study of ageing. *Psychosomatic Medicine* 75 (2): 161–170.

Ulrich, R.S., Zimring, C., Zhu, X. et al. (2008). A review of the research literature on evidence-based healthcare design. *HERD* 1 (3): 61–125.

Yuen, B. (2019). *Ageing and the Built Environment in Singapore*. Cham: Springer.

Further reading

Cornally, N., Cagney, O., Burton, A. et al. (2019). *Evaluation of the Irish Hospice Foundation Design & Dignity Programme*. Cork: University College Cork.

Harrison, S.L., Dyer, S.M., Laver, K.E. et al. (2017). Physical environmental designs in residential care to improve quality of life of older people. *Cochrane Database of Systematic Reviews* (12): CD012892.

12

Working with persons' beliefs and values

Suzanne Martin[1], Lisa Luhanga[2], and Catherine Wells[1]

[1] *Ulster University, Northern Ireland, UK*
[2] *Queen Margaret University, Edinburgh, Scotland, UK*

Contents

Fundamentals of Person-Centred Healthcare Practice, First Edition. Edited by Brendan McCormack, Tanya McCance, Cathy Bulley, Donna Brown, Ailsa McMillan and Suzanne Martin.

Learning outcomes

- Develop an understanding of what beliefs and values are.
- Explore how personal and professional beliefs and values impact on how we practise.
- Appreciate beliefs and values within the context of the Person-centred Practice Framework.

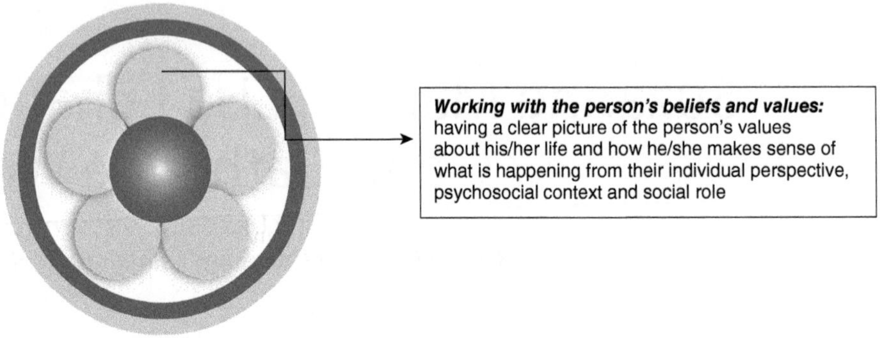
Working with the person's beliefs and values:
having a clear picture of the person's values about his/her life and how he/she makes sense of what is happening from their individual perspective, psychosocial context and social role

Introduction

Beliefs and values impact on everything we say and do. They influence how we perceive the world and how we respond to people and events around us. The Oxford Dictionary defines a belief as 'something one accepts as true or real, a firmly held opinion' and a value as the 'principles or standards of behaviour, one's judgement of what is important in life' (Oxford English Dictionary 2019). In this chapter we will explore beliefs and values and how these are relevant to our understanding of the Person-centred Practice Framework.

Beliefs, values and person-centredness

Our beliefs may emerge from our internal understandings of the external world, whilst values can be established by others, for example a professional body. Values often form part of our inner sense of what is right and wrong. Beliefs and values develop from birth, shaped and influenced by those around us and our life experiences. Beliefs and values are ubiquitous, we bring them with us as we strive to connect within the therapeutic relationship and develop rapport as the nurse or therapist and the service user.

To facilitate person-centred practice and ensure the best interests of the service user are upheld, staff (you and I) need both clarity and awareness of our beliefs and values and an understanding of the influence they exert on our clinical practice (Levy 1976; Rabow et al. 2010). Earlier chapters highlight the importance of understanding and connecting with ourselves as human beings with feelings, emotions, thoughts and desires as an essential component of being human (McCormack and McCance 2017). In bringing all of ourselves into our working lives, we bring with us our beliefs and values.

Beliefs and values impact on everything we say and do. They influence how we perceive the world and how we respond to people and events around us. Let us take a moment to think about our beliefs and values to start to understand what motivates us. This is part of developing the skill we need to be a reflective practitioner. This is discussed further in Chapter 29.

Activity

Fifteen-minute reflection: Take a blank page and brainstorm your beliefs and values in relation to legalisation of non-regulated drugs, Do you feel strongly about this? What influences your views on this?

Personal beliefs and values

As people, we change over time depending on our experiences. You may have previously held the belief that the legalisation of non-regulated drugs would be a positive change for society. However, if you have friends or family who have had castastrophic events from using drugs, this view may have changed. Both Piaget and Kohlberg defined set stages of moral development in which our understanding and development of social norms and values are progressed (Carpendale 2000). During childhood, we learn to respond to the cultural rules of 'good', 'bad', 'right' and 'wrong' and as we grow older, we develop a more complex understanding of the laws that govern behaviour in society, progressing to an understanding and awareness of ethical principles.

The development of our values is based on our specific culture and society, influenced by our parents or primary carers (Grusec et al. 2000). The quality of attachment and relationship between parent and child has been shown to be a vital component of setting the standard against which we see the world and develop our own relationships and connections as we grow through childhood into adulthood (Marone 2014). We adopt the ways of thinking and behaving specific to our cultural norms, through interactions with parents/caregivers and those more knowledgeable than ourselves, for example an older child or sibling and our peers (Doherty and Hughes 2014). As young children, we generally reflect our parent's values which are often time and place specific; for example, what may be seen as important in one culture may not be in another culture or another time period. Traditional long-held family beliefs and values can be strong, making it a challenge to change or move away from these intergenerational cycles. As we grow and move into our professional careers, we assimilate and blend our own personal and professional beliefs and values.

Professional values

There may be overlap and blending between personal and professional values, particularly in a healthcare profession where we are required to bring so much of our physical, psychological and emotional selves into the caring relationships and our professional roles. It is also important to recognise that to work effectively in healthcare involves personal growth and development. Routinely, we evolve as human beings through continuous development. You might find it helpful at this point to revisist Chapter 5 on Flourishing. As mentioned earlier, our beliefs and values may be challenged by many things such as exposure to people from different backgrounds, academic learning at odds with our own perspectives, observations of practice and the experiences we accumulate over time. Following these challenges, we emerge with our worldview altered.

Once an individual embarks on a professional role, the values of the professional group will inform their practice and govern expected standards of behaviour. Sometimes there may be conflict between our professional and personal values. In order to maintain our registration to practise, we are all required to adhere to standards of ethical practice set by our regulatory and professional bodies. Professional values can unite us globally and yet our cultural differences can be helpful within our local communities to enable us to practise in ways that meet the needs of our specific communities and services. However, challenges can arise; for example, the global mobility of healthcare staff and international needs can lead to the economic migration of a significant volume of healthcare staff. As we work in person-centred ways, it is important to be aware of our own values and beliefs and yet remain open to experiencing different views and perspectives. Working with persons from different backgrounds (staff or service users) can help us to see the world through a different lens and prevents us from being stuck in our views and ways of being or doing.

Activity

Three nursing, occupational therapy and physiotherapy students have been working together on an acute medical ward in a busy hospital. The person in charge has asked them to work together on the care planning, intervention and home discharge plan for a young man aged 35 who has been admitted to the ward. The man lives with his aged parents. He has been admitted with heart failure and pressure sores. He has a Body Mass Index [BMI] of 42 and is described as morbidly obese, requiring bariatric care. When you go to the coffee area at break time, you hear some of the other staff laughing about the size of the man, and you see staff from other wards come to have a look at the 'giant'.

How does this make you feel? How do you respond? What actions can you take?

Looking at the code of standards and ethics related to your professional body (for example Nursing and Midwifery Council, Chartered Society of Physiotherapy, Royal College of Occupational Therapy, Society of Radiographers, etc.), think about what values this highlights for you What is the code asking you to do?

Respecting all beliefs and values

Respecting our beliefs and values (McCormack and McCance 2017) and respecting those of our service users are core to person-centred practice. Actions and behaviours will flow from these. It is clear therefore that we must be true to ourselves (authentic) to avoid internal conflict and possibly even the manifestation of personal disease or illness (Mate 2011). Many persons live a life unaligned with their own beliefs and values and without the knowledge they are doing so. This is one of the many reasons why self-reflection is of such importance (see Chapters 4 and 29). When we are aware of our true nature, we can live a life in alignment with ourselves, allowing our actions to arise from a place of authenticity. This can help avoid internal conflict. Living a life unaligned with our beliefs and values can not only cause an emotional disconnect leading to mental ill health, but can also lead to a multitude of physical health issues (Mate 2011). Therefore, the concept of living aligned with and valuing the true self also feeds into self-care. It is important as healthcare staff that we value our own well-being. The old adage 'You can't pour from an empty cup' has never been more relevant than in today's busy healthcare context. If we don't take care of ourselves, how can we be expected to bring our whole selves to caring for others? As healthcare staff, we have significant knowledge about the promotion of physical and mental well-being and we have a duty of care to use this knowledge and truly value ourselves, so that we can better serve others. As reflective practitioners, we should notice when our beliefs and values are impacting on the care decisions we make for ourselves and other people.

Contemporary considerations and challenges

If our actions and decisions don't align with our beliefs and values, it is possible we may experience dissatisfaction. Living a life aligned with our beliefs and values can instil a sense of meaning, fulfilment and happiness. As healthcare staff, we are also exposed to the beliefs and values of service users. Having an increased awareness of self and others is a vital component of being person-centred. In other chapters, different ways of aiding this have been explored, for example, reflexivity and using skills of sympathetic listening. A knowledge of service users' values and what underlies or influences their values and beliefs could support and inform shared decision making, as these may explain behaviours, choices and decisions (Schwartz 2012).

An underlying factor that can often influence a person's beliefs and values is spirituality, which is an important dimension of healthcare. This concept is often thought of as a uniquely religious experience, which is a very limited view. Spirituality in the healthcare field has been defined by Gardner et al. (2020) as finding meaning in life in a way that connects the inner sense of meaning with a sense of something greater. This concept recognises that individuals express meaning and purpose in diverse ways. For some people, it could be through religion, but for others it's playing with their child, connecting with friends, walking in nature or watching their favourite football team. Investigating what is meaningful to a person in a spiritual sense can give us a better understanding of what informs their beliefs and values. Indeed, anything that connects us with other people and ourselves when life is tough or the future is uncertain can be framed as spiritual.

There is no doubt that spirituality is a complex and delicate topic and yet within person-centred practice there is most definitely a need to explore this for both ourselves and users of healthcare services. We need to build both our confidence and knowledge on how to have conversations with service users about spirituality (Meredith et al. 2012). We must listen without necessarily knowing, act with an intention of service and embrace the mystery of the person (McColl 2016). We can serve most effectively when we enter into the service user's spiritual understanding of the world, and set aside our personal beliefs and values if they are conflicting with those of the client.

Working with a person's values and beliefs can be challenging when they are different from our own. Some deep-rooted values and beliefs are formed as part of the culture and society within which we live. One example of this is gender. Gender is argued to be socially and culturally constructed. Over time, gender roles can become deeply engrained in society. Throughout history, different views about gender have emerged, developed and changed. This can be seen in fashion trends that either have kept to the traditional expectations of female and male trends or have tried to cross boundaries of socially accepted norms (Farvid 2017; Woodward 2017). It could be argued that in today's society we are becoming less restrictive and moving away from the social norms and rethinking values in terms of gender roles, identity and images, for example governments and schools actively increasing access for more girls to have careers in science and technology. There is a growing number of high street shops now selling 'gender neutral' clothes, and toy suppliers being pressured into reducing and eliminating the gender labelling of toys and games.

Challenging established norms and values is not always easy and may be difficult for some to accept. As discussed earlier, when a person's own identity or values are not perceived to align with those of society in general, there can be huge challenges that can affect health and well-being. One current issue is the categorisation of gender other than through the traditional two binary categories (male and female) to a number of identities from lesbian, gay, bisexual, transgender and a growing number of people who identify as non-binary (non-binary describes gender/sex as continuous or irrelevant) (Hyde et al. 2019).

There is a reported disparity for non-binary persons in healthcare access and outcomes, for example higher mental health issues and substance misuse (Clark et al. 2018). There have been positive developments in government policies and recognition of persons in society, for example to improve barriers to healthcare in education and communities (Government Equalities Office 2018). There remains a need, however, for a more person-centred approach in relationship building and working with all persons. Values can be compromised and challenged when a person is labelled and not seen as a person. This is very apparent in our working environments when we will perhaps work with others who may not share the same person-centred values as us.

Activity

Jo is a 24 year old who identifies as non-binary. Jo is currently seeking support for significant mental health issues, which have impacted on Jo's ability to work. The staff in the outpatients clinic where Jo is attending are talking about Jo in the staff room. You hear one member of staff joking that they are not sure what to call Jo – 'he or she?' – and laughingly say 'I wonder what toilet he/she is going to go into!'.

How might you react to this? How can you respond if thinking about working with Jo in a person-centred way? How might you challenge the labelling of others to think differently and recognise the person?

Beliefs and values in person-centred practice

For a variety of reasons, for example external pressures or job demands, service users often experience an interaction or care that is rushed, depersonalised and emotionally detached, and yet when we are at our most vulnerable, our greatest human need is for loving kindness and compassion (Youngson and Blennerhassett 2016). Aside from the moral drive to fulfil this basic human need, studies have shown that care provided within the framework of person-centredness improves clinical outcomes and can give meaning, joy and job satisfaction to healthcare staff. For a healthcare worker, integrating these concepts into our interactions does not need to be time consuming or expensive.

Person-centred practice provided within the Person-centred Practice Framework enables us to humanise healthcare. By bringing our whole self to the healthcare space, we bring compassion and a humane response to human suffering – this is how we support healing (Youngson and Blennerhassett 2016). Watson (2009) says we need a deep, philosophical values-based approach in addition to healthcare staff who are capable of having loving, caring, kind and sensitively meaningful personal connections with an increasingly enlightened public.

Conclusion

Our professional values form the foundation of person-centred practice. We bring our personal values and beliefs into our practice when we bring our whole self into the person-centred space. While we develop as persons, our beliefs and values are shaped, challenged, refined and reviewed through reflection and meaningful engagement with others. Placing our beliefs and values at the centre of our reflective activities ensures an engagement with practice that is evidence informed and shaped through meaningful connections with others.

Summary

- Beliefs and values form the foundation of our being and doing as person-centred practitioners.
- Whilst our beliefs and values are shaped and formed from an early age, as we grow and move into our professional careers, we assimilate and blend our own personal and professional beliefs and values.
- The biggest challenge we face as person-centred practitioners is that of aligning the values we espouse with our everyday practices, engagements and behaviours.
- Working from a values-driven approach enables practitioners to experience meaningful engagements with others and access our potential for compassion in care.

References

Carpendale, J.I. (2000). Kohleberg and Piaget on stages of moral reasoning. *Developmental Review* 20: 181–205.

Clark, B.A., Veale, J.F., Townsend, M. et al. (2018). Non-binary youth: access to gender-affirming primary health care. *International Journal of Transgenderism* 19 (2): 158–169.

Doherty, J. and Hughes, M. (2014). *Child Development. Theory and Practice 0–11*, 2e. London: Pearson.

Farvid, P. (2017). Saying goodbye to binary gender. www.youtube.com/watch?v=DW5YctpK7pM

Gardner, F., Tan, H., and Rumbold, B. (2020). What spirituality means for patients and families in health care. *Journal of Religion and Health* 59: 195–203.

Government Equalities Office (2018). LGBT Action Plan: Improving the Lives of Lesbian, Gay, Bisexual and Transgender People. www.gov.uk/government/publications/lgbt-action-plan-2018-improving-the-lives-of-lesbian-gay-bisexual-and-transgender-people

Grusec, J.E., Goodnow, J.J., and Kuczynski, L. (2000). New directions in analyses of parenting contributions to children's acquisition of values. *Child Development* 71 (1): 205–211.

Hyde, J.S., Biglar, R.S., Joel, D. et al. (2019). The future of sex and gender in psychology: five challenges to the gender binary. *American Psychologist* 74 (2): 171–193.

Levy, C.S. (1976). Personal versus professional values: the practitioner's dilemmas. *Clinical Social Work Journal* 4 (2): 110–120.

Marone, M. (2014). *Attachment and Interaction: From Bowlby to Current Clinical Theory and Practice*, 2e. London: Jessica Kingsley.

Mate, G. (2011). *When the Body Says No: The Cost of Hidden Stress*. Canada: Vintage.

McColl, M.A. (2016). Client-centred care and spirituality. In: *Spirituality and Occupational Therapy. A Model for Practice and Research* (ed. T. Keiter Humbret), 167–174. Bethesda: AOTA Press.

McCormack, B. and McCance, T. (2017). Underpinning principles of person-centred practice. In: *Person-Centred Practice in Nursing and Healthcare Theory and Practice*, 2e (eds. B. Mc Cormack and T. Mc Cance), 13–35. Oxford: Wiley Blackwell.

Meredith, P., Murray, J., Wilson, T. et al. (2012). Can spirituality be taught to health care professionals? *Journal of Religion and Health* 51 (3): 879–889.

Oxford English Dictionary (2019). www.oed.com/

Rabow, M.W., Remen, R.N., Parmelee, D.X., and Inui, T.S. (2010). Professional formation: extending medicine's lineage of service into the next century. *Academic Medicine* 85 (2): 310–317.

Schwartz, S.H. (2012). An overview of the Schwartz theory of basic values. *Online Readings in Psychology and Cullture* 2 (1): 11.

Watson, J. (2009). Caring science and human caring theory: transforming personal and professional practices of nursing and health care. *Journal of Health and Human Services Administration* 31: 466–482.

Woodward, J. (2017). Skirts for men! Elizabeth Hawes and challenging fashion's gender binary. *Journal of Popular Culture* 50 (6): 1276–1292.

Youngson, R. and Blennerhassett, M. (2016). Humanising healthcare. *BMJ* 355: i6262.

Further reading

Pirsig, R. (1991). *Zen and the Art of Motorcycle Maintenance: An Inquiry into Values*. London.: Vintage Books.

Stichter, M. and Saunders, L. (2019). Positive psychology and virtue: values in action. *Journal of Positive Psychology* 14 (1): 1–5.

Wiles, K., Bahal, N., Engward, H., and Papanikitas, A. (2016). Ethics in the interface between multidisciplinary teams: a narrative in stages for inter-professional education. *London Journal of Primary Care* 8 (6): 100–104.

13

Engaging meaningfully and effectively

Ailsa Espie[1], Georgios Tsigkas[1], and Donna Brown[2]

[1] Queen Margaret University, Edinburgh, Scotland, UK
[2] Ulster University, Northern Ireland, UK

Contents

Fundamentals of Person-Centred Healthcare Practice, First Edition. Edited by Brendan McCormack, Tanya McCance, Cathy Bulley, Donna Brown, Ailsa McMillan and Suzanne Martin.

Learning outcomes

- To explain the term 'engaging authentically', identifying what it means to you to engage meaningfully with others, as a precursor to human flourishing.
- Use critical reflection to develop your understanding of human agency and consider participatory strategies to overcome challenges outlining your own learning and develop an action plan.
- Draw on examples from practice learning to develop your understanding of times when engaging authentically and meaningful has or has not occurred.

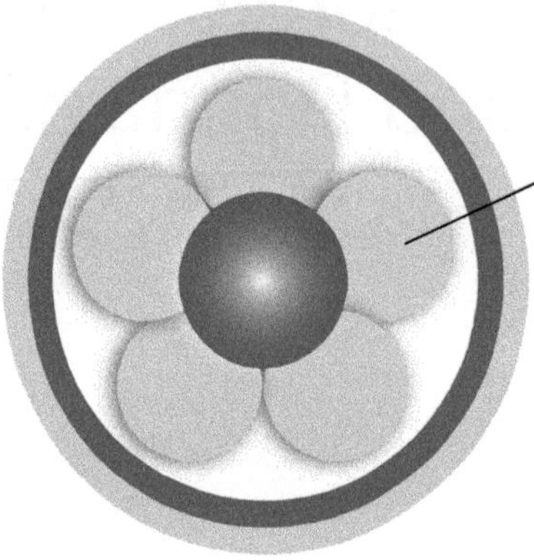

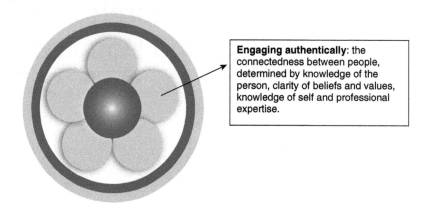

Engaging authentically: the connectedness between people, determined by knowledge of the person, clarity of beliefs and values, knowledge of self and professional expertise.

Introduction

In the context in which we practise, we are required to communicate with many different people to share and receive complex information. This requires good interpersonal connections in order to provide care and ensure optimal team working. The interconnectedness of person-centred practice requires us all as people to engage meaningfully and effectively in all our interactions. This chapter will focus specifically on the person-centred process of 'engaging authentically' which you will have seen in Chapter 3. We will guide you to explore different ways of understanding how we engage meaningfully and what this means for human agency and working with people.

Engaging authentically

Engaging authentically is a complex interrelational process and one that can be best described as a way of being and becoming (see Chapter 29). It is not a static state but rather a dynamic approach to being in relationship with another person or persons. To engage meaningfully with another person means to accept them as they are. This involves us being open to learning more about our self and others and to exploring and sharing beliefs and values. Within the context of the Person-centred Practice Framework, engaging authentically is one of the person-centred processes required for a good care experience and a healthful culture.

Just saying you are person-centred does not necessarily mean that you are. Being truly person-centred is about being authentic. Authenticity requires you to be genuine, open and honest and in touch with your own feelings and reality, while also being aware of the needs of others (Heron 1999). Consequently, it is not just about what you say, it's about what you believe and value about yourself and other people, and how you connect with others. That said, because we live in a world where we are interconnected with others, it is easy to be influenced by the context in which we work. This has significance as engaging authentically requires us to recognise this and accept that we have freedom and are accountable for the choices we make (Lawler and Ashman 2012). This may require us to unlearn ways of being or perhaps question assumptions that we make about others and ourselves. As you learn more about yourself and understand that your own self-concept is built from the beliefs you hold and how others respond to you, then you will be able to consider others in any relationship. You may like to look back on Chapter 1 where you had the opportunity to explore the person in person-centred practice.

To engage authentically, you need to connect as a person so that you have some understanding of where the other person is coming from and what matters both to you and to them at that time. Accepting this, with every individual interaction you can be developing yourself and be working in a way which keeps the principles of person-centred practice at the forefront of your interactions (the activity below will provide an opportunity to explore this). We recognise this is an ongoing process and one that requires skills of personal critical reflection and evaluation of your interactions and communications with other people.

Levels of engagement

McCormack (2003) suggests there are three different levels of engagement: full engagement, partial engagement and complete disengagement. Full engagement is experienced when people work in partnership, sharing decisions and unconsciously working with one another's values. Partial engagement can occur when for some reason a relationship is interrupted and altered, for example due to a difference of opinion. Complete disengagement is the period of time that elapses as you objectively consider the available options and reassess the values that support the relationship and decision making (McCormack and McCance 2017). This is the point at which people working in a variety of care settings need to ask themselves what they need to do better next time to avoid disengagement at any level and decide on a course of action to re-establish the relationship.

Activity

Emma is a community practitioner who is visiting Frank for the first time, in his own home. She engages him in conversation as she tries to get to know him better. During the conversation, Frank tells Emma that he finds it upsetting when the community team discuss his care needs. Working with her own beliefs and values, at first Emma considers that this is a trivial matter and wonders how discussing care needs could cause anyone anxiety. However, on exploring the issue further, Frank, reveals that the conversations often take place in his home, when his daughter, grandchildren or visitors are present. Frank is a proud, private man and he considers the discussion about his care needs makes him seem vulnerable. Emma realises that she had not considered the impact her own care agenda and workload would have on Frank. Her normal care practice was at odds with what was right for Frank.

You are encouraged to discuss the above activity with your peers. Do you think Emma could develop a better shared understanding about Frank's needs and ensure that his views are equally respected by all members of the care team in the future? In your discussion, think about different or creative ways that may be used to engage authentically with Frank. Reflect on issues of privacy, confidentiality, honesty, trust and record keeping, for example.

We are always learning to become (see Chapter 29) and as persons we are both fortunate and challenged by the human frailty which we bring into our daily lives and the interactions and actions with others. However, if you want to engage meaningfully in a person-centred way in every interaction, you will need to try and work towards full engagement. One way to develop this skill is to be prepared to invest in developing yourself as a person and to role model positive behaviours and interactions with and for others (see Chapter 4). This requires you to reflect on the way you are and the decisions you make. You need to challenge yourself and consider if you have been your best self in this interaction. Perhaps you could have viewed the situation from a different perspective, negotiated with that person better or challenged the assumptions that you made. These are important questions to ask and reflect on if you aspire to engage authentically with others.

Reflection offers a mechanism to explore and learn from the uncertainties, muddles and anxieties of working in complex and unpredictable environments (Bolton 2013). Being person-centred and engaging more meaningfully is something that can be practised and that you can get better at. One way to do this is to try being fully aware of your agency and how through this you can indeed shape the social structures around you. The next section will provide an overview of the key concepts of human agency and reflexivity.

Human agency and reflexivity

Health and social care settings are dynamic environments. They are deemed to be open systems where situations may vary and change from time to time. This change can influence or be influenced by a person's activity which, in sociological terms, is called human agency (Elder Vass 2013). Drawing from this perspective, human agency is usually explored through a person's ability and power to make decisions through various activities which are typically guided and shaped by their desires, beliefs and values and these may influence social structures (Archer 2010). Social structures are social arrangement networks and places where the interweaving of the interactions of people, in a more or less repetitive and stable way, usually takes place. People are an integral part of these social arrangements or social order, and it is these structures that influence human agency and where human agency also exercises its own influence. Although a person's agential activity can be really powerful and may dramatically affect the way a social structure functions, social structures are generally viewed as independent entities which can in turn heavily influence and sometimes frame our agential activity. An example of this is the engagement between Peter and Tom outlined in the activity below.

Activity

Peter is a final-year student who is on practice learning in a rehabilitation centre. The centre is extremely busy and Tom, one of the healthcare assistants, asks Peter if he could help him walk an older man to the toilet. Peter responds abruptly and in an aggressive way, saying that this is not his responsibility as he is currently very busy working with another client.

To be able to work together in a person-centred way, Tom and Peter need to be able to engage meaningfully and effectively with each other.

Take some time to consider Tom and Peter's situation and how human agency and social structures may have influenced this interaction. You are encouraged to consider what factors may have influenced Tom to ask Peter for help. What social structures are at play here and how may Peter's view of his role and the environment he is working in have influenced his actions? Can you think of any approaches Tom and Peter could use to gain a better understanding of each other's perspectives? For example, perhaps they could talk through what happened in a reflective conversation or ask another person to facilitate them in a discussion to consider what has occurred and why.

Now think of a situation where you and another person were challenged to engage meaningfully and effectively. Try to evaluate your own actions and those of the other person, giving consideration to perceived hierarchies and established systems of care. Having read this chapter and considered the situation again, would you engage in a similar manner in the future?

Going back to the focus of this section, some may argue that the constant interplay between human agency and social structures can determine the ways in which we collaborate and engage with others from a personal and professional point of view. The quality and nature of personal and professional relations can also be affected by this interaction between our agential existence and social structures. This is a crucial point to consider, as you will engage with a variety of people – colleagues, clients, relatives and students – in different clinical and community settings, such as acute or rehabilitation wards and health centres. Whether this engagement is meaningful and effective, or not, can fundamentally depend on the outcome of the interaction between human agency and the social structures within that care environment. This does not necessarily mean that you are person-centred in your approaches, as you may often make assumptions about a situation or make a decision which is not consistent with the spirit of person-centredness nor completely in line with other people's beliefs and values. There might also be occasions where the practice setting dramatically shapes your agential activity, resulting in adopting approaches and behaviours which are not person-centred.

Archer (2010) has argued that there would be no such thing as society if people were not reflexive persons. Reflexivity is being able to critically evaluate your own beliefs and values, systematically examining factors which led you to act in a certain way and the impact they had on a situation. It is about your ability to recognise how your presence can influence that situation and how the context may affect you. In other words, reflexivity is about taking a step back and thinking deeply about what, why and how a situation has happened. Your agency can be affected by your ability to reflexively evaluate key aspects of your activity in various social contexts. It is generally believed that awareness of your agential activity is influenced by your ability to reflexively evaluate your worldview and influence on and by social structures. Reflexivity can act as a mediator between human agency and social structures which could then enable you (or Peter in the earlier scenario) to approach similar situations differently in future.

Challenging the status quo and non-person-centred practices

Developing an understanding of authenticity requires us to have an awareness of the authentic self and to be authentic. Once achieved, this can enhance effective communication not only with service users and their family but with other people in the multidisciplinary team. Collaborative and participatory approaches that enable better communication and co-operation will help promote an environment in which everybody can flourish, be respected and be equally heard; you can learn more about this in Chapter 8.

To be authentic and to engage meaningfully, we need to recognise that working in different environments may sometimes challenge our beliefs and values. You are likely to encounter a range of challenging experiences and be exposed to complex situations with a wide range of people, all with their own perspectives and worldviews. Persons are social beings with a need to belong, so there is often a strong desire when in a new environment to be accepted by others. Where those people share your beliefs and values and you are able to connect, it can be a very rewarding experience. Nevertheless, on occasion, you may find yourself in a situation where the ways of working and the beliefs and values of the team or those you are caring for are at odds with your own. This can be a stressful time as you learn new skills and practices and you may feel overwhelmed as you try to settle in and align your moral principles with what is happening around you.

Understanding behaviours or interactions of others which are at odds with the principles of person-centred practice is an important skill to develop. Receiving and giving feedback will involve developing your self-awareness, paying attention to what is happening with others and noticing what is going on in the wider context. To engage meaningfully you will also need to be sensitive to both sides of the relationship and be able to see other perspectives, including any challenges this presents to your practice.

Activity

Terry is a pre-registration learner who has just started in a busy unit. On his first day, he is warmly welcomed by his practice supervisor, Omnia, who introduces herself. She appears confident and friendly and puts Terry at ease. During his first formal feedback interview with Omnia, she highlights to Terry that while he is progressing well, she has become aware that he constantly refers to the people by their bed number rather than their name. Omnia uses a soft tone of voice to discuss the issue with Terry. She is kind and considerate as she explains what is required in order for Terry to work in a more person-centred way. Terry feels very uncomfortable, because the use of bed numbers, rather than each person's name, was the norm in his previous practice learning area. He feels disappointed because he wants to create a good impression with his practice supervisor and the clinical team.

Drawing on all you have read and learned in this chapter, you are invited to consider what person-centred principles you think Omnia is role modelling. As a human agent in this environment, how has the social structure of Terry's previous environment influenced his ability to engage authentically? Look back at Chapter 5 to think about ways in which Terry could enhance his potential for human flourishing.

Conclusion

In this chapter, we have explored the importance of developing interpersonal connections with others, in order to engage meaningfully and effectively across multiple health and social care settings. It has been identified that for us to engage authentically, we need to be open to learning about ourselves and be able to value what matters to others. Drawing on notions of the constant interplay between human agency and social structures, we have outlined some challenges you might experience as you attempt to live out person-centred ways of being when working in complex and fast-paced environments. Reflexive activities provide opportunities for reflection into ways of developing deep connections with others and to facilitate insight into becoming a more authentic person. Engaging meaningfully and effectively is one of the person-centred processes and it requires us to develop and use our ongoing knowledge, experience and increased awareness of self to work authentically with others in the complex environment of health and social care.

Summary

- To be able to engage meaningfully and effectively, you have to be authentic in all interactions with others.
- Being authentic is a process of becoming.
- Human agency and social structure influence the way we engage with others.
- Creative reflective practices are a useful way to explore self, open ourselves to different perspectives and flourish as persons.

References

Archer, M. (2010). Routine, reflexivity and realism. *Sociological Theory* 28 (3): 272–303.

Bolton, G. (2013). *Reflective Practice: Writing and Professional Development*, 4e. London: Sage.

Elder Vass, D. (2013). *The Reality of Social Construction*. Cambridge: Cambridge University Press.

Heron, J. (1999). *The Complete Facilitators Handbook*. London: Kogan Page.

Lawler, J. and Ashman, I. (2012). Theorizing leadership authenticity: a Sartrean perspective. *Leadership* 8 (4): 327–344.

McCormack, B. (2003). A conceptual framework for person-centred practice with older people. *International Journal of Nursing Practice* 9: 202–209.

McCormack, B. and McCance, T. (2017). *Person-Centred Practice in Nursing and Health Care: Theory and Practice*, 2e. Chichester: Wiley Blackwell.

Further reading

Archer, M. (2003). *Structure, Agency and the Internal Conversation*. Cambridge: Cambridge University Press.

Dewing, J. and McCormack, B. (2015). Engagement: a critique of the concept and its application to person-centred care. www.fons.org/library/journal/volume5-person-centredness-suppl/article6

Rogers, C. (1967). *On Becoming a Person: A therapist's View of Psychotherapy*. London: Constable.

Seedhouse, D. (2017). *Thoughtful Healthcare: Ethical Awareness and Reflective Practice*. London: Sage.

Starr, S. (2008). Authenticity. A concept analysis. *Nursing Forum* 43 (2): 55–62.

14

Sharing in decisions

Jean Daly Lynn[1], Assumpta Ryan[1], and Fiona Kelly[2]

[1] Ulster University, Northern Ireland, UK
[2] Queen Margaret University, Edinburgh, Scotland, UK

Contents

Fundamentals of Person-Centred Healthcare Practice, First Edition. Edited by Brendan McCormack, Tanya McCance, Cathy Bulley, Donna Brown, Ailsa McMillan and Suzanne Martin.

Learning outcomes

- Be able to explore the application of shared decision making (SDM) with service users.
- Have an understanding of the opportunities and challenges associated with SDM in the promotion of more person-centred approaches to practice.
- Examine SDM from the perspectives of a range of service users.

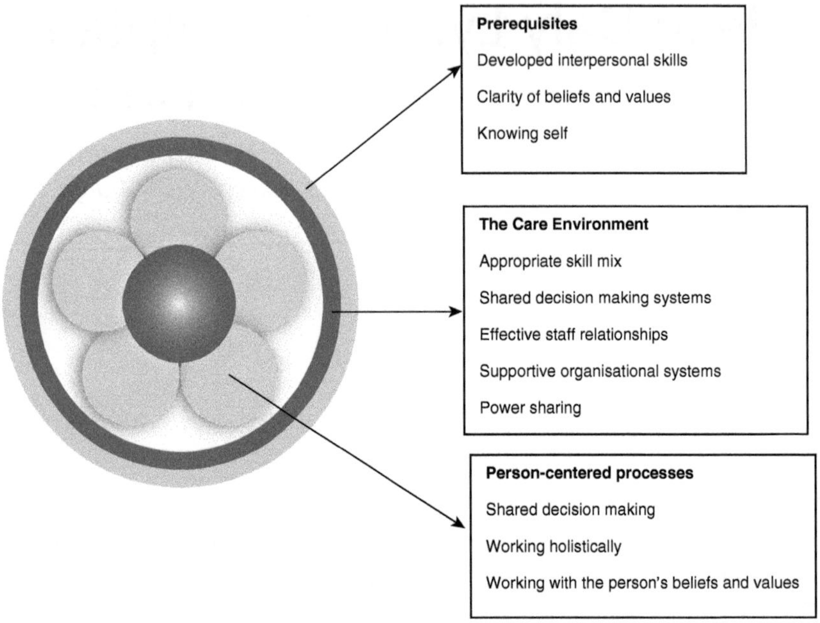

Prerequisites
Developed interpersonal skills
Clarity of beliefs and values
Knowing self
The Care Environment
Appropriate skill mix
Shared decision making systems
Effective staff relationships
Supportive organisational systems
Power sharing
Person-centered processes
Shared decision making
Working holistically
Working with the person's beliefs and values

Introduction

This chapter will focus on shared decision making (SDM) which sits within the person-centred processes domain of the Person-Centred Practice Framework. You will have seen that the Person-Centred Practice Framework set out in Chapter 3 describes shared decision making as 'the facilitation of involvement in decision making by patients and others significant to them by considering values, experiences, concerns and future aspirations'. Chapter 9 reflected on person-centred decision making and as a result you will have an understanding of decision making from the service user's perspective, as well as from the professional and organisational standpoint. This chapter complements the learning from Chapter 9 and helps to build a picture of the complexities around this important skill. SDM enables self-determination for service users and is embedded in characteristics such as partnership working, mutuality, authenticity, honesty and respect (McCormack and McCance 2010). We want to illustrate to you that this concept of SDM is interwoven through all aspects of practice.

Shared decision making with service users

Shared decision making is defined by Coulter and Collins (2011) as 'a process in which clinicians and patients work together, sharing information about options with the aim of reaching agreement on the best course of action'. SDM is at the core of the Person-Centred Practice Framework and is described as a 'negotiated approach' by McCormack and McCance (2017, p. 22). As described in Chapter 9, previously the service user–practitioner relationship was largely paternalistic, with practitioners making decisions on behalf of people in the belief that they, as experienced and knowledgeable practitioners, knew best. However, in recent years, there has been a significant shift away from this type of thinking and a move towards a more person-centred approach to practice. This move from paternalism to person-centredness is characterised by a new emphasis on empowerment, partnership, mutuality, respect, information and autonomy.

Service users generally want to be more involved in their own healthcare decisions but remain unsure of how to achieve this (O'Neill et al. 2020). Despite this, there is evidence that SDM is not widely practised (Lee and Emanuel 2013). Ryan and Cunningham (2014) highlight four key reasons to engage in SDM.

- A legal imperative
- An ethical obligation
- The right thing to do
- Wanted by service users

Shared decision making involves a number of essential stages (Makoul and Clayman 2006; Ryan and Cunningham 2014) as you will see in our case study example in Section 14.3.

Shared decision making in action

An example of the stages in SDM is illustrated through a case study of two parents with spinal cord injuries (SCI) navigating maternity services. For the purposes of this story we will call them Mary and John. They were wheelchair users living with SCI expecting their first baby together and they wanted a natural birth, meaning they wanted to avoid or minimise medical intervention.

1. *Explain the issue in layman's terms.*
   Due to Mary's disability, the pregnancy was considered high risk and therefore consultant-led care was necessary. This was explained to the parents.
2. *Present all options, including the option of doing nothing. The service user should be made aware of a position of equipoise or balance, where there is no right or wrong decision, only a preferred choice.*
   From the first consultant appointment, a collaborative approach was taken to ensure a healthy pregnancy and natural birth. At the initial appointment, both the medical team and the parents expressed their wish for a healthy pregnancy and a natural unmedicated birth. The options of assisted birth and caesarean section were discussed. Current research was consulted by the parents and the medical team to ensure an informed, evidence-based approach was taken.
3. *Discuss the pros and cons including the benefits, risks and cost of each option. These should be explained together with the respective probabilities, if known, as service users often find it easier to weigh up choices they can quantify.*
   A major SDM process was around a water birth. Early in the process, Mary's desire to have a water birth was considered to be too risky. However, after further discussions, with all parties drawing on the pros and cons, the risk was reduced as the midwives were sent on a manual handling course in advance so they could support Mary into the birthing pool using a hoist.

4. *Clarify the service user's values and preferences by exploring their attitudes to, concerns about and expectations of each option.*
   The consultants were led by the desires and wishes of Mary and John. A birth plan was developed by Mary and John and discussed at each appointment to identify how these care desires could be met collaboratively.
5. *Discuss the service user's ability and self-efficacy. The service user should be made aware that they do not need to make this decision alone. Family members and friends can be invited to participate where appropriate and subject to the consent of the service user. It is important to remember that some service users may not wish to make the decision themselves and it may be counterproductive to force them to do so.*
   At the start of the third trimester, Mary and John had a tour of the delivery suite to ensure it was accessible and met their needs. During this time, they met the ward sister who supported them by walking them through a person's typical experience in the delivery suite.
6. *Present what is known and make recommendations. The practitioner should present the best available evidence together with their clinical experience and counsel the service user in the SDM process.*
   At each appointment, Mary and John and the medical team reviewed the birth plan. Mary and John were kept informed about multidisciplinary meetings held to discuss their desires and the possible outcomes. Following the tour of the delivery suite, a collaborative conversation between Mary, John and the ward sister was held to present the information they had and identify any future needs. It was decided that a second bed was to be brought into the suite for John and a over-bed pole was to be fitted to Mary's bed.
7. *Clarify the service user's understanding and provide opportunities to ask questions and to request more information and more time if necessary.*
   Mary and John had numerous opportunities to ask questions through regular appointments with the specialist team and these were answered honestly and thoroughly.
8. *Make or explicitly defer a decision. Some service users will make the decision at the consultation but for others, it will be appropriate to defer making the decision until they have had more time to consider all the options. A follow-up appointment should be arranged in most cases.*

During the birth, decisions had to be made quickly because the medical team identified that Mary had acquired an infection. Complications during labour meant she was unable to use the birthing pool and it was not possible to achieve aspects of the birth plan such as where Mary would labour and the positions she would like to be in. However, Mary and John were given choices within the changing circumstances which enabled them to have a sense of control over the natural birth of their baby. The preparation in advance of the birth had equipped the parents and the medical team to make decisions quickly. The consultants came to visit John, Mary and baby Michael after the birth and discussed the experience with them. This process contributed to the positive physical and psychological experience and provided a sense of empowerment over the birthing of their baby.

Unlike the example above, you may have experienced situations where the service user does not engage in decision making, either because they do not want to, do not feel equipped to or because they lack the capacity. Some service users choose to devolve decision making to a significant other, or indeed to the practitioner. In the latter case and acknowledging the principles of person-centred practice, as the practitioner you should not force the service user to engage in SDM but it is important to demonstrate reasonable steps to attempt to do so and to ensure that the service user is sufficiently well informed for consent to be valid. Strategies such as the therapeutic relationship, sympathetic presence and motivational interviewing can promote SDM with service users.

Activity

What has been your experience of SDM?

What impact did this experience have on your ability to provide a person-centred approach to practice?

Opportunities and challenges with shared decision making

You may now be starting to realise that SDM brings with it a range of opportunities and challenges for service users and care providers. We have listed some of these in Table 14.1.

The process of sharing information, taking steps to build a consensus about treatment and reaching decisions together presents an opportunity to build strong relationships between service users and practitioners (Chewning et al. 2015). This moves away from a hierarchical approach, where the practitioner knows best, to a position of empowerment for the service user. You can develop mutuality with the service user when you develop genuine partnerships within the SDM process (McCormack and McCance 2017). SDM can provide service users with a sense of control in an uncontrollable situation, as with the parents in the case study, offering a clear focus and strategy for coping.

Service users value information being shared with them in a clear, simplified manner as this reduces the uncertainty of what is to come. Complete information about the pros and cons of a treatment or intervention must be given before an informed decision can be made. This means that practitioners must provide accessible information in lay terms and adjust how they deliver their information to enable collaborative working. It is important that you learn how to communicate information in the easiest and clearest way possible.

A major challenge with SDM can be the complexity of the decision that needs to be made. Within a healthcare setting, terminology, diagnosis and treatment plans are inherently complicated. This can make the entire SDM process overwhelming for a person with a new diagnosis

Table 14.1 Opportunities and challenges with shared decision making

Opportunities	Challenges
• Working in partnership • Improved service user knowledge • Reduced anxiety • Improved self-esteem • Greater autonomy and control • Greater satisfaction • Develop good communication • Can foster trusting relationships • Generating appropriate information to share • Using lay terms about treatment • More accurate risk perception • Mutual respect	• Complexity of information and decisions • Not everyone feels competent • All participants need the skills • The type of condition • The type of treatment • Ongoing process • Reaching a mutual decision • Takes more time • Not all service users want it • Not all consultations are suited to it (e.g. emergency situations) • Lack of training • Cognitive impairment

or new to a service. SDM requires a person receiving a service to actively engage in decisions about their care but in order to do so, they need education and support in SDM to participate in their own care. Peer support, particularly online forums, can provide invaluable support to persons navigating complex information to inform their decision. This can bring a host of issues in itself but can be very beneficial. Additionally, third party organisations and charities can act as an advocate for service users during this process. While for some knowledge means power, for others this information overload can provoke high levels of anxiety. You should also note that after a significant diagnosis, service users may not want additional information or to engage in SDM (Chewning et al. 2015). Equally, as a care provider you might find this process of providing information in simple non-medical terms challenging; don't worry, it is a skill that develops with practice. The inherent complexity of organisational decision making and the culture that impacts SDM, as explored in Chapter 9, are further challenges that need to be negotiated.

Activity

Think of a time when you have been in a healthcare setting and you felt SDM did or would have worked well. Consider this interaction and write down what worked well and what didn't work so well.

The personality and characteristics of the person in receipt of treatment or services can affect the dynamics of the SDM. Service users may differ in the degree to which they wish to participate in SDM. Additionally, the personality and characteristics you bring as a healthcare provider can impact the SDM dynamic and you may need to have more interactions with some service users in order to make collaborative decisions. Keeping this in mind, the unique perspectives of a service user and a practitioner are presented here to illustrate the differing points of view that can be experienced.

> On reflection, when I go into a hospital setting, I often feel vulnerable and powerless. Even though I am an expert in my circumstances and a confident person, in a healthcare setting I seem to change. I don't always say what I feel or need to. I sometimes come away from appointments feeling that I have not been listened to. I have been to appointments even though I have tried to articulate how unnecessary I feel that would be. I comply because I don't want to miss out on service provision which might happen if I refuse an appointment. When I feel listened to and understand where the practitioner is coming from, I am happy to compromise. Working in partnership and as part of a team to create a care plan for me helps me feel motivated and engage in self-care.

> As a practitioner, I really love it when I can work in collaboration with people. When it goes well it is such a natural process. It is not always an easy process and sometimes it can go in a direction I am not happy with. I understand it is not appropriate to enforce my views and decision on people, but I also think people should be aware of the guidelines, policy and procedures I have to work within. This can make my job more challenging, particularly when someone wants something done in a particular way that is outside my control. However, I do feel having more people involved in decision making, the

person, family members and even third party advocates, helps the process and results in strong consensus about treatment and care.

The type of condition a person is living with can bring challenges to the SDM approach. A person living with multiple diagnoses can make decision making very challenging. Additionally, if the intervention requires a rapid decision or if it can be deliberated on over some time, this can impact on SDM. You might have a very strong opinion about a treatment plan in the best interest of the service user, while the service user may have a very different viewpoint based on the quality of the life they wish to live. This may lead to dissatisfaction with the process by some members of the SDM team. SDM is often viewed as a snapshot of a point in time but it should be seen as an ongoing, fluid process, evolving in response to the changing needs and circumstances of service users.

Shared decision making and cognitive impairment

Autonomy is the capacity to make an informed, uncoerced decision and may be compromised or challenged for people with cognitive impairment. The powerful call from groups such as the Scottish Dementia Working Group, or individuals living with dementia such as Kate Swaffer and Christine Bryden, to do 'nothing about us without us' has shifted the practice of 'doing to' to 'working with', and this extends to decision making. This concept of 'working with' persons is a core component of your work as a healthcare provider, particularly with your mandatory requirement for co-production within service provision and delivery. 'Working with' persons is also a key principle of legislation such as the Adult Support and Protection (Scotland) Act 2007 (Scottish Parliament 2007), which mandates providing adults at risk of harm with as much relevant information and support as is necessary to enable them to participate as fully as possible. The Act also stresses the importance of 'ensuring that the adult is not, without justification, treated less favourably than the way in which any other adult (not being an adult at risk) might be treated in a comparable situation'.

In relation to supporting SDM with persons with a cognitive impairment such as dementia, the eight stages detailed above also apply. However, as cognitive impairment progresses, the challenges (see Table 14.1) may be more acute and the practitioner will need advanced observation and communication skills to arrive at a decision that best meets the person's desires and needs.

One way in which practitioners can support decision making with persons living with dementia is to recognise and support selfhood. Within the field of dementia care, the Selfs framework evolved with the work of Sabat and Harré (1992), who argued against the dominant assumption of loss of self as dementia progresses. Sabat (2001) subsequently included three aspects of Self (Selfs 1–3), providing a useful framework for exploring visual and verbal expressions of self of people with dementia in long-term care. This work is explained in detail in Chapter 1. Sabat's work implicates the actions and attributions of others – informal and formal carers, members of the public, etc. – in positioning persons living with dementia (Sabat et al. 2004; Sabat 2006) and in contributing to the construction or deconstruction of their selfhoods (Sabat and Harré 1992).

The key to successfully interacting with persons living with dementia is not only recognising aspects of self, but also responding to and supporting expressions of self (Kelly 2013). Here is an example from practice where an aspect of self is recognised but not supported.

> Charlie is up again, walking. . . He approaches the staff nurse. Charlie reaches out and the staff nurse asks him what he wants. Charlie's speech is difficult to make out and the staff nurse says: 'If I can help you, I will', but he's still walking. Charlie follows him for a few steps; hand outstretched, but the nurse is too quick and he's away.

In this example, the nurse recognised Self 1 by referring to Charlie *as 'you'* but by withholding his need for contact, the nurse failed to support Self 1. Although the nurse half-heartedly offered to help, the absence of a therapeutic relationship or sympathetic presence meant the opportunity to explore Charlie's wishes and feelings was lost. Consequently, the opportunity to work with Charlie to explore options to comfort him was also lost.

Here is another example of lack of recognition and, therefore, lack of support of another aspect of self: Self 3.

> Nora is served her soup but she is unhappy with the soup spoon. She stands up to go to clean it but is intercepted by the staff nurse who takes it from her, looks at it and explains that it only has soup on it. The nurse then puts the spoon into the bowl and brusquely tells Nora to sit down. Nora refuses to eat her soup. She slips into ill-being.

Nora was a proud woman and liked things to be neat and tidy. Had the nurse allowed Nora to wash her spoon, or helped her to choose another one, she would have supported her wish to take control over an unsatisfactory situation and co-constructed with Nora her desired role of home-maker (Self 3). Instead, by disempowering her, by not supporting her to participate in her desired role, the nurse contributed to Nora's increasing ill-being.

The principles of SDM, while time-consuming and requiring skilled communication, can be simplified and applied in these two examples. For example, in Nora's case, the nurse could have listened to Nora's complaint that the spoon was dirty and given Nora the option of choosing another spoon. By doing so, she would have worked with Nora in the way that any other adult would expect – with mutuality, authenticity, honesty and respect (McCormack and McCance 2010).

Activity

There is a woman living with dementia in your practice setting and you notice she starts to become restless as dusk falls. Using the Selfs framework to support SDM, how could you work with her to reduce her restlessness and foster well-being?

In relation to decision making and the idea of autonomy – the desire to make one's own choices or the freedom to make choices – it is clear that one way to facilitate this is to recognise a person's needs, wishes, or preferences and support these by whatever means possible. Using Sabat's selfhood framework can assist this in a way that is meaningful for the person living with dementia and fulfilling for practitioners.

Conclusion

This chapter has explored the centrality of shared decision making in the provision of person-centred care to a broad range of persons across diverse settings. We have described the opportunities that SDM brings, including benefits for service users such as improved knowledge and a sense of control and empowerment. The benefits for practitioners have also been highlighted, with a particular focus on the role of SDM in the promotion of a greater therapeutic alliance between those who provide care and those who receive it. Recognising that SDM can be challenging in certain contexts or conditions, we have suggested that careful consideration of the person's needs, wishes, preferences, verbal and non-verbal expression, a positive attitude towards risk and recognition of the need for review should result in decisions that are meaningful and acceptable to the individuals involved.

Summary

- Shared decision making is characterised by partnership working, empowerment, autonomy, mutuality, authenticity, honesty and respect.
- As a practitioner, you are required to work in partnership with a person to navigate the opportunities and challenges that can be presented.
- The skills you require as a partner in shared decision making include communication skills, openness, understanding, respect and honesty.
- The Selfs framework can support your approach to SDM with people in a real-world setting.

References

Chewning, B., Bylund, C., Shah, B. et al. (2015). Patient preferences for shared decisions: a systematic review. *Patient Education and Counseling* 86 (1): 9–18.

Coulter, A. and Collins, A. (2011). *Making Shared Decision-Making a Reality. No Decision About Me Without Me*. London: King's Fund.

Kelly, F. (2013). Bodywork in dementia care: recognising the commonalities of selfhood to facilitate respectful care in institutional settings. *Ageing and Society* 34 (6): 1073–1090.

Lee, E.O. and Emanuel, E.J. (2013). Shared decision making to improve care and reduce costs. *New England Journal of Medicine* 368: 6–8.

Makoul, G. and Clayman, M.L. (2006). An integrative model of shared decision making in medical encounters. *Patient Education and Counselling* 60: 301–312.

McCormack, B. and McCance, T. (2010). *Person-Centred Nursing: Theory, Models and Methods*. Oxford: Wiley Blackwell.

McCormack, B. and McCance, T. (2017). *Person-Centred Practice in Nursing and Health Care*, 2e. Oxford: Wiley Blackwell.

O'Neill, M., Ryan, A., Tracey, A., and Laird, E.A. (2020). 'You're at their mercy': older people's experiences of moving from home to a care home: a grounded theory study. *International Journal of Older People Nursing* 15: e12305.

Ryan, F. and Cunningham, S. (2014). Shared decision making in healthcare. *Faculty Dental Journal* 5 (3): 124–127.

Sabat, S. (2001). *The Experience of Alzheimer's Disease: Life Through a Tangled Veil*. Oxford: Blackwell.

Sabat, S. (2006). Mind, meaning and personhood in dementia: the effects of positioning. In: *Dementia: Mind, Meaning and the Person* (eds. J. Hughes, S. Louw and S. Sabat), 287–302. Oxford: Oxford University Press.

Sabat, S. and Harré, R. (1992). The construction and deconstruction of self in Alzheimer's disease. *Ageing and Society* 12: 443–461.

Sabat, S., Napolitano, L., and Fath, H. (2004). Barriers to the construction of a valued social identity: a case study of Alzheimer's disease. *American Journal of Alzheimer's Disease and Other Dementias* 19 (3): 177–185.

Scottish Parliament (2007). *Adult Support and Protection (Scotland) Act 2007.* www.legislation.gov.uk/asp/2007/10/section/2

Further reading

Bunn, F., Goodman, C., Russell, B. et al. (2018). Supporting shared decision making for older people with multiple health and social care needs: a realist synthesis. *BMC Geriatrics* 18: 165. https://doi.org/10.1186/s12877-018-0853-9.

National Institute for Health and Care Excellence (England). *Shared Decision Making.* www.nice.org.uk/about/what-we-do/our-programmes/nice-guidance/nice-guidelines/shared-decision-making

Slade, M. (2017). Implementing shared decision making in routine mental health care. *World Psychiatry* 16 (2): 146–153. https://doi.org/10.1002/wps.20412.

The Health Foundation (2013). *Implementing Shared Decision Making: Clinical Teams' Experiences of Implementing Shared Decision Making as Part of the MAGIC Programme.* London: The Health Foundation www.health.org.uk/sites/default/files/ImplementingSharedDecisionMaking.pdf.

15

Being sympathetically present

Tanya McCance[1], Brendan McCormack[2], Karl Tizzard-Kleister[1], and Lynn Wallace[2]

[1] Ulster University, Northern Ireland, UK
[2] Queen Margaret University, Edinburgh, Scotland, UK

Contents

Fundamentals of Person-Centred Healthcare Practice, First Edition. Edited by Brendan McCormack, Tanya McCance, Cathy Bulley, Donna Brown, Ailsa McMillan and Suzanne Martin.

Learning outcomes

- Understand the concept of sympathetic presence and be able to distinguish this concept from other related concepts, such as empathy and contemplation.
- Consider the challenges posed for people in operationalising the concept in practice.
- Reflect on the place of contemplative practices in sympathetic presence and how they can be integrated with everyday practices.
- Understand the need to be reflexive on one's own ways of being as a person in order to be present in the moment.

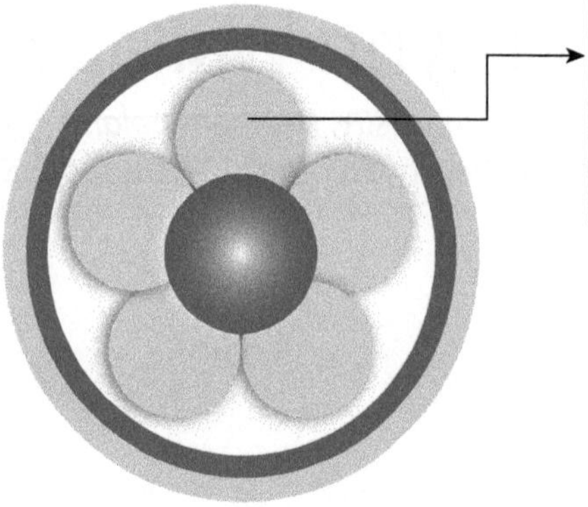

Being sympathetically present: an engagement that recognises the uniqueness and value of the person, by appropriately responding to cues that maximise coping resources through the recognition of important agendas in their life

Introduction

This chapter will explore the concept of sympathetic presence, one of the five person-centred processes within the Person-centred Practice Framework. The emergence of the concept will be described, and we will examine how it differs from the related concept of empathy. The importance of being sympathetically present and its fundamental impact on human beings, their relationships and their care experience will be considered, alongside the significant challenges experienced when trying to operationalise the concept in our everyday practice. This chapter will also consider contemplative practices as a way of enhancing a person's ability to know self and to use that knowledge to be sympathetically present.

On reading the poem on the next page you might think: how could a person act in this way? You might feel that it resonates with similar experiences you have had or observed in practice. How difficult was it to identify a contrasting experience that reflected different levels of engagement? Did you describe very different actions going on in the encounters or were you able to place them on a continuum of engagement? Consider the skills that were displayed or lacking and consider your own development in terms of being present with a person.

Activity

Read the poem presented below and describe the interaction it captures in 100 words. Then consider and describe a contrasting experience you have observed when a person in practice was intentionally engaging with a patient or family member. Compare your two descriptions and try to draw out the actions that were important.

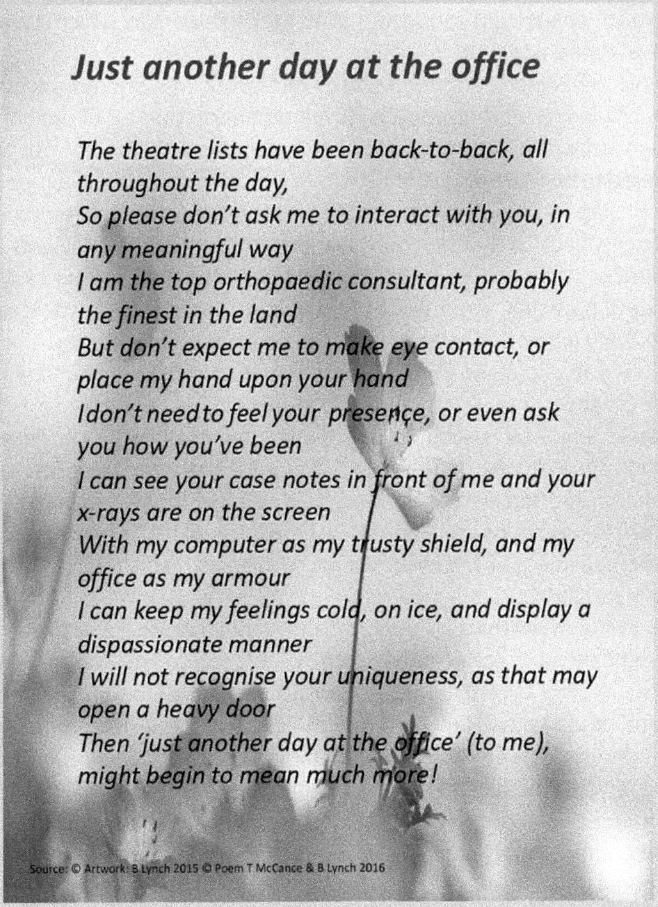
Just another day at the office
The theatre lists have been back-to-back, all throughout the day,
So please don't ask me to interact with you, in any meaningful way
I am the top orthopaedic consultant, probably the finest in the land
But don't expect me to make eye contact, or place my hand upon your hand
I don't need to feel your presence, or even ask you how you've been
I can see your case notes in front of me and your x-rays are on the screen
With my computer as my trusty shield, and my office as my armour
I can keep my feelings cold, on ice, and display a dispassionate manner
I will not recognise your uniqueness, as that may open a heavy door
Then 'just another day at the office' (to me), might begin to mean much more!

Source: © Artwork: B Lynch 2015 © Poem T McCance & B Lynch 2016

Understanding sympathetic presence

Sympathetic presence describes a way of being with people that is consistent with person-centredness but is also achievable in a practice context. Sympathetic presence borrows from the idea of sympathy, particularly in how sympathy does not require you to place your own ideas or 'understanding' over another person's. It is both a recognition of another's personhood (McCormack 2001) and an availability towards them (McCance 2003). Being sympathetically present is a way of being that recognises the uniqueness and value of the individual and reflects the quality of the relationship between practitioner and patient. It relates to working with the person's beliefs and values and having some insight into what is important to them in their life. To have a person accept the other, and sympathetically understand their situation, is to build a healthful relationship. It asks you to pay attention to another's feelings, experiences, characteristics and any other elements that may contribute to their identity in that current moment (McCormack and McCance 2010, 2017). Being sympathetically present is something more than just being physically present, reflecting the ability of a person to be available in that moment. It is an openness and connection with the other person, which is emotional, cognitive, rational, and, at times, physical.

As authors of the Person-centred Practice Framework, McCormack and McCance have continually been challenged throughout its development on the use of the concept of sympathy rather than empathy. The argument frequently presented is: why not use the term 'empathy', often considered to be more appropriate within a healthcare context? Empathy can be defined as an ability to step into another's shoes, to accurately perceive their unique feelings and to communicate this back to that person (Mearns and Thorne 2007; Williams and Stickley 2010, p. 752). McCormack and McCance (2017) reject the idea that anyone can fully comprehend another person's particular experience. To illustrate this, they use the example of loss and bereavement. They argue that even if you have also experienced bereavement, this leaves you no closer to being able to 'stand in that person's shoes' and to understand what that experience truly feels like for them.

In many cases empathy is seen as a cure-all to the struggles in interpersonal care facing healthcare staff (Hojat 2009a; Jeffrey 2017). Empathy has been used in a concerted effort to address the many reported instances of less than compassionate care in the UK (Health Service Ombudsman 2011; Cummins and Bennett 2012; Francis 2013), but it has also been confusingly used alongside, or in place of, related concepts such as sympathy and compassion (Hojat 2009a; Bramley and Matiti 2014).

Reflecting on the move towards person-centred practice, there has been a reconsideration of empathy in healthcare. For example, Jeffrey (2017) suggests that to address the empathy gap that exists in clinical care, empathy should be considered and applied as a more relational concept. Meanwhile, Heggestad et al. (2018) explore the difficulty experienced by healthcare undergraduates with the emotional work of care. Their findings advocate for more teaching and engagement with what they call 'affective' empathy rather than 'cognitive' empathy, arguing that 'a proper balance between affective and cognitive empathy is what professionality is about' (Heggestad et al. 2018, p. 12). This suggests the concept of empathy is being seen less as an intellectual understanding of another person and more as an emotional and holistic understanding. This also links to the notion of emotional intelligence, which is discussed in greater detail in Chapter 18. As Williams and Stickley's study of empathy in nursing concludes, 'The meaning of empathy that is most relevant to nursing practice relates to the significance of the quality of the presence that a nurse may bring to the moment' (2010, p. 755). This shift is much more aligned to being sympathetically present. Furthermore, Hojat describes empathy and sympathy as overlapping processes. For him, 'Empathy involves an effort to *understand* the patient's experience without joining them, whereas sympathy involves an effortless feeling of *sharing* or joining the patient's pain and suffering' (2009a, p. 12).

Nonetheless, the following are some of the contrasting features that separate the two concepts:

- empathy is a feeling whereas sympathy is an active state, that is, being 'with' in order to understand what needs to be done
- sympathetic presence is *relational,* meaning that it happens between people

- unlike empathy, being sympathetically present does not require one person to *understand or feel* another person's emotions, pains, thoughts or perspective, but instead to *recognise* these as important features of that person at that moment.

How we learn the practice of being sympathetically present can be challenging because it requires us to learn about 'self'. The activity below is drawn from the field of applied drama to help create an experience of sympathetic presence between people. It is difficult to explain sympathetic presence using words or by just thinking about it – understanding it is much easier after you experience it. We recommend you try this activity and then re-read this section to see if it makes more sense and also reconsider what you have read previously on knowing self in the context of being sympathetically present.

Activity

Exercises to explore sympathetic presence can't really be conducted on your own. To really explore what sympathetic presence feels like, you need another person to be present or, better yet, a small to mid-sized group of people.

In pairs, person A closes their eyes and person B places their hand on their partner's shoulder, elbow or wrist – or otherwise maintains whatever physical contact is possible and comfortable for each pair. Person B then leads person A around the room in complete silence and very slowly to begin with. Person B must be very aware of where they are leading person A, as well as the movements person A is able or unable to do – perhaps they have sore knees and cannot bend them easily or maybe they cannot use their arms when getting to the floor and up again. Person B should also be aware of the other people or objects around them, ensuring that person A is safe and won't bump into anything. Most importantly, person B must be acutely aware of how person A is feeling. For instance, are they nervous, confident, tired, happy, in pain, worried or perhaps excitable? Person B must recognise these feelings, and adapt how they lead person A. If person A doesn't quite trust person B yet, person B should keep a slower pace, be conscientious and build that trust with their partner before trying more complex and quicker movements. As discussed above, person B needn't feel or understand the pain or anxiety of their partner to 'care for' them, but they should recognise this and adapt their actions with sympathetic presence. After a short while, stop, have a short discussion, swap roles and repeat the exercise.

It always helps to finish off doing an exercise like this with a group discussion. Be open with each other and consider asking and answering questions like: How did this exercise make you feel? Did you trust your partner? Why? How could you have felt more cared for? What did you notice about how your partner moved? How did the room feel when everyone was walking slowly? Is this how the atmosphere of a care environment feels? And so on. Perhaps consider how much attention you paid to the needs of your partner, and whether your own needs were attended to. Also consider whether you could feel the presence of the others in the room with you. Maybe if it is possible to feel sympathetic presence through this simple exercise, you can see how to apply this in other contexts too.

Being present in the moment

Contemplative approaches can enrich the interconnectedness between practitioner and service user that is so fundamental to sympathetic presencing. Contemplation is about looking thoughtfully at something, observing, paying attention and increasing awareness. Mindfulness is one contemplative approach that cultivates awareness in the present moment. It is gaining popularity within healthcare, both as a therapeutic option in clinical care and as a professional life skill for the health and well-being of healthcare staff.

Young (2016) uses the term 'present-centredness' when discussing the meaning of mindfulness. In the UK, as well as being offered in the NHS, mindfulness now features as a secular extracurricular practice in universities. It is even being included within some healthcare degree programmes. Mindfulness as defined by Kabat-Zinn (1994) is about paying attention, in a particular way, on purpose in the present moment and non-judgementally. This is achieved through a range of meditative and movement practices.

Cottrell (2018) provides a useful starter guide for learners interested in mindfulness practice. There are also recognised foundation mindfulness programmes available for those wishing to have a more formal and comprehensive grounding. Programmes vary in their focus, for example, from mindful living, self-compassion and stress reduction to cognitive therapy. For some healthcare professionals undertaking a foundation programme, sustaining regular mindfulness practice might be possible and desirable to help boost personal resilience as well as influencing practice. Even just becoming aware of the attitudinal foundations of mindfulness and applying these in your practice could help to enrich sympathetic presencing.

In the field of nursing, Barratt and Wagstaffe (2018) introduce mindfulness for professional practice, illustrating how the seven attitudinal foundations of mindfulness can be integrated into care: adopting a beginner's mind; non-striving; letting go; acceptance; non-judging; patience; and trust. These all contribute to cultivating mindful awareness. By paying attention in the present moment, staying curious and being open to experience, you can be more mindful of your engagement with service users. In a busy practice environment you may experience being so focused on what you are 'doing' that you become distracted from being fully aware of self and others. It is easy to go on 'auto-pilot', perhaps becoming 'mindless' of some aspects of what is happening. For example, this might manifest in not paying full attention when performing a familiar routine procedure, not being aware of another person's body language reflecting their emotions, or not fully listening to them as they express distress or suffering.

The application of mindfulness to strengthen sympathetic presencing in moments of care helps by cultivating a deeper level of awareness of self and being able to reflect on the needs of others. A nice example of such application is the G.R.A.C.E. process (Halifax 2014). This encourages practitioners to open up to and stay present with their service users' experiences. The process involves a number of stages: gathering attention; recalling intention; attuning to self and others; considering, through insight, what care would best serve; and engaging fully (being mindful in entering and ending clinical encounters). Finding space, time and the environment in which to mindfully pause may be challenging. There are times when it is necessary to physically pause and be still and silent and present. Alternatively, capturing mindful moments 'on the go' in the sometimes frantic pace of care situations, by accepting things just as they are, is possible and can be helpful.

A list of contemplative practices to facilitate meaningful engagement is presented in Table 15.1. At this stage we encourage you to reflect on what you read in Chapter 4 on knowing self, and how engaging in contemplative practice can contribute to achieving the conditions for human flourishing.

Table 15.1 Contemplative practices to engage with service users

• Deep listening • Three-minute breathing space • Mindful movement, e.g. walking, walking in nature, simple stretching, yoga, qigong • Mindful eating • Journalling, story telling	• Poetry (reading or writing) • Music (listening to, singing, playing instrument) • Beholding (looking out the window, at a picture or work of art) • Drawing or painting

You may be new to the notion of mindfulness or you may have engaged in some of the contemplative practices presented above. Regardless of your experience, we encourage you to undertake the activity below.

Activity

Use the following weblink to access a series of six short films produced by the Royal College of Nursing: http://rcn.org.uk/mindfulness

- Watch one of the videos, which feature different stages of the working day. Follow the mindful practice offered. Make some reflective notes about your experience and how being mindful could be useful in your clinical practice.
- Take time over the next few weeks to watch the remaining films in the series, repeating the experiential and reflective activities suggested in Activity 1.

What did you learn from reflecting on your mindfulness experiences? How did you feel after participating in mindfulness? What ideas do you have for incorporating contemplative practices such as mindfulness or the suggestions in Table 15.1 into your daily practice? In your discussion you may have considered your awareness of thoughts, feelings, emotions and sensations in the body, experiencing greater focus, attention and concentration, or a feeling of calm.

Conclusion

In this chapter we have explored the concept of being sympathetically present and placed it in the context of other related concepts, such as empathy. We described sympathetic presence as a way of being that recognises the uniqueness and value of persons and reflects the quality of the relationship between persons. In simple terms, sympathetic presence is remaining *available* to and being *present* for other persons in a particular moment. We acknowledged the challenges in learning the practice of being sympathetically present, particularly within busy clinical environments. We offered activities drawn from applied drama and contemplative practice that help create an experience of sympathetic presence between persons. We have also made links with other chapters in this book, including knowing self and creating the conditions for human flourishing.

Summary

- Being sympathetically present is a way of being that recognises the uniqueness and value of people and reflects the quality of the relationship between persons. It relates to knowing the person and having some insight into what is important to them in their life.
- Sympathetic presence is *relational*, i.e. it happens between people, and is an active state that is about being with in order to understand what needs to be done.
- Learning the practice of being sympathetically present can be challenging because it requires us to learn about 'self'. It is often difficult to learn through conventional teaching approaches but is more conducive to active learning.
- Contemplative approaches such as mindfulness can enrich the interconnectedness between people that is fundamental to sympathetic presencing.

References

Barratt, C. and Wagstaffe, T. (2018). Nursing and mindfulness. In: *Coping and Thriving in Nursing: An Essential Guide to Practice* (ed. P.J. Martin), 62–80. London: Sage.

Bramley, L. and Matiti, M. (2014). How does it really feel to be in my shoes? Patients' experiences of compassion within nursing care and their perceptions of developing compassionate nurses. *Journal of Clinical Nursing* 23 (19–20): 2790–2799.

Cottrell, S. (2018). *Mindfulness for Students*. London: Palgrave.

Cummins, J. and Bennett, V. (2012). *Compassion in Practice: Nursing, Midwifery and Care Staff, Our Vision and Strategy*. www.england.nhs.uk/wp-content/uploads/2012/12/compassion-in-practice.pdf

Francis, R. (2013). *Report of the Mid Staffordshire NHS Foundation Trust Public Inquiry: Executive Summary*. London: Stationery Office.

Halifax, J. (2014). G.R.A.C.E for nurses: cultivating compassion in nurse/patient interactions. *Journal of Nursing Education* 4 (1): 121–128.

Health Service Ombudsman (2011). *Care and Compassion? A Report of the Health Services Ombudsman on Ten Investigations into NHS Care for Older People*. www.ombudsman.org.uk/sites/default/files/2016-10/Care%20and%20Compassion.pdf

Heggestad, A.K.T., Nortvedt, P., Christiansen, B., and Konow-Lund, A. (2018). Undergraduate nursing students' ability to empathize: a qualitative study. *Nurse Ethics* 25: 1–10.

Hojat, M. (2009a). *Empathy in Patient Care: Antecedents, Development, Measurement, and Outcomes*. New York: Springer.

Jeffrey, D. (2017). Communicating with a human voice: developing a relational model of empathy. *Journal of the Royal College of Physicians of Edinburgh* 47 (3): 266–270.

Kabat-Zinn, J. (1994). *Wherever You Go, There You Are*. London: Piatkus.

McCance, T. (2003). Caring in nursing practice: the development of a conceptual framework. *Research and Theory for Nursing Practice* 17 (2): 101–116.

McCormack, B. (2001). *Negotiating Partnerships with Older People: A Person-Centred Approach*. Aldershot: Ashgate.

McCormack, B. and McCance, T. (2010). *Person-centred Nursing: Theory, Models and Methods*. Oxford: Blackwell Publishing.

McCormack, B. and McCance, T. (2017). *Person-centred Nursing and Health Care: Theory and Practice*. Chichester: Wiley Publishing.

Mearns, D. and Thorne, B. (2007). *Person-Centred Counselling in Action*. London: Sage.

Williams, J. and Stickley, T. (2010). Empathy and nurse education. *Nurse Education Today* 30 (8): 752–755.

Young, S. (2016). What is mindfulness? A contemplative perspective. In: *Handbook of Mindfulness in Education* (eds. K.A. Schonert-Reichl and R.W. Roeser), 29–45. New York: Springer.

Further reading

Hojat, M. (2009b). Ten approaches for enhancing empathy in health and human services cultures. *Journal of Health and Human Services Administration* 31 (4): 412–450.

Williams, M. and Penman, D. (2012). *Mindfulness: A Practical Guide to Finding Peace in a Frantic World*. London: Piatkus.

16

Providing holistic care

Neal F. Cook[1] and Michelle L. Elliot[2]

[1] *Ulster University, Northern Ireland, UK*
[2] *Queen Margaret University, Edinburgh, Scotland, UK*

Contents

Fundamentals of Person-Centred Healthcare Practice, First Edition. Edited by Brendan McCormack, Tanya McCance, Cathy Bulley, Donna Brown, Ailsa McMillan and Suzanne Martin.

Learning outcomes

- Define holism within the context of person-centredness.
- Reflect on what it means to be holistic and person-centred in practice.
- Identify strategies for practising within a holistic, person-centred context.

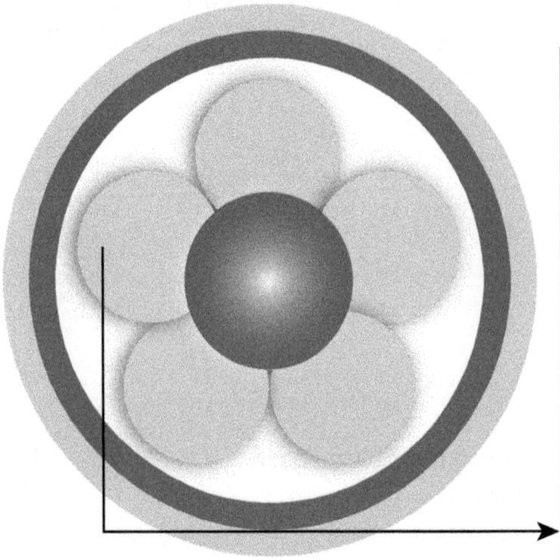

Working with the person's beliefs and values: having a clear picture of the person's values about his/her life and how he/she makes sense of what is happening from their individual perspective, psychosocial context and social role.

Sharing decision making: engaging persons in decision making by considering values, experiences, concerns and future aspirations.

Engaging authentically: the connectedness between people, determined by knowledge of the person, clarity of beliefs and values, knowledge of self and professional expertise.

Being sympathetically present: an engagement that recognises the uniqueness and value of the person, by appropriately responding to cues that maximise coping resources through the recognition of important agendas in their life.

Introduction

The focus of this chapter is on holistic care, which McCance and McCormack (2017, p. 58) define as:

> the provision of treatment and care that pays attention to the whole person through the integration of physiological, psychological, sociocultural, developmental and spiritual dimensions of persons.

Within the Person-centred Practice Framework, providing holistic care is one of five constructs of person-centred processes. In this regard, the definition above is set within the context of practice. This is important as it means that holism and its translation to practice are not theoretical. Rather, they are lived out through the application of values in working with and addressing the needs of the whole person and their support networks.

The concept of holism

The concept of holism is not new to healthcare practices or contexts. In fact, the concept of considering and working with a person as a whole, rather than as a sum of their parts, has existed for millennia, crossing cultures and associated practices globally. In addition to the alignment with the Person-centred Practice Framework, this sense of holism is compatible with the views of Neuman (1995) and is captured in Figure 16.1.

Similar to the Person-centred Practice Framework, you will see in this figure that while components of holism can be identified and separated into different elements, it is the bringing together of these elements that represents authentic holism. The ability to integrate these can be considered a practised craft. You may have great abilities and insight into some elements; over time, as you develop your practice, you will further enhance your skills to focus on all the elements of being within personhood (see Chapter 1). This is achieved, in part, through tailoring your practice to ensure that the relevance and importance of each element are considered. Understanding that holism is an integration of these elements and not separate facets of persons is a skilled and sensitive form of working that is both art and science, requiring continual practice and attention. As you learn and develop, it is a journey that will require you to be continually reflective and reflexive in order to stand back and consider how authentically you are practising holistically (see Chapters 10, 13 and 29).

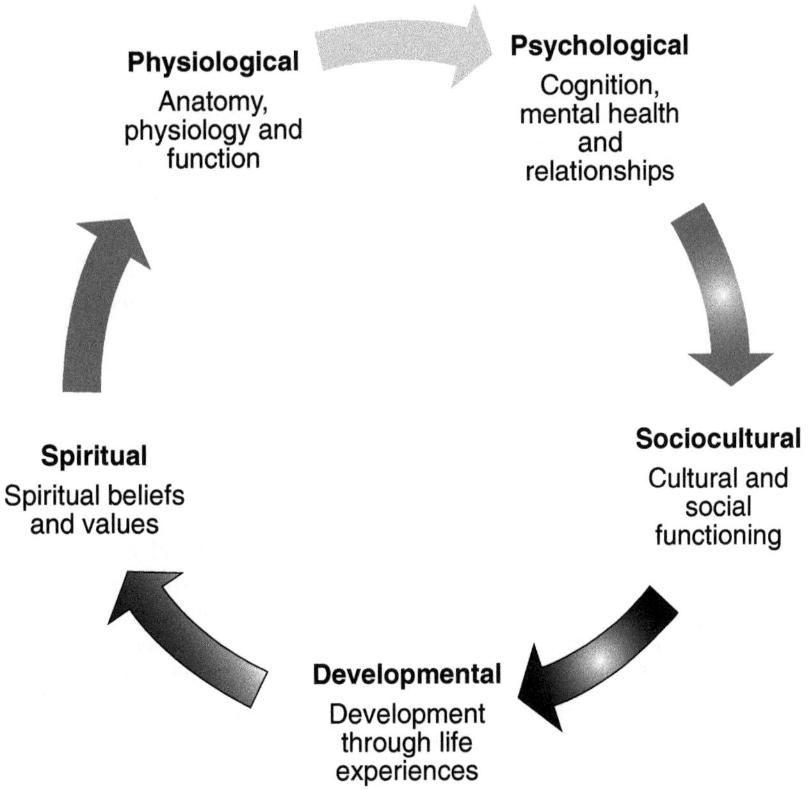

Figure 16.1 Elements of holism. Source: Adapted from Neuman (1995) and McCormack and McCance (2017).

When we address only one aspect of a person in our work, we are being reductionistic, meaning we reduce a person to a singular issue rather than see them as a dynamic and multifaceted being. For example, if we meet a young person newly diagnosed with type 1 diabetes mellitus, we need to consider the possibility that any difficulty with controlling their blood sugar levels may relate to issues beyond their diet and medication. They may like to take part in high-energy sport, or frequent cafes with their friends, or they may be concerned with how their peers view them and how their diabetes may impact on such social networks at a very formative time in their life. Alternatively, the young person and their family may have beliefs about medication or limited financial means to address the new dietary requirements of the diagnosis.

Working holistically means staying aware of and being attentive to a multitude of interrelated elements of a person's everyday life, in partnership with the individual themselves. It also requires effective team working; no single professional group is responsible for ensuring that all aspects of a person's life are maintained or considered. There may be social factors that need to be addressed (e.g. access to healthy foods), mental health issues impacting on effective self-care management, a need for nutritional education and advice, or consultation on medication schedules may be required. Each of these aspects of the person's life might be the focus of a different team member, yet the broader understanding of how the issues exist in relation to the wider sense of personhood and health must be retained. This is at the heart of holistic care and the ethos of working in a person-centred manner.

Activity

To learn more about the concept of holism, please read the Further Reading articles of McMillan et al. and Michaelson et al. at the end of the chapter. Then reflect on the following questions.

- How effective are current healthcare systems and structures in facilitating holistic care?
- What challenges do people working in healthcare face in being holistic in their practice?
- What have you learned that you will take forward to practise more holistically?

People, healthcare and holism

A first step to providing holistic care is to consider those in your care as people; seeing them as 'patients' or 'clients' can establish a relationship where you and your colleagues hold the power. If we are to avoid dividing aspects of health and disease, we must see the whole person (Woods 2015), including their concerns, strengths and personal contexts. In order to understand health within the context of all the elements of holism, we need to be able to establish a therapeutic relationship that enables us to engage fully with a person (see Chapters 10 and 26). Working in a holistic way means we must be aware of what 'everyone brings' to the healthcare practice. While we may have (or be learning) specialised knowledge and skills, it is important to remember that all people involved in providing, accessing and receiving healthcare possess unique and valuable knowledge and experiences. Holistic care therefore means working with a respectful and inclusive approach to address all facets of personhood (see Chapter 1).

People's experiences of healthcare, holism and person-centred practice

In being holistic in our practices, the insights and needs of the people we work with are central. The nature of our engagement impacts on whether we can engage in holistic processes and recognises that if we create barriers to therapeutic relationships, seeing and understanding people, health and context as a whole becomes challenging.

The Public Health Agency (PHA) (2017) in Northern Ireland engaged with people (10 000 voices) who accessed unscheduled care to learn from their experiences, identifying that people feel the need to be treated with courtesy, by professionals who engage authentically with them. It is full engagement that enables us to realise the interrelationship between the elements of holism for that person. Holistic care is therefore not only what we *do* but how we *are* together. Consequently, we must first attend to the conditions that affect the establishment of the therapeutic relationship, factors that are evident in the Care Environment elements of the Person-centred Practice Framework.

Factors influencing holistic provision of care

In learning about the elements of the Person-centred Practice Framework within this book, you will have considered that healthcare and your practice with an individual person (or groups of people) do not occur within a vacuum. How we practise will influence how effective we are at practising holistically. For example, attending to an injury in an emergency department without understanding the full context of the injury for that person can fragment a holistic approach if we do not work in an integrated way. The injury may be part of a pattern of events connected to social circumstances, a wider medical issue, connected to the individual's mental health and have social implications for maintaining an income, managing the care of children or being in a safe environment.

The Person-centred Processes section of the Person-centred Practice Framework identifies that we need to engage authentically, be sympathetically present and to work within a model of shared decision making (see Chapters 10, 14 and 15). We therefore need to engage with the person authentically to understand their health within the context of their life, and work with others in a supportive, positive process to facilitate them towards health. In the example given, this could include linking in with social workers to source greater support at home, or identifying aids and self-management strategies with the occupational therapist and physiotherapist to enable independence where possible. None of this occurs in isolation of working with the person to share in decision making with them, as opposed to for them. Through engaging authentically, making the time to focus on being sympathetically present, and sharing the decision-making process with others, we begin to fashion an integrated approach to care. In doing so, we seek to have full-sightedness, gaining perspective, and we foster collaborative working to provide care that acknowledges the relationship between personhood, health and care.

Being resilient is central to delivering holistic care as it underpins our ability to retain our values and principles of working. Resilience aligns to the prerequisites of the Person-centred Practice Framework in that it influences knowing self (see Chapter 4), having clarity of beliefs and values and being professionally competent. Jackson et al. (2007, p. 3) define resilience as the 'ability of an individual to adjust to adversity, maintain equilibrium, retain some sense of control over their environment, and continue to move on in a positive manner'.

Table 16.1 Enablers and inhibitors to holistic care

Enablers	Inhibitors
Knowing self, your values and principles and applying these to practice	Lack of clarity about your values and principles or not applying them to practice
Being receptive to the wider aspects of the person in your care	Responding to only a single aspect of a person's health (e.g. treating a condition rather than a person)
Engaging authentically with people to understand their perspective and experience of health, demonstrated through active listening	Not being receptive or actively listening to the person, or not engaging with them to understand (e.g. placing the responsibility on a person, who may be vulnerable, to provide this perspective)
Working with others to provide integrated care	Working in isolation
Facilitating people to be champions of their own health, facilitating empowerment and independence	Being paternalistic (e.g. doing to/for people and making decisions for them and without them)
Being resilient in order to work around challenges to holism and positively influence a culture of holism	Avoiding challenges to practices that are not holistic or changing how you practise to fit in with the culture of practice

You may encounter others in practice who do not follow through on holistic care. As a student, this can be particularly challenging as the care you witness may not live up to the values and principles you are learning. Being resilient is essential to working in adversity to influence practice and work around the challenges you encounter, to still deliver what you can towards a holistic care experience. As you develop, you will learn to advance the craft of providing holistic care and will recognise that being political and strategic in developing and advancing ways of working facilitates a wider approach to the provision of holistic care.

Leadership and being an effective change agent is central to creating a culture that enables holism to be realised in care processes. Table 16.1 provides a summary of key enablers and inhibitors to holistic care. This list is not exhaustive but should help you to focus on the key factors.

Providing holistic care

The Person-centred Practice Framework intentionally includes the 'doing' of holistic care within a person-centredness philosophy (see Chapters 1–3). The concept of holism, including its focus on personhood, should not be just a concept or ideal that we claim unless we live it out in our practice. It must become a way of working collectively, at all levels, in all contexts and with all people. This means that holistic care that supports health is about what we do, how we see and hear, how we read and listen, and how we are with people in our everyday practices. 'Health, and what makes people healthy, can only be fully understood by exploring the myriad of interactions and influences that emerge out of the complexities of human experience and the various inter-relationships of the mind, body and society' (Yuill et al. 2010, p. 14).

This is not to say it is easy; quite the contrary, as health and social care contexts and interactions are often complex. They perhaps occur in busy, resource-limited settings, and therefore prioritisation of the 'problem', 'issue' or 'symptom' becomes the focus and this culture is normalised. To give an example, a person needing assistance with attending to their personal hygiene and dressing needs will have developed a preferential way of addressing these over their lifetime. However, in a busy care setting, there may be many people who need assistance in these activities and so it is easier to go from one to the other, washing and dressing them. This is not holistic care but a practice influenced by resources (time, equipment and people). The same can occur in a busy setting where people need support to eat their meals. It is quicker to feed these people rather than take the time to facilitate them to maintain or move towards independence.

The challenge comes back to how we practise, how we live out holism. Facilitating a person to use an adaptive aid that enables independence in everyday occupations such as washing, dressing or eating may take more time today. However, we must remember that it meets their needs, is the focus of what and how we 'do and be' person-centred, and is ultimately a more effective use of time.

Upholding the holistic gaze

Working with people – in receipt of care, in teams, within systems, for the 'greater good' – is work. It takes time, energy, commitment, and continual learning and reflection on successes, failures and opportunities that could be realised. Providing holistic care within the framework of person-centredness is not an endpoint. It is a reference point for us to return to as a guide for our practice and as a foundation from which our work is built. The discussion below offers an example of responding to the broader concept of health in a specific clinical setting.

In practice – a critical reflection by a Canadian occupational therapist

On the wall of the day programme therapy room in a hospital-based eating disorder clinic was a piece of paper, a testament to the clinic's approach to care and a reflection that the illness had a far-reaching impact on many facets of daily life. The small poster mentioned:

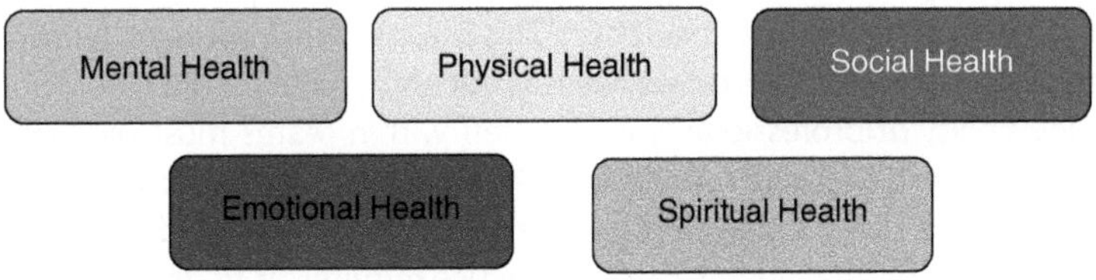

A new member of the interdisciplinary team recognised that the various therapeutic approaches offered and people from different disciplines working at the clinic embodied the first four domains. However, it was not clear where or how spiritual health was being considered. The team took its holistic care message seriously, thus the promotion of a message that was not upheld in practice became an opportunity for action. Spiritual health may not have the same centrality for all members of the team to explore within the treatment context. However, if it was considered an important aspect of health and recovery, then a duty of care existed to ensure it was being addressed and supported.

In partnership with the interfaith chaplains who provided pastoral support across the hospital, spirituality was incorporated into the group therapy programme facilitated by the occupational therapist. Its relevance and significance to the illness experience and recovery journey was respectfully acknowledged and the spiritual domain was returned to the holistic representation of health and well-being – in theory and in practice.

Words matter

Despite people in health and social care aligning themselves with holistic practice over the years, there is still a tendency for a biomedical approach to dominate. Our professions might communicate in this language and therefore we must become fluent, or at least be 'conversational' in it. It is important that you can translate this 'professional' language into words and approaches that are more widely understood and personally relevant to those you are working with. Similarly, we must also ensure that we retain holism and humanity at the heart of how we work and communicate. For instance, we work with *people* and *families* not 'unique cases' or 'conditions'. While assessment findings are documented in records with acronyms and shorthand, we need to ensure we can discuss these in other ways. They are reference points for care and not the sum total of who a person is. Furthermore, our descriptions of behaviours or responses need to be carefully considered. For example, describing someone as 'non-compliant' with a treatment approach is different than if the same person is understood to be having difficulties with the expectations/requirements of that approach.

Context matters

Why might a radiographer care about independence with dressing or a nurse about a person returning to the football pitch? Why might an occupational therapist care about antibiotic resistance? These examples reflect ways in which people delivering healthcare may acknowledge the boundaries of their scope of practice. However, our scope of practice must not limit the fullness of our view of the person. When we work holistically, we see the person 'in context', not merely within our profession-specific context. This means that each member of a team understands that their contribution exists within a system and not a hierarchy.

This understanding extends not only to the provision of holistic care to service users and families, but equally must be adopted between ourselves as persons working in health and social care (McCormack and McCance 2017). This is especially important for the demonstration of a unified value of holistic care; do we live this out and understand our contribution to holistic care? The invisibility of professional support staff within teams must be challenged. The dismissal of occupational therapists as the people who 'keep patients busy' must be challenged. The reasons behind the unanswered call bell must be challenged. The impatience with a worried family must be challenged. Holistic practice requires us to develop the attributes, skills and confidence to be that person who challenges, but does so in a way that creates momentum and fosters a culture that continues to grow in delivering on holistic practice. We are all part of the systems; we are part of the whole and we are all persons within the framework aspiring to enable health and well-being.

Activity

Using reflection, create a written journal, poetry, collage, images or alternate creative expression to consider:

- What situations you have experienced/observed that 'felt' holistic?
- What words or images reflect that 'feeling?'
- What contributed to this sense of holistic care?
- What tools enabled you to ensure that the 'whole' person is considered?

Working with a small group of your peers, review what you have created above. Discuss how well you think your reflection reflects a holistic representation of the individual, family or community? What might be overlooked? What are the strengths?

Conclusion

In this chapter we have learned about what holism is and its centrality to person-centred practice. In adapting the definition of holism by McEvoy and Duffy (2008), quoted below, this chapter has shaped a definition of care.

> Holistic care collectively embraces the mind, body and spirit of the person, in a culture of healthcare relationships that are collaborative, and grounded in harmony and healing. Holistic care is person led and focused in order to provide integrated care that is tailored to the whole of the person.

We have learned that holistic care is not an abstract concept; rather, it is a way of working and being with others. Living out holism in practice requires effort, resilience and a commitment to shaping a culture where systems and teams work in an integrated way to facilitate holistic care. It is therefore challenging to achieve holism but this challenge is superseded by facilitating positive experiences of healthcare where all involved flourish.

Summary

- Being holistic is to treat and care for a person in a way that integrates the physiological, psychological, sociocultural, developmental and spiritual dimensions of that person in an authentic, whole and insightful manner. It is person led and focused.
- Seeing those in your care as people rather than patients and establishing a therapeutic relationship with them is foundational to holistic care.
- Becoming holistic is a journey that we must embark on at the start of education and continue throughout our career. It is underpinned by the ability to be reflexive and reflective.
- Holism does not occur passively in practice; it requires leadership, critical insight and advocacy skills to create the dynamics and culture that enable holism to flourish through person-centred practices.
- In order to champion and realise authentic holistic practice, we need to be conscious of the enablers and inhibitors to holism.

References

Jackson, D., Firtko, A., and Edenborough, M. (2007). Personal resilience as a strategy for surviving and thriving in the face of workplace adversity: a literature review. *Journal of Advanced Nursing* 60 (1): 1–9.

McCance, T. and McCormack, B. (2017). The person-centred practice framework. In: *Person-Centred Practice in Nursing and Health Care – Theory and Practice*, 2e (eds. B. McCormack and T. McCance), 36–66. Chichester: Wiley Blackwell.

McCormack, B. and McCance, T. (eds.) (2017). *Person-Centred Practice in Nursing and Health Care – Theory and Practice*, 2e. Chichester: Wiley Blackwell.

McEvoy, L. and Duffy, A. (2008). Holistic practice – a concept analysis. *Nurse Education in Practice* 8 (6): 412–419.

Neuman, B. (1995). Neuman's systems model. In: *Analysis and Evaluation of Conceptual Models of Nursing* (ed. J. Fawcett), 217–276. Philadelphia: FA Davis.

Public Health Agency (Northern Ireland) (2017). *10,000 Voices – Unscheduled Care Report*. Belfast: PHA.

Woods, S. (2015). Holism in health care: patient as person. In: *Handbook of the Philosophy of Medicine* (eds. T. Schramme and S. Edwards), 1–17. Dordrecht: Springer.

Yuill, C., Crinson, I., and Duncan, E. (2010). *Key Concepts in Health Studies*. London: Sage.

Further reading

Brown, T. (2013). Person-centred occupational practice: is it time for a change of terminology? *British Journal of Occupational Therapy* 76 (5): 207–208.

McMillan, E., Stanga, N., and van Sell, S. (2018). Holism: a concept analysis. *International Journal of Nursing and Clinical Practices* 5: 282.

Michaelson, V., Pickett, W., and Davison, C. (2018). The history and promise of holism in health promotion. *Health Promotion International* 34 (4): 824–832.

SECTION 3

Person-Centredness in Health and Social Care Systems

In many ways, writing a book about person-centred concepts and theories is 'easy' and it is also relatively easy to convince the reader of the value of these concepts and theories. To many of us who have been working with person-centredness, these ways of thinking are enshrined in our ways of being. But what about our ways of doing? How easy is it to transfer the principles of person-centredness into everyday practices, in different contexts and with a variety of different factors that either help or hinder their adoption? We know from previous research that implementing person-centred principles in organisations is a challenging process and in some cases it is never really achieved. However, we also know of many individuals, teams and organisations that have successful developed health and social care cultures that embrace person-centredness. In these teams and organisations, a continuous approach to implementation is adopted and person-centred practices are normalised as everyday work. So we know it is possible and we know that many excellent examples of it do exist.

In this section of the book, we address the many different contexts in which person-centredness manifests. We have tried to embrace contexts that represent a variety of client groups (such as mental health, long-term conditions, children and maternity services) and a range of settings in which people experience health and social care (such as acute care, community, nursing homes), so as to unpick the many issues that need to be addressed. We know that whilst the 11 chapters in this section provide a rich landscape of exploration, it is not exhaustive. Given that the context of healthcare provision is always changing, it is important not to see these chapters as isolated 'stand-alone' examples, but parts of a rich landscape of health and social care that collectively illustrate how person-centred practice can be brought to life.

Fundamentals of Person-Centred Healthcare Practice, First Edition. Edited by Brendan McCormack, Tanya McCance, Cathy Bulley, Donna Brown, Ailsa McMillan and Suzanne Martin.

17

Sociopolitical context in person-centred practice

Deborah Baldie[1], Tanya McCance[2], and Brendan McCormack[3]

[1] NHS Tayside and Queen Margaret University, Edinburgh, Scotland, UK
[2] Ulster University, Northern Ireland, UK
[3] Queen Margaret University, Edinburgh, Scotland, UK

Contents

Fundamentals of Person-Centred Healthcare Practice, First Edition. Edited by Brendan McCormack, Tanya McCance, Cathy Bulley, Donna Brown, Ailsa McMillan and Suzanne Martin.

Learning outcomes

- Have an awareness of the different aspects of the sociopolitical (macro) context that impact on health and social care systems.
- Understand the potential impact of the macro context at different levels within the system.
- Identify and describe the challenges encountered by healthcare staff in operationalising person-centredness at a practice level arising from the influences of the macro context.

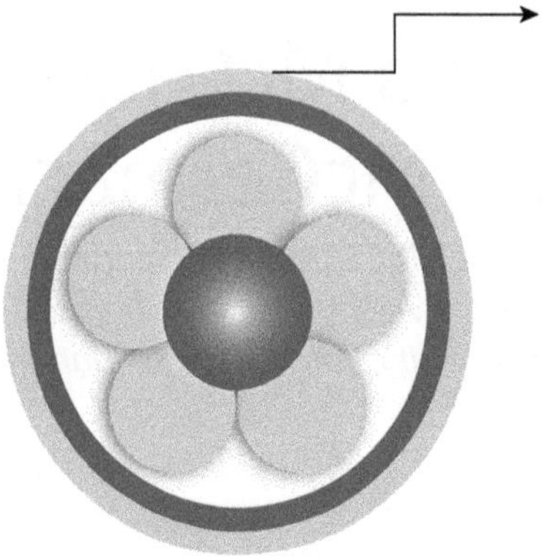

Strategic leadership: Engagement of key stakeholders in the development, implementation and sustainability of strategies for person-centred cultures.

Health and social care policy: International, national and local policies with a vision, mission and time frames to guide the development and evaluation of person-centred cultures.

Strategic frameworks: International, national and local frameworks that are focused on implementing policy directions with the intention of influencing the development of person-centred cultures.

Workforce developments: International, national and local models and frameworks that guide the development and sustainability of staffing models as well as learning and support systems for person-centred cultures.

Introduction

Engaging in person-centred practice is an intentional way of being. It operates at the individual and collective level and therefore requires individual practitioners to continually be reflexive, not only aware of their own practice but also how it can be influenced by the sociopolitical context within which they work. In the Person-centred Practice Framework, the macro context within which healthcare operates influences the development of person-centred health systems. Sociopolitical factors operate across healthcare systems, at all levels of an organisation, within and between practitioners, and between practitioners, service users and families. In the Person-centred Practice Framework, there are four key sociopolitical influencing factors that sit within the macro context. How each of these factors influences the development of person-centred cultures and practice will be explored in this chapter, alongside the implications these have for individual staff, teams and organisations.

Strategic leadership

Leadership theory has previously highlighted the power of authentic leadership (taking a values-based approach) in building effective work relationships and productivity in the workplace (Avolio et al. 2004). There is now systematic review-level evidence (Alilyyani et al. 2018) that staff outcomes are improved through authentic leadership. This leadership style encompasses many of the domains of person-centred ways of being, including working in a values-based way; enabling healthy relationships; supporting individuals and teams to flourish; and continually critiquing personal and collective practices and cultures.

Links between leadership and more distant outcomes such as patient outcomes have until more recent years been lacking. Pioneering work undertaken by Lyubovnikova (2015) in the United Kingdom has, however, demonstrated correlations between effective teams and better outcomes, including mortality. Additionally, many years of research have shown that practice development efforts aimed at enhancing person-centred cultures and care have been consistently more effective when supported by strategic leadership (Watling 2015).

Evidence supporting the positive influence of leadership is further validated through numerous examinations of care system failures. Repeatedly, the erosion of leadership values associated with person-centred practice in favour of other strategic priorities such as cost containment and meeting targets for waiting times has been cited as a core cause for such failures (Francis 2013; Godlee 2018). In such environments, over time, practitioners find it not only difficult to work in person-centred ways but increasingly difficult to provide safe care. When viewing this through the lens of the Person-centred Practice Framework, one could argue that in these cases many of the prerequisites for staff and the enabling characteristics of the practice environment were not present. Strategic leadership support for safe, effective person-centred cultures is therefore crucial to achieving person-centred practice. Strategic leaders, of course, also have responsibility to ensure the health and safety of all. Quality and health and safety are all governed by national and local policies and as such are subject to scrutiny internally within organisations and externally by regulatory bodies.

Taking a values-based approach to governing and leading healthcare organisations to provide safe working environments creates the conditions for staff to feel empowered to continually seek to enhance high standards of care and care cultures. These principles can be applied to all components of the system to ensure people are growing, learning and safe in the workplace. Through their authenticity and honesty, leaders who work in person-centred ways create an atmosphere of trust and develop relationships that build commitment and energy in themselves and others. In cultures such as this, innovation thrives, the need for control and bureaucracy decreases and outcomes for those working in such cultures and those receiving/experiencing services are improved (Laloux 2014; West et al. 2014).

Health and social care policy

In the UK and most other developed countries, health and social care are publicly funded and therefore healthcare models and provision are strongly influenced by strategic policies that set out ambitions and timelines for improved services and improved population health. Over the last decade or so, policies have increasingly included a focus on patient-centred care (see Chapter 2 for differences between patient- and person-centred care). The Health Foundation in the UK has been influential in generating support for person-centredness in healthcare organisations (Kitson et al. 2013). At a global level, the World Health Organization (WHO) has promoted person-centred approaches underpinned by human rights principles. Focusing on 'people-centred and integrated healthcare systems', the WHO has adopted a population-level approach to promoting person-centred principles in health systems design. Such influence has led to a range of person-centred focused policies such as the Patient Rights Act in Scotland (2011) (Scottish Government 2011), the national experience surveys in the USA (HCAHPs 2019), the UK (Care Quality Commission 2018) and most of Europe, and the Health and Social Care Standards for people receiving health and/or social care in communities in Scotland (Scottish Government 2016).

Previously, criticism of the approaches taken at a policy level has included their focus on patient-centred care and a lack of attention to the creation of person-centred cultures (McCormack et al. 2015). More recently, however, health and social care policies have also included ambitions that more closely relate to person-centred cultures. While that term may not be visible in such policies, they do pay attention to some core underpinning principles of person-centredness such as healthier workplace cultures and their relationship with high-quality care. Staff surveys, for example, are widely used to assess workplace cultures and thus create an opportunity for teams to reflect on and improve their cultures so they become increasingly person-centred.

So why does this matter, you might ask? Well, it matters because such policies influence the strategic frameworks within which leaders work, they influence the focus and volume of nationally supported work programmes, and in turn what strategic and operational priorities managers are asked to deliver on and demonstrate progress with. Managers therefore must pay attention to the policy framework and work with relevant stakeholders to enable and support practitioners to deliver and model care in accordance with overall ambitions. This often requires a 'taking stock' of how healthcare practice is experienced and increasingly working with the public to review and redesign services so that they better meet people's needs and preferences.

Activity

A central strategy in the development of person-centred services is that of improving the 'patient experience'. Consider what policies and frameworks are in place in your organisation that aim to ensure a positive care experience for service users and others significant to them. For example, how is service user feedback managed? What is the policy for handling complaints?

Strategic frameworks

Health and social care policies typically come with a governance framework and a strategic work programme. These are designed to enable the ambitions set within policy to become a reality in practice. While few people have formally assessed the extent to which strategic frameworks influence how person-centred organisations are, we can see patterns that highlight the significant influence of such frameworks. The work of Gerteis (1993), for example, led to an articulation of seven domains of person-centred care. This in turn was adopted by the Picker Institute in 2004 (Picker Institute 2014), used to assess person-centred practice across the US and Europe, and by the Institute of Medicine (2001) and integrated into their framework for quality – Crossing the Quality Chasm. While this has been influential in developing strategy and frameworks for healthcare, some commentators have highlighted a lack of associated governance arrangements and work programmes supporting its implementation. This, they argue, has limited the adoption of principles of person-centred practice in the everyday care that patients experience (Kitson et al. 2013).

More recently, we have seen a significant increase in such work programmes and governance arrangements that place person-centred care in a more prominent position. In the UK alone, there are more resources than ever before to help all healthcare stakeholders become more person-centred in their approach to practice. Examples of this include the Health Foundation resource on person-centred practice (The Health Foundation 2019); the Health Care Improvement Scotland resources on person-centred care and enhancing patient experience (HIS 2019);

and academic modules on working in person-centred ways or leading the development of person-centred cultures (Queen Margaret University 2019).

Despite this, there is still a significant way to go to ensure users of services are kept truly at the centre of their care. Alongside frameworks that seek to enhance person-centred cultures and care, there are those designed to increase efficiency, cut costs and reduce variability and risk. While none of those are individually bad for patient care and experience, they can work in unintended ways that do not enhance the care experience. Instead, they can limit the time that professionals have with persons receiving healthcare and curtail the choices people are offered. Furthermore, they can reinforce ritualistic routines based on the belief that such rituals are more economical and effective than those that place users at the centre of care. Many of these frameworks are tightly governed and therefore hold a higher legitimacy in services that are often increasingly subject to managerial rather than professional logic.

It is argued that for health services to become truly person-centred will require a sea change in the minds of professionals and users of services (McCormack et al. 2015). McCormack et al. (2015) suggest it is time to move away from solely person-centred care to person-centred cultures, because without this it is impossible to consistently achieve person-centred care. This will require staff at all levels to engage in systematically reviewing how they lead and work together in large interconnected systems. This will enable the development of new ways of being that give people closest to practice the autonomy to engage with service users and others to make shared decisions that are right for them and not predominantly determined by the system or the resources that they have at their disposal. However, for this to happen in a way that doesn't morally compromise staff, joined-up healthcare policy and strategic implementation plans are needed as well as effective leadership.

Activity

Building on the previous activity, locate your organisation's Patient Experience Strategy. Identify one component of that strategy (e.g. quality and patient safety priorities; patient and significant other feedback strategy) What do you see as the key challenges in your particular part of the organisation to making this component everyday practice?

Workforce developments

Workforce models adopted at national and regional levels hugely influence the ability of individual staff and teams to work in person-centred ways. Such models often use the language of 'skill mix', meaning the number of staff in a team with the requisite knowledge, skills and expertise to provide safe and effective care. Workforce models aren't just about 'numbers', though. They need to reflect the complexity of the care and treatment needs of service users in particular settings. For example, they need to include emotional support in direct care calculations; ensure sufficient time for indirect patient care activities (such as record keeping) that go beyond 'getting ready to provide care'; include time for continuous professional development; consider quality and performance data; as well as account for innovation and practice-based learning and development.

When such activities are not featured in workload models and associated assessment tools, they are not factored into staffing ratios or calculations. Time for teams to meet and reflect on their performance and how they work together is crucial to creating person-centred cultures.

Without this, it becomes very difficult to make collaborative decisions and co-design, test and evaluate improved practices. Lack of time for these activities has recently been cited by healthcare staff as a key reason for failure to improve or engage in improving services (Hignett et al. 2018). For example, 'lack of time' is often cited by staff as a reason for not being able to be person-centred in practice. Effective organisational leaders are those who work with teams to transform the workplace culture and create more time for such activity. Some have, for example changed shift patterns, changed routines in practice or used approaches to make necessary tasks leaner. Essentially, leaders who value and make quality a key work issue find the time to engage their team and as such reap the benefits in staff well-being, patient experiences and outcomes.

We have found that when leaders invest in developing the skills in staff to take a transformational learning approach to their work, the barriers previously experienced are largely overcome. Let's look at a specific case study.

Case study

Leaders in a Scottish healthcare setting providing acute inpatient care to young adults with severe mental health conditions did just that and the results were amazing. They invested in staff skills and knowledge in practice development and quality improvement. Those staff then helped the whole team collectively develop a vision and values for the service and to continually engage with the young people and their families to enhance the care experience. To enable this, the leader created three 'awaydays' per year for the whole team. This feels impossible to most managers but they ran the same 'awayday' on two consecutive days to ensure all staff were able to attend, learn and contribute. Their efforts led to increased work-based learning and reflection in practice; developing and evaluating care plans with the young people; enhanced skills across the whole team to ensure adequate access to therapy and support; and changes to roles with the creation of new role (within existing resources) for family support and a clinical academic position.

Learning in this place is not seen as privileged for some, unnecessary or routine. It is active, happening as and when challenges in practice are faced. It consists of a combination of structured times to reflect on and learn the evidence associated with issues as well as opportunistic, real-time learning in practice. An example of opportunistic learning is the use of reflective triads and dissenting voices methods. In both methods, a practitioner can seek out others during the working day to discuss an issue that is concerning them. Others are actively invited to challenge their thinking with either the dissenting voices method or a reflective triad where one person asks enabling and challenging questions of the reflector and the other provides feedback to the enabler on how they helped the person reflect. Decisions are made by the practitioner and the issue is either more deeply explored or the learning is directly applied to practice. Issues being raised are shared with the whole team in order to share learning and ensure best practice. These activities take 15 minutes and have therefore been sustainable in a busy clinical settings.

There needs to be a commitment to time for learning if such powerful and sustainable learning in practice is to be achieved. Investment in staff development of skills in facilitating reflection and a commitment by all, including strategic managers, to staff having time to consider the quality of care and treatment they provide is also essential. Doing so in the setting described above has resulted in enhanced performance on nationally agreed quality criteria (most recent external review had no improvement recommendations) and enhanced staff well-being and team working – validated by enhanced team culture scores and improved attendance at work.

Activity

What is done in your area when people don't work consistently to ensure a positive experience for service users or others – how is that addressed? Is it a learning opportunity? What could you and others do to make such instances better learning opportunities?

Developments like revalidation in nursing and midwifery in the UK are another example of change that has enabled some core learning processes, critical to person-centred practice. It has created an expectation that healthcare staff will engage in learning and development through such processes as personal reflection, seeking feedback on their technical competence and relational care from a range of people, including users of services and families, and integrating their learning into their future ways of working. It therefore theoretically helps staff to pay attention to their personal contribution to person-centred cultures and care. If holistically embraced by organisations, such a development could be a key to creating more healthful cultures (the ultimate outcome of person-centred practices). Organisations could, for example, use routinely collected data such as complaints and patient feedback to enable people to engage in collective learning and reflection on their personal practice.

Workforce developments can also be orientated to all staff and managers and not specific to those involved in direct care giving. In many developed countries, there are now work programmes aimed at creating healthier workplaces. Such programmes aim to ensure people's workplace experiences are positive and are ones where they feel treated fairly, listened to and supported. In Scotland, for example, there is the iMatter staff experience continuous improvement tool to help individuals, teams and health boards understand and improve staff experience (NHS Scotland 2019). In Ireland, there is a staff engagement programme to help leaders learn the skills to engage staff in quality improvement and a staff voices section focused on listening to and acting on staff experiences and views (HSE 2019).

Wider workforce development programmes have focused on developing a capacity for learning in large complex systems. Clinical governance, risk management, significant incident review, the IHI patient safety programme and reformed approaches to managing and responding to complaints are a few of the most significant developments in recent healthcare reform that have fundamentally shaped how we learn in the workplace; how we learn and how person-centred we are with each other and with people receiving health and social care services. Box 17.1 provides a short description of each.

We have moved into an era where we are expected to welcome critique, to examine our systems and processes to understand underlying causes for variance and errors and to work in ways that make it easier to seek and offer peer and managerial feedback. Such developments don't, of course, take immediate effect and the degree to which organisations embrace the underlying principles of adult learning and learning in the workplace is significantly moderated by the leadership and aspects of quality that are given value in an organisation.

Health and social care organisations need to invest in work-based learning. Previously, learning has been mainly the realm of educators in distinct roles but getting time away from providing clinical care to attend a clinical skills laboratory or lecture theatre is challenging and not always most meaningful. Helping clinical leaders and mentors build confidence and competence in work-based learning means learning is closely linked to practice, in real time and therefore ensures that skills and practice are developed to meet the needs of patients and families. Such an approach still requires organisational support, with educators and facilitators enabling the growth of skills in others to facilitate work-based learning See Timlin et al. (2019) for an example of how this has been undertaken in one large organisation.

Box 17.1 Approaches to developing capacity for learning in complex systems

Clinical governance

A systematic approach to maintaining and improving the quality of patient care within a health system. Normally consists of reporting mechanisms and structures to provide understanding of quality and for sharing best practice.

Risk management

A system that ensures risks to patients, staff and the organisation as a whole are identified, prioritised and managed so that their impact is reduced.

Significant incident review

An investigation process that seeks through inclusion of all stakeholders to find the reasons for a significant event (error) and to develop a plan to avoid such errors in the future. Plans normally include sharing of learning or changes in standard processes.

Institute of Healthcare Improvement [IHI] patient safety programme

An international programme with a set of measures and methods to reduce variation and harm in healthcare.

Changes to managing and responding to complaints

Processes that seek feedback proactively and enable early resolution of concerns. They also are designed to enhance and share learning through using feedback and complaints trends to identify areas for improvement and best practice.

Activity

Continue to use the example of enhancing patient experience. What is the organisational support for work-based learning at team level? What is enabling work-based learning to be usual and meaningful, and what is inhibiting this?

Positive associations between person-centred cultures and patient and staff outcomes are now well evidenced. Person-centredness is, however, not a stable state in health and social care settings. It is in a constant state of change, sometimes being positively influenced by policy, strategy, frameworks and/or workforce developments. Other times, the ability to be person-centred can be challenged by policies or frameworks that focus on things other than person-centredness, such as improving efficiency of services or rationing of budgets.

Conclusion

In this chapter, we have shared how sociopolitical developments at international and national levels influence activity in health and social care organisations. More recent developments have sought more explicitly to promote person-centred care and there are increased efforts through staff well-being programmes to improve workplace cultures. Implementing policy into practice is dependent on effective strategic and operational leadership. Authentic leaders play an important role in connecting policy, strategic frameworks and workforce developments with how teams work together, practise and thus engage with service users, families and each other.

Person-centred practice is not just a personal choice of practitioners who are driven to work in values-based ways or by those who seem particularly heroic or brave. It should be the right of every service user to receive care in ways that are meaningful to them and it should be the right of staff to be able to provide care in such ways. Being able to practise in person-centred ways is, however, significantly influenced by the contexts in which people work. Staff need to understand how to use relevant frameworks to enable their personal development, evaluate their practice and the service quality, mobilise resources to address gaps in the provision of person-centred services and align local developments so that they become not only safer and more effective but also increasingly person-centred.

Summary

- Increasingly healthcare policies pay attention to person-centred care but few pay attention to person-centred cultures.
- Authentic leaders can enable the workforce to engage with such programmes in ways that are meaningful and enhance person-centredness.
- Person-centredness is not a reality for all – some policies that aim to increase efficiency or reduce variation in practices can threaten the uniqueness of each person receiving healthcare.
- Organisations need to invest in work-based learning to enable people to continually critique how they work and how that can be changed to create person-centred cultures.
- Staff need to be aware of the strategic context in which they work and how the values of person-centredness can be enhanced.

References

Alilyyani, B., Wong, C.A., and Cummings, G. (2018). Antecedents, mediators, and outcomes of authentic leadership in healthcare: a systematic review. *International Journal of Nursing Studies* 83: 34–64.

Avolio, B.J., Gardner, W.L., Walumbwa, F. et al. (2004). Unlocking the mask: a look at the process by which authentic leaders impact follower attitudes and behaviors. *Leadership Quarterly* 15: 801–823.

Care Quality Commission (2018). *Adult inpatient survey 2018.* www.cqc.org.uk/publications/surveys/adult-inpatient-survey-2018

Francis, R. (2013). *Report of the Mid Staffordshire NHS Foundation Trust Public Inquiry.* London: Stationery Office.

Gerteis, M., Edgman-Levitan, S., Daley, J., and Delbanco, T. (1993). Medicine and health from the patient's perspective. In: *Through the Patient's Eyes* (eds. M. Gerteis, D.J. Edgman-Levitans and T. Delbanco), 1–15, 29. SanFrancisco: Jossey-Bass.

Godlee, F. (2018). Lessons from Gosport. *BMJ* 362: k2923.

HCAHPs (2019). *Patient Perspectives of Care Survey.* www.cms.gov/Medicare/Quality-Initiatives-Patient-Assessment-Instruments/HospitalQualityInits/HospitalHCAHPS.html

Health Improvement Scotland (2019). *Person-centred care.* www.healthcareimprovementscotland.org/our_work/person-centred_care.aspx

Hignett, S., Lang, A., Pickup, L. et al. (2018). More holes than cheese. What prevents the delivery of effective, high quality and safe health care in England? *Ergonomics* 61 (1): 5–14.

HSE (2019). *Leadership skills for engaging staff – Valuing Voices.* www.hse.ie/eng/about/who/qid/staff-engagement/valuing-voices/leadership-skills-for-engaging-staff-valuing-voices.html

Institute of Medicine (2001). *Committee on Quality of Health Care in America. Crossing the Quality Chasm.* Washington, DC: National Academy Press.

Kitson, A., Marshall, A., Bassett, K., and Zeitz, K. (2013). What are the core elements of patient-centred care? A narrative review and synthesis of the literature from health policy, medicine and nursing. *Journal of Advanced Nursing* 69: 4–15.

Laloux, F. (2014). *Reinventing Organizations: A Guide to Creating Organizations Inspired by the Next Stage in Human Consciousness.* Brussels: Nelson Parker.

Lyubovnikova, J., West, M.A., Dawson, J.F., and Carter, M.R. (2015). 24-Karat or fool's gold? Consequences of real team and co-acting group membership in healthcare organizations. *European Journal of Work and Organizational Psychology* 24 (6): 929–950.

McCormack, B., Borg, M., Cardiff, S. et al. (2015). Person-centredness – the "state" of the art. *International Practice Development Journal* 5: 1–15.

NHS (2019). *Scotland Staff Governance – iMatter*. www.staffgovernance.scot.nhs.uk/monitoring-employee-experience/imatter Viewed 23rd October.

Picker Institute (2014). *Discussion Paper 2 Key domains of the experience of hospital outpatients*. www.picker.org/wp-content/uploads/2014/10/Discussion-paper-. . .-hospital-outpatients.pdf

Queen Margaret University (2019). *Postgraduate programme in person-centred practice.* www.qmu.ac.uk/study-here/postgraduate-study/2020-postgraduate-courses/msc-pgdip-pgcert-person-centred-practice

Scottish Government (2011). *The Patient Rights (Scotland) Act.* www.legislation.gov.uk/asp/2011/5/contents

Scottish Government (2016). *Carers (Scotland) Act 2016.* www.legislation.gov.uk/asp/2016/9/contents/enacted

The Health Foundation (2019). *Person-centred care.* www.health.org.uk/topics/person-centred-care

Timlin, A., Hastings, A., and Hardiman, M. (2019). Workbased facilitators as drivers for the development of person-centred cultures: a shared reflection from novice facilitators of person-centred practice: critical reflection on practice development. *International Practice Development Journal* 8 (1): 8.

Watling, T. (2015). Factors enabling and inhibiting facilitator development: lessons learned from essentials of care in South Eastern Sydney Local Health District. *International Practice Development Journal* 5 (2): 3.

West M., Eckert, R., and Pasmore, B. (2014). *Developing collective leadership for health care.* www.ctrtraining.co.uk/documents/DevelopingCollectiveLeadership-KingsFundMay2014.pdf

Further reading

Lynch, B.M., McCance, T., McCormack, B., and Brown, D. (2018). The development of the person-centred situational leadership framework: revealing the being of person-centredness in nursing homes. *Journal of Clinical Nursing* 27 (1–2): 427–440.

Perlo, J., Balik, B., Swensen, S. et al. (2017). *IHI Framework for Improving Joy in Work.* Cambridge, MA: Institute for Healthcare Improvement.

The Buurtzorg Model of Care. www.buurtzorg.com/about-us/buurtzorgmodel

18

Being person-centred in the acute hospital setting

Christine Boomer[1], Bill Lawson[2], and Robert Brown[3]

[1] *Ulster University, Northern Ireland, UK and South Eastern Health and Social Care Trust*
[2] *Queen Margaret University, Edinburgh, Scotland, UK*
[3] *Western Health and Social Care Trust, Derry, Northern Ireland, UK*

Contents

Fundamentals of Person-Centred Healthcare Practice, First Edition. Edited by Brendan McCormack, Tanya McCance, Cathy Bulley, Donna Brown, Ailsa McMillan and Suzanne Martin.

Learning outcomes

- Understand the impact of the acute care environment on being person-centred in this setting.
- Recognise what constitutes person-centred moments and explore what can enable a more consistent approach to practice to enhance people's experiences of care.
- Develop an understanding of improvement methodologies and approaches utilised in acute settings to enhance the care experience and develop more healthful cultures.

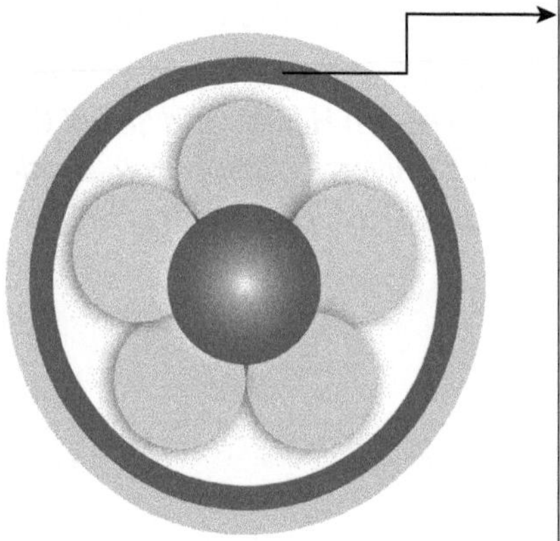

Appropriate skill mix: the number and range of staff with the requisite knowledge and skills needed to provide a quality service relevant to the context

Effective staff relationships: interpersonal connections that are productive in the achievement of holistic person-centred care

Physical environment: healthcare environments that balance aesthetics with function by paying attention to design, dignity, privacy, sanctuary, choice/control, safety, and universal access with the intention of improving patient, family and staff operational performance and outcomes (adapted from HfH 2008)

Supportive organisational systems: organisational systems that promote initiative, creativity, freedom and safety of persons, underpinned by a governance framework that emphasises culture, relationships, values, communication, professional autonomy, and accountability

Introduction

This chapter will explore person-centredness in the acute hospital setting. First, an overview of the evidence base will be shared. The idea of person-centred moments versus the consistent delivery of person-centred practice will be discussed. The practice environment has been highlighted in the literature as key in acute care, therefore attention will be given to how this domain of the Person-centred Practice Framework impacts on being person-centred in this setting. Finally, approaches that support the development of person-centred practice in acute hospital settings will be explored in relation to developing healthful cultures.

An overview of person-centredness in the acute hospital setting

McCormack et al. (2011) proposed that the biggest challenges to the development of person-centredness in acute care are the organisational culture, learning culture and the care environment itself. Hospital missions and visions express the desire to deliver person-centred care, often articulated as delivering quality, safe and compassionate care that pays attention to the patient experience. The reality experienced by service users, however, can often be quite different. This is highlighted in several public inquiries looking at failures in care, which exposed where, how and when the person-centred experience went awry (Francis 2013; MacLean 2014).

The complexity of acute contexts and the challenges associated with being person-centred in these settings are highlighted in the literature. Acute hospital environments provide challenges for staff in terms of being person-centred and for patients, families and staff in terms of experiencing person-centredness (Boomer and McCance 2017). Person-centredness in acute settings has been explored extensively in the literature, including people with long-term conditions (Burton et al. 2017), older people (Grealish et al. 2019) and people with dementia (Clisset et al. 2013). The emergent themes in this literature emphasised the positive value of person-centred practice, and the challenges in undertaking it in the acute setting.

The level of analysis of impact can focus on very specific aspects; for example, a study by Bolster and Manias (2010) focused on person-centred interactions during medicine rounds. Contextual, professional and attitudinal factors were identified as influencing the degree to which person-centred care was realised. Walker and Deacon (2016) examined nurses' experience of caring for the suddenly bereaved in adult acute and critical care settings. Their study identified barriers to establishing nurse–family relationships. These included the demands of caring for acutely ill patients; the busy environment; workforce, resource and care delivery issues. The nature and brevity of encounters between practitioners and patients led to what McCormack et al. (2011) referred to as 'person-centred moments', in contrast to occasions arising where routine practices and tasks took precedence. The practical aspects of care took priority over the wider components of holistic care. Additionally, the establishment and maintaining of a rapport with families was influenced by the organisation of care, shift patterns or personal choices involving staff. Research by Bolster and Manias (2010) highlighted that care by nurses was more orientated to task and routine and away from individualised assessment, management and patient participation. The two main reasons cited focused on communication challenges within the multidisciplinary team and time constraints.

McCance et al. (2013) described the constant tussle between conflicting priorities experienced by staff when engaged in a programme aimed at promoting person-centredness in a range of acute care settings. In fact, much of the international literature highlights the barriers to person-centred practice in acute hospitals, which include complexities and challenges in the practice environment. The impact of an unsupportive (ward) culture can be significant and may include poor staff relationships, lack of role modelling, leadership and skill mix challenges. These may be as a result of the conditions in which staff work, both in terms of the physical environment itself and the quality of the learning environment, for example, whether or not there are opportunities for reflective practice and shared practice-based learning.

Person-centred moments versus consistent person-centred practice

Evidence suggests that what people actually experience in acute hospital settings is person-centred 'moments' (McCormack and McCance 2010; McCormack et al. 2011). This can be experienced by staff as those moments when there was real satisfaction and sense of a job well done, resulting in positive feedback and well-being. Patients in acute hospitals are exposed to vulnerability in hospital wards (Laird et al. 2015). Within the acute hospital setting it has been argued that healthcare staff do not always grasp every opportunity to make their practice person-centred (Clisset et al. 2013). However, a person-centred culture needs to be in place allowing staff to experience person-centredness and be enabled to work in a person-centred way (McCormack et al. 2015). Thus, the challenge for people working in the acute setting is how we join up these individual moments to develop effective person-centred cultures. If we can start to understand what makes these moments person-centred, then we can try to promote a regular pattern within practice settings. It is argued within the person-centred literature that this can only be developed and sustained by commitment to facilitated culture change within teams and across organisations.

Activity

Building on the notion of person-centred moments, this activity aims to enable you to conceptualise what a person-centred moment looks and feels like in your field of practice. Think back to your last shift in the acute setting – were there any interactions that went well? Write down what was happening, why they were positive and person-centred. Using the Person-centred Practice Framework (if possible enlarge it) and some Post-It notes (you could get colours to match the constructs of the framework), use the notes to map your findings to the domains and constructs of the Person-centred Practice Framework.

Secondly, consider if there were any missed opportunities in relation to being person-centred during this shift. What were you (or others) doing and what was happening at these times? What could or would have made these interactions more person-centred? It may be useful to discuss this with another practitioner, your mentor/supervisor or fellow students to unravel person-centred moments further.

The impact of the practice environment on person-centredness in acute settings

The practice environment focuses on the context in which care is delivered (see Chapter 3). Within the current acute hospital setting, increasing patient acuity alongside high patient turnover is the norm. This is compounded by the effects of an ageing population with associated co-morbidities, set within an era of high public expectations and funding limitations (Kelly et al. 2019). Thus, this setting is inherently complex, with people converging in an environment that is often frenetically busy, noisy and intimidating. The complexities of the hospital environment have already been highlighted and as such, the questions surrounding the formation of the practice environment are many and varied. For example, what is deemed to be an appropriate skill mix? How are effective staff relationships developed and what actions are in place to ensure shared decision making?

Slater et al. (2015) claim that the factors needed to help develop and sustain person-centred practice are already present in acute hospitals. While this was a study focusing on nurses and midwives, the authors demonstrated that staff band (grade) and length of time in post (experience) have a positive impact on person-centred practice. This has implications where staff skill mix, experience and expertise are not at optimal levels, a situation currently faced by many professional groups in acute hospitals. Ross et al. (2015), however, raised the argument that the (nursing) profession needs to look beyond the discourse of busyness, of being short-staffed and underresourced in order to practise person-centredness. This argument was further highlighted by Nilsson et al. (2019), who stated that person-centred practice needs to be delivered despite fluctuations in staff–patient ratios.

Acute hospitals and healthcare facilities have been designed and built with clinical efficiency rather than person-centredness in mind (McCormack et al. 2011). Added to this, across the globe, acute hospital environments are changing. Increasingly, we are seeing new buildings made up of 100% single rooms, a departure from the 4–6-bed bays with a limited number of side rooms. Additionally, therapy rooms are often isolated from wards and departments. These changes to the physical environment are affecting how people experience care (Kelly et al. 2019). While the 100% single room environment raised concerns from staff regarding patient visibility and safety (Maben et al. 2015; Kelly et al. 2019), patients had an increased sense of control, privacy and satisfaction, for example by being able to go to the toilet in a single room. However, this was predicated on a recognition that the organisation of care has had to be reconfigured (e.g. intentional rounding and open visiting) to reduce the sense of isolation felt by some. Considerations for this increasingly common environmental configuration include orientating patients to the whole ward, thinking how to make rooms feel more homely and where to locate the staff bases. Multiple factors need to be recognised when maximising potential within the physical environment, including the role of shared decision making, sense of isolation for both staff and patients, balancing visibility with privacy with safety.

The experience of care and the nature of the relationships between persons will not be improved by changes to the physical environment alone. This will only take place if the engagement with culture and person-centredness has also been established. For the person-centred approach to be successful, there needs to be a change of mindset (Moore et al. 2017). Ross et al. (2015) noted that providing person-centred care takes effort, and requires a shared team and organisational philosophy of care developed from the prerequisites and practice environment. This raises the question, what can you do in your own practice environment to move beyond these perceived and actual barriers?

The focus on the relationship between persons is of course fundamental, but it is not the only association that should be considered. The Person-centred Practice Framework supposes that we should pay attention to how we develop positive relationships with others (McCormack and McCance 2017). The high level of complexity within hospitals and increasing acuity of patient care means that we work with a range of people across the multidisciplinary spectrum. Support within these teams, to include sharing responsibility and supporting each other, were key factors highlighted in enabling person-centredness (Nilsson et al. 2019). Moore et al. (2017) suggested that a power shift and a change in mindset is required, and that staff committed to person-centred practice can motivate others across professional groupings, teams and practice settings.

Looking at this through the lens of an experienced manager, we suggest that those who fulfil a leadership role in hospital settings, such as, but not exclusively, the ward manager, clinical lead or team leader, have both opportunity and responsibility to shape the culture in their setting. To do so requires an understanding of the Person-centred Practice Framework and facilitation of its application in practice. This is encouraged through establishing ways of knowing self, knowing others and an awareness of our own and others' limitations and knowing the environment. Establishing a team philosophy of person-centred practice, we believe, could help to promote consistency in care giving.

The Person-centred Practice Inventory for staff (PcPI-S) (Slater et al. 2015) offers a means for staff and teams to measure person-centred practice. Subsequently inventory findings can be used to guide team members in reflective practice, facilitate shared decision making, create healthful or therapeutic relationships and involve people in an authentic way from the onset. That initial connection affords the first opportunity and often lasting impression of the effectiveness of relationships between people. In fact, the relationships between the provision of person-centred practice and a positive experience, alongside a clear link between the provision of person-centred care and patient outcomes, was evidenced by Parlour et al. (2014) using the PcPI-S.

The role of effective leadership and facilitation in achieving a healthful ward culture is paramount. This requires leadership throughout the organisation, from the boardroom to the bedside in a way that demonstrates clarity of intent facilitated by the establishment of trust, autonomy and ways of creating innovative practices supported through learning in and from practice. To do so, the organisational system needs to be supportive at the strategic level (overcoming barriers to meaningful relationships such as conflicting priorities, working to achieve adequate staffing and resources for continuous approaches to practice development [PD]), as well as at the individual practitioner and team leader level (establishing trusting relationships, creating effective team working, enabling patients and practitioners to flourish). Leadership for person-centred practice requires persons to understand what matters to patients, families and team members. This is about acknowledging the values, choices and preferences of people, articulated by Dewing and McCormack (2017) as a certain type of nurse–patient relationship, one that is always compassionate and giving in nature.

Activity

Often when we are caught up in the busyness of everyday practice, we are unable to see what is really going on and consider the culture. In order to step back, we invite you to complete this visualisation/observation exercise.

Find yourself a quiet, safe space, get comfortable and close your eyes. Take a few mindful deep breaths, in and out, to relax and focus. Think about your busiest day in recent weeks. Now take yourself on an imaginary walk (keep your eyes closed). Go to the doors of the ward/clinic/department. Open the doors and walk in, walk around all the areas and mentally note what you see, hear, smell and feel. Once you have visited everywhere, walk back out, open your eyes and when ready note down your observations in a narrative.

Note down key elements and/or issues from your observation narrative on Post-It notes – just one per note – and stick these on the relevant domains and constructs of the framework. What are you starting to see emerge about person-centredness in the acute hospital environment?

How can we move beyond person-centred moments in acute hospital settings?

It has become clear that developing person-centred practice requires a sustained commitment to the facilitation of multiple aspects of culture change in clinical settings and organisations. Achieving sustained practice improvement and effective cultures appears to be dependent on an organisational (preferably) or at least a team infrastructure that nurtures authentic engagement with people, the ability to understand and work with challenging contexts. Key to this is engagement in active learning, the process of learning through everyday practice (Dewing 2010).

The principles of quality improvement (QI) and PD are employed as ways of working and culture development. They can be seen as vehicles of change to enhance the delivery of care. What do these methodologies contribute to the delivery of person-centred care in the acute care setting? From a QI perspective (Bowie et al. 2015), 'person-centred practice' is commonly referred to in a somewhat similar way to the definition we have become used to in the field of PD. For example, the Institute for Healthcare Improvement (IHI) articulates person and family-centred care as 'putting the patient and the family at the heart of every decision and empowering them to be genuine partners in the care' (IHI 2015). Both are continuous processes that require a sustained commitment from organisations and teams, they are dependent on skilled facilitation, are outcome driven and require an awareness of the importance of culture and context.

However, there appear to be important conceptual as well as practice improvement differences in the way in which the theory and practice underpinning PD and QI are applied. QI methodology indicates a tendency towards technical approaches to practice improvement. From this perspective, person-centred care is viewed as developing care pathways in a co-designed way with individuals, ensuring that people's preferences are understood and honoured, collaborating with people to improve engagement, shared decision making and compassionate care, and working to ensure people are supported to stay healthy and to provide care closer to home. In contrast, person-centred practice developed through an emancipatory PD approach focuses on the ongoing process of developing a person-centred culture (Manley et al. 2008). This enables individuals and teams to develop person-centred cultures where satisfaction, involvement and such things as feelings of well-being for patients, teams and families become commonplace.

In busy acute hospital settings, QI methods are utilised in a range of ways, such as to reduce the number and injury impact of people who fall or develop a pressure ulcer. A strong evidence base has emerged for how evidence-based bundle interventions and cycles of change can lead to rapid and sustained improvement (Wood et al. 2019). Taking the incidence of pressure ulcers as an example, QI methods will ensure that interventions are undertaken with patients such as a reliable assessment of risks associated with being in hospital; that they have a care plan that documents this assessment and the resulting actions required to promote their safety; and that staff receive appropriate education and training and work together to promote a safe environment of care.

The importance of person-centred PD approaches to improvement reflect the need to work with the values and beliefs of people. This focuses on understanding from the person rather than the practitioner's perspective, 'what matters to them', rather than 'this is what matters to us'. It is an approach that nurtures respect and dignity, compassion and commitment to working in a person-centred way. Working in a person-centred way, for example, to reduce the incidence of pressure ulcers will ensure the QI cycle is implemented in an individualised way, respectful of choices, beliefs and values.

Conclusion

The positive impact of person-centred practice on the delivery of care is increasingly demonstrated across a wide range of settings and specialities, including in the acute care hospital setting. The influences and challenges associated with the acute practice environment on the potential to implement and build person-centred practice are also recognised and acknowledged. This should not inhibit but, indeed, act as a spur for an organisation (ward) to examine its culture, practices and environment. This will provide the means and momentum to shape 'moments' of person-centredness into established patterns and ways of working.

Summary

- Acute hospital practice environments can lead to problem- or task-based rather than people- or person-focused approaches. Building relationships and focusing on using every interaction as an opportunity can make a real difference to the practice experience for all.
- Acute hospitals are dynamic complex organisations and we collectively need to rise to the challenge of moving beyond person-centred moments and missed opportunities within the complexities to make a concerted effort to develop healthful cultures and enhanced experiences.

References

Bolster, D. and Manias, E. (2010). Person-centred interactions between nurses and patients during medication activities in an acute hospital setting: qualitative observation and interview study. *International Journal of Nursing Studies* 47: 154–165.

Boomer, C. and McCance, T. (2017). Meeting the challenges of person-centredness in acute care. In: *Person-Centred Practice in Nursing and Health Care: Theory and Practice* (eds. B. McCormack and T. McCance), 205–214. Chichester: Wiley Blackwell.

Bowie, P., McNab, D., Ferguson, J. et al. (2015). Quality improvement and person-centredness: a participatory mixed methods study to develop the 'always event' concept for primary care. *BMJ Open* 5: e006667.

Burton, C.D., Entwistle, V.A., Elliott, A.M. et al. (2017). The value of different aspects of person-centred care: a series of discrete choice experiments in people with long-term conditions. *BMJ Open* 7 (4): e015689.

Clisset, P., Porock, D., Harwod, R., and Gladman, I. (2013). The challenges of achieving person-centred care in acute hospitals: a qualitative study of people with dementia and their families. *International Journal of Nursing Studies* 50: 1495–1503.

Dewing, J. (2010). Moments of movement: active learning and practice development. *Nurse Education in Practice* 10 (1): 22–26.

Dewing, J. and McCormack, B. (2017). Editorial: tell me, how do you define person-centredness? *Journal of Clinical Nursing* 26: 2509–2510.

Francis, R. (2013). *The Mid-Staffordshire NHS Foundation Trust Public Inquiry*. London: Stationery Office.

Grealish, L., Simpson, T., Soltau, D., and Edvardsson, D. (2019). Assessing and providing person-centred care of older people with cognitive impairment in acute settings: threats, variability, and challenges. *Collegian* 26 (1): 75–79.

Hospice Friendly Hospitals (HfH) Programme (2008). *Design and Dignity Guidelines for Physical Environments of Hospitals Supporting End of-Life Care*. Dublin: Irish Hospice Foundation.

Institute for Healthcare Improvement (2015). Overview. www.ihi.org/Topics/PFCC/Pages/Overview.aspx

Kelly, R., Brown, D., McCance, T., and Boomer, C. (2019). The experience of person-centred practice in a 100% single room environment in acute care settings – a narrative literature review. *Journal of Clinical Nursing* 28 (13–14): 2369–2385.

Laird, E., McCance, T., McCormack, B., and Gribben, B. (2015). Patients' experiences of in-hospital care when nursing staff were engaged in a practice development programme to promote person-centredness: a narrative analysis study. *International Journal of Nursing Studies* 52 (9): 1454–1462.

Maben, J., Griffiths, P., Penfold, C. et al. (2015). One size fits all? Mixed methods evaluation of the impact of 100% single-room accommodation on the staff and patient experience, safety and costs. *BMJ Quality and Safety* 25 (4): 241–256.

MacLean, L. (2014). *The Vale of Leven Hospital Inquiry Report*. https://hub.careinspectorate.com/media/1415/vale-of-leven-hospital-inquiry-report.pdf

Manley, K., McCormack, B., and Wilson, V. (eds.) (2008). Introduction. In: *Practice Development in Nursing: International Perspectives*, 9. Oxford.: Blackwell.

McCance, T., Gribben, B., McCormack, B., and Laird, E. (2013). Promoting person-centred practice within acute care: the impact of culture and context on a facilitated practice development programme. *International Practice Development Journal* 3 (1): 2.

McCormack, B. and McCance, T. (2010). *Person-centred Nursing: Theory, Models and Methods*. Oxford: Blackwell Publishing.

McCormack, B. and McCance, T. (eds.) (2017). *Person-Centred Practice in Nursing and Health Care: Theory and Practice*. Chichester: Wiley Blackwell.

McCormack, B., Dewing, J., and McCance, T. (2011). Developing person-centred care: addressing contextual challenges through practice development. *Online Journal of Issues in Nursing* 16 (2): 3.

McCormack, B., Borg, M., Cardiff, S. et al. (2015). Person-centredness – the 'state' of the art. *International Practice Development Journal* 5 (Suppl): 1.

Moore, L., Britten, N., Lydahl, D. et al. (2017). Barriers and facilitators to the implementation of person-centred care in different healthcare contexts. *Scandinavian Journal of Caring Sciences* 31: 662–673.

Nilsson, A., Edvardsson, D., and Rushton, C. (2019). Nurses' descriptions of person-centred care for older people in an acute medical ward – on the individual, team and organisational levels. *Journal of Clinical Nursing* 28: 1251–1259.

Parlour, R., Slater, P., McCormack, B. et al. (2014). The relationship between positive patient experience in acute hospitals and person-centred care. *International Journal of Research in Nursing* 5 (1): 27–36.

Ross, H., Tod, A., and Clarke, A. (2015). Understanding and achieving person-centred care: the nurse experience. *Journal of Clinical Nursing* 24 (9–10): 1223–1233.

Slater, P., McCance, T., and McCormack, B. (2015). Exploring person-centred practice within acute hospital settings. *International Practice Development Journal* 5 (Suppl): 9.

Walker, W. and Deacon, K. (2016). Nurses' experiences of caring for the suddenly bereaved in adult acute and critical care settings, and the provision of person-centred care: a qualitative study. *Intensive and Critical Care Nursing* 33: 39–47.

Wood, J., Brown, B., Bartley, A. et al. (2019). Reducing pressure ulcers across multiple care settings using a collaborative approach. *BMJ Open Quality* 8: e000409.

Further reading

Beardon, S., Patel, K., Davies, B. et al. Informal carers' perspectives on the delivery of acute hospital care for patients with dementia: a systematic review. *BMC Geriatrics* 18: 23.

Hirshon, J.M., Risko, N., Calvello, E.J.B. et al. (2013). Health systems and services: the role of acute care. *Bulletin of the World Health Organization* 9 (1): 386–388.

19

Person-centred rehabilitation

Jackie Gracey[1] and Ailsa McMillan[2]
[1] Ulster University, Northern Ireland, UK
[2] Queen Margaret University, Edinburgh, Scotland, UK

Contents

Fundamentals of Person-Centred Healthcare Practice, First Edition. Edited by Brendan McCormack, Tanya McCance, Cathy Bulley, Donna Brown, Ailsa McMillan and Suzanne Martin.

Learning outcomes

- Be able to describe how to enable person-centred rehabilitation.
- Share this understanding with others who may participate in or facilitate rehabilitation in a range of contexts.
- Be able to facilitate person-centred goal planning, while working with a person's beliefs and values.

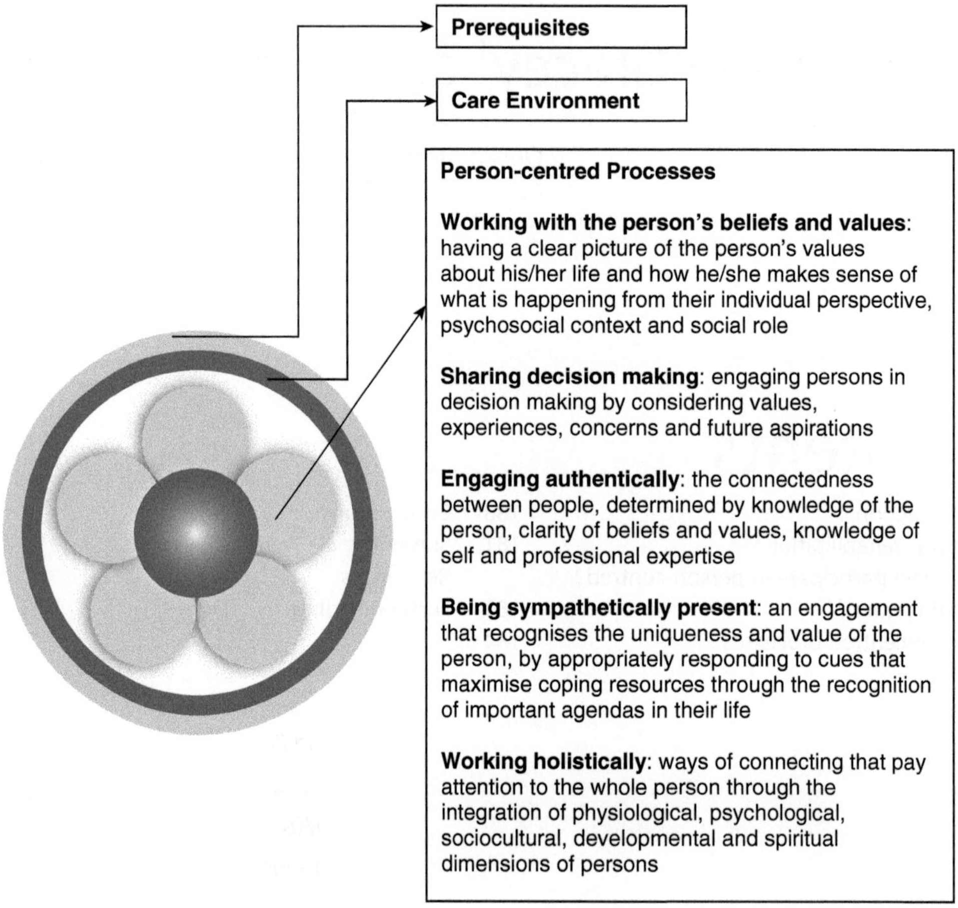

Prerequisites
Care Environment
Person-centred Processes
Working with the person's beliefs and values: having a clear picture of the person's values about his/her life and how he/she makes sense of what is happening from their individual perspective, psychosocial context and social role
Sharing decision making: engaging persons in decision making by considering values, experiences, concerns and future aspirations
Engaging authentically: the connectedness between people, determined by knowledge of the person, clarity of beliefs and values, knowledge of self and professional expertise
Being sympathetically present: an engagement that recognises the uniqueness and value of the person, by appropriately responding to cues that maximise coping resources through the recognition of important agendas in their life
Working holistically: ways of connecting that pay attention to the whole person through the integration of physiological, psychological, sociocultural, developmental and spiritual dimensions of persons

Introduction

This chapter will introduce the concept of person-centred rehabilitation and consider how it can be facilitated in any work environment. We will specifically focus on the person-centred processes in rehabilitation, but we will also consider how the prerequisites and care environment influence practice. In Chapter 3 the idea of person-centredness as humanistic caring with therapeutic intent was articulated and in the context of rehabilitation, the relationships developed with people will influence the outcome of their rehabilitation. We will guide you through some reflections that will help you understand this connection between relationships and rehabilitation practices. In addition, the chapter will identify different interventions and models relevant to rehabilitation practice; we are sure you will experience or identify some synergy between these interventions and models and the Person-centred Practice Framework. This will help you reflect on being person-centred in your practice. We will share some ideas about definitions of rehabilitation, use the person-centred processes as a framework to help increase understanding of person-centred rehabilitation, provide vignettes to illustrate person-centred rehabilitation and offer some critical questions for reflection.

What is rehabilitation?

The World Health Organization (WHO) defines rehabilitation as:

> a set of interventions needed when a person is experiencing or is likely to experience limitations in everyday functioning due to ageing or a health condition, including chronic diseases or disorders, injuries or traumas. (WHO 2017)

There are many other definitions of rehabilitation based on, for example, the Social Model of Disability or the International Classification of Functioning (ICF) (Dean et al. 2012) and individual professions will provide more detailed definitions or examples of their role in rehabilitation. The Social Model of Disability was developed in the 1970s and 1980s by people who have a disability. It recognises that barriers to participation occur within communities rather than the person and can be viewed through an environmental, attitudinal, communication or organisational lens. For example, a person who is unable to manage their finances independently because all banking is electronic should be enabled to do this in other ways, perhaps through support from financial institutions or care agencies. People who are labelled by society and the subsequent challenges or assumptions they may face as a consequence of this can prevent or minimise participation in activities.

The ICF is used to consider a person's health and functioning in association with personal and environmental factors. Rehabilitation practitioners don't ignore what illness or injury may have caused the disability, but they don't privilege it either. This is a different approach from the medical model which would privilege the disease or injury over the person.

However, defining rehabilitation is as challenging as catching a wave yet when you catch the wave the outcome can be exciting and transformational. Person-centred practice captures all that is essential in rehabilitation. Co-production of goals with a person is fundamental and key to rehabilitation.

The evolution from the medical model of disability (seeing the person as the 'problem') to the social model (seeing the person as the solution) is a welcome move in our practice. The biopsychosocial model may be one that you are familiar with, therefore engaging with the Person-centred Practice Framework will, we hope, feel like a natural progression. Being able to consider rehabilitation in concert with human flourishing (which was presented in Chapter 5) could move us from thinking of the success of rehabilitation being defined by recovery or getting 'back to normal' in a physical sense, to the growth of the person from a psychological perspective (Buetow 2019; Buetow et al. 2020). Acknowledging the loss or difference a person may feel or experience and enabling them to engage positively with this may be one aspect of flourishing in the presence of challenges. If we recognise and engage with the psychological conditions apprehension, appetite, attitude, ambiguity, autonomy, accountability and ambiopia, we could co-design interventions and ultimately optimise human flourishing (Buetow et al. 2020).

The challenge of defining the goals for rehabilitation and establishing the individual's perception of their needs is central to our role in rehabilitation. Remember that many people will benefit from rehabilitation whether they have a life-limiting illness such as cancer or motor neuronedisease, a degenerative condition such as Parkinson's disease or dementia or an acquired injury or illness such as a brain injury or trauma.

Practice environment

You might think that rehabilitation only takes place in specialist rehabilitation centres or by staff who have received a specialist qualification in rehabilitation practice. However, the reality is that all of us can and do participate in and enable rehabilitation. When we work with a person to co-design interventions that will address their impairments, activity limitations and restrictions, enabling them to live a full and active life in the way they want to live it, we are engaging in rehabilitation practice. Rehabilitation can take place in primary, secondary or tertiary services, in a person's home, place of employment, or leisure spaces. The practice environment can therefore be anywhere and with a whole range of different constructs. For example, the decision-making and staff relationships may be with a person's employers or in a third sector organisation.

Getting to know someone, engaging with their beliefs and values and sharing decision making is fundamental to the positive outcomes of rehabilitation. The key consideration is for the multiprofessional team to work together in partnership with the person. For some people, their rehabilitation goal may be to return to their previous level of function and for others it may be more complex. Opportunities may emerge that would not be predicted and creatively addressing challenges and thinking beyond the obvious can lead to flourishing. Ultimately, the aim is to enhance the person's quality of life through shared decision making, active listening and personalised goal setting (Gracey et al. 2016).

Activity

As we progress through the next section, we will consider some of the questions in relation to Ewan and his family.

Ewan was diagnosed with multiple sclerosis six months ago and has been in a rehabilitation unit for assessment for the last two weeks. He is ataxic, has altered sensation in his hands and when he gets tired his speech is dysarthric. He lives in a first-floor flat with his husband Neil and their 4-year-old daughter Eilidh. Ewan is a primary school teacher in the town where they live while Neil is self-employed and works from home. Ewan enjoys cooking, painting and park running, amongst other activities. He is keen to be discharged home and wants to talk with you about returning to work and his relationship with Neil. Ewan is feeling guilty about the anxieties Neil has expressed but doesn't want him to fuss. Ewan wants to return to work as soon as possible and has asked you to help him work out how to do this.

Who can participate in person-centred rehabilitation?

There is not a defined list of people who would be involved in rehabilitation. The person and those important to them are key. The seamless working of interprofessional teams is the key component in effective person-centred rehabilitation. Thereafter, any professionals, volunteers or representatives from the community might participate in setting and facilitating rehabilitation goals. We would encourage you to always think of what you can do as an individual and as part of the team to facilitate rehabilitation. Remember that sometimes making small changes to the environment can make a significant difference to a person's independence. So, for example, ensuring the person can reach their belongings, setting up a space to enable a person to be independent, taking time to be with a person rather than rushing to do something for them are all rehabilitative practices. An occupational therapist and nurse may collaborate to enable a person to be independent in their personal care, but they may also work together with a person to plan their return to employment or parenting.

For example, if Ewan developed issues with his continence, the nurse, occupational therapist and physiotherapist might consider the influence his work environment may have – if there are two hours between breaks in teaching, can Ewan remain continent for that time or is his classroom near a toilet? If he is tired and the pupils struggle to understand him, what other resources might help, can the order of the day be adjusted to help? Take some time to consider which of the lenses of the Social Model of Disability could inform goal setting for Ewan and how you might start a conversation about the goals.

An occupational therapist, psychologist and social worker may work with Ewan and Neil to support ongoing rehabilitation at home. If you blend your knowledge of multiple sclerosis with Ewan's beliefs and values, you can work together to use the person-centred processes to set goals. Ewan and Neil had hoped to have another child but they are now concerned about how the family will manage. Think about the conversations you might have with them all.

We should try not to be inhibited by a predefined list of people who may be able to engage in rehabilitation. Teams and communities vary and can offer a range of opportunities for activities and support for people. Third sector organisations often supplement and complement tertiary services and participants in rehabilitation.

Activity

Think about the community you live in and the different activities you participate in. How do you think this would change if you were unable to attend the group or participate in the activity? How could the activity or environment be adapted and who might you ask to help with this?

The scope of rehabilitation is dependent on the people involved in it. How each person views their 'disability' or the things that restrict their participation in activities is unique. In the same way that person-centredness does not pathologise people, widening the concept of rehabilitation to include human flourishing as an unconscious outcome could enhance our experiences and complement our practice (Buetow et al. 2019). Successful and effective rehabilitation is reliant on a person being in control of their priorities and maximising their strengths. The person needs the opportunity in an empathetic environment to be listened to and to set their personal goals through shared decision making. Person-centredness embodies this and to achieve it, we should strive to understand the person's perspective, share power and responsibility, and develop therapeutic alliances with persons receiving services (Bishop et al. 2019). To help make this a reality, we draw upon the 'person-centred processes' of the framework described in Chapter 3.

Person-centred processes

Working with a person's beliefs and values in rehabilitation

In Chapters 2 and 3, you were encouraged to consider ways of getting to know people and develop an understanding of what person-centredness is. A person's beliefs and values are a core component of the approach you can use to help persons create rehabilitation goals. You might do this by encouraging them to share what is important to them and talk about the roles they have in life and how they participate in them. Your skills of noticing and attending to a person's narrative will help you ask questions. Goals can seem small or large, short term or long term. If we think about Ewan, being curious and interested in his life and his roles will help you identify together what his goals might be and how they can be achieved. Ewan might ask you about his sexual and sensual relationship with Neil – think about how you might respond. If he has been courageous enough to discuss this with a relative stranger, how would you engage authentically with Ewan?

If a person has participation limitations, this may prove increasingly challenging, therefore working with others who are important to that person can make a difference. There is of course a unique balance to be reached between privacy, insight and ethics. Who has the right to speak on behalf of another person? How do we know we are doing what is best? If a person shares goals that seem to be unreasonable or unsafe, how can we work together? A person may have cognitive impairment and, as a consequence, limited insight into their needs and safety. Understanding what might influence cognitive functioning and any legislation about supporting people who have impaired capacity is essential in rehabilitation. Taking time to get to know a person is a critical part of successful rehabilitation and creating an appreciation of their connections and relationships will add value to that experience.

Being able to invite a person to share their narrative is far more satisfactory and beneficial than systematically completing the questions on an admission document. For example, the documentation may ask you to identify if a person is at risk of falling and to do this categorise intrinsic, extrinsic and behavioural risk, yet the fear of falling is also important. Taking time to actively listen to a person and notice any fear will enrich your assessment and relationship with them. In rehabilitation settings, a person will often share much more about themselves and for us, this is a great privilege. One of the great joys of rehabilitation practice is pushing the boundaries while developing and maintaining a therapeutic alliance. The notion of a therapeutic alliance emerges from psychodynamic theory and represents the unique constellation of personal connections, professional and family collaboration (Bishop et al. 2019). This alliance or relationship is as nuanced as each person's beliefs and values, yet the benefits can have a positive influence on outcomes.

Shared decision making in rehabilitation

Sharing decisions is not just about being together when a decision is made or inviting a person to a goal-setting meeting. As you develop communication skills that become increasingly facilitative and enabling, then any person is more likely to participate in conversations and therefore decision making. As we create person-centred cultures, communication and team-work can develop and positively influence decision making. Relationships with people during rehabilitation can create many challenges, not least when there may be a conflict of interests, wishes or ethical considerations. Being able to hold the space in these moments can be challenging and impact on our relationships with persons in our care. Think about a time when you have advocated for a person even though their wishes may have been in conflict with your own beliefs and values.

McCormack and McCance (2010) discuss the three stances of engagement that professionals may experience in their relationship with a person: full engagement, partial disengagement and complete disengagement. In rehabilitation, if you are fully engaged with a person, partnership exists and collaboration between you and them is fluid and reflects both your values. You are aware of external influencers but are able to blend them with your practice. However, if a dilemma emerges then you may move to partial disengagement while you consider the disruption, then to complete disengagement to create space to critically reflect and consider re-engagement. The movement between these three stances will enable you to engage in critical reflexivity, consider the ethical implications of your practice and remain connected with a person's beliefs and values.

Activity

Read this short history and take some time to consider the conversations you might have with Stevie and his parents to enable Stevie to meet his goals. Think about the relationships and Stevie's rights as a person.

> Stevie is 19 and has just finished second year at university. Three months ago, he was celebrating the end of exams with his friends when he fell from a wall. Stevie fractured his femur and sustained a moderate traumatic brain injury. The rehabilitation team have said that Stevie would manage back at university with some support. He will also have ongoing community rehabilitation. Stevie wants to live in the flat he shares with his friends and return to university in September. His mum and dad want him to stay in the family home and take a year out. Some of the team feel that Stevie should live with his parents, but he asked you how you would feel having to go back home and not have your own space and this has made you think.

If you were supporting Stevie, you might believe that returning home to his parents would be unhelpful as he would lose his independence, go back a year in university and have to get to know a whole new cohort, yet being at home might mean he would eat well, his parents would take him to appointments and encourage him to participate in rehabilitation activities. Living in a flat with his mates might mean that he has good company and fun, continues with his studies and doesn't lose his friends group, or he might disengage from rehabilitation, go to parties, drink alcohol and take risks. Our own life experiences and roles may influence our decision making so stepping back and looking in on a situation can help us ask challenging and enabling questions. Being aware of the assumptions we make about people and situations will also help in decision making.

Engaging authentically

Engaging authentically in rehabilitation is a complex process, but essentially it encourages us to be ourselves. Yet in practice we are required to be professional and sometimes discouraged from becoming attached to a person. We are sure you will have had experiences that bring to the surface your profession's code of conduct and duty of candour and the ethical implications of breaching this.

The early chapters of this book will help you understand personhood and person-centredness, while Chapter 13 will guide you through engaging meaningfully and effectively. Being able to balance all these concepts and responsibilities requires us to engage authentically with each other and ourselves, acknowledging the uniqueness of each person in relationships and creating the conditions for rehabilitation to take place.

Activity

Imagine you are invisible and able to walk around your place of work unnoticed. Listen to the way that everyone is speaking to each other, no matter who they are. Think about the words that they use and the way they speak. Are they kind? Are people listening? Then think about yourself and write a description of how you communicate. What assumptions do you make, what words do you use, what does your communication look and sound like?

It may be helpful to draw or create a visual picture of your thoughts and feelings at the end of this activity. Stepping back from our culture and paying attention to what we see, hear and imagine might be going on is a helpful way to reflect on our practice. What might other people feel when they step into our place of work? Do we welcome them in, or do we reach out?

Being sympathetically present

Having a sympathetic presence is described as 'an engagement that recognises the uniqueness and value of the individual, by appropriately responding to cues that maximise coping resources through the recognition of important agendas in daily life' (McCormack 2001). The material in Chapter 15 will inform your understanding of sympathetic presence and its influence in rehabilitation. Being sympathetically present in rehabilitation is about being alongside and working with a person, their values and beliefs and their goals. In rehabilitation, we don't 'do to' or 'do for' a person, therefore the time spent in doing activities or being with a person can be far greater but can result in a person developing a new independence in an activity, being enabled to generate their own solutions and have a sense of ownership of their recovery or improvement.

Working holistically

Working holistically in rehabilitation requires us to consider the physiological, psychological, sociocultural, developmental and spiritual dimensions of persons. You may already have some knowledge of human development and have encountered the work of, for example, Erikson as he described the different life stages. If these stages are interrupted by illness or injury, we must still consider the dimensions of a person when engaging in rehabilitation practice. How we develop and progress through different ages and stages of life varies according to our individual priorities and life plan.

Different professions use different models; for example, the Canadian Model of Occupational Performance and Engagement (CMOP-E) (www.thecopm.ca) or the Model of Human Occupation (MOHO) (www.moho.uic.edu/default.aspx) are occupational therapy conceptual models that can be used in a variety of contexts (e.g. palliative care or neurological rehabilitation). Both these models are centred on what is important to the person and when used by practitioners, will enable a broad and integrative analysis of human occupation.

The recovery model used in mental health nursing and psychology is focused on the person and the idea of connectedness, social support and the individual's strengths. A different approach to assessment is the FIM + FAM measure; this is used by multiprofessional teams to assess neurological disability and can then be used as a framework to create goals and plan activities and interventions with a person. You will notice when you look at these models or measures that they also talk about holistic practice, empowering people and valuing their stories. These approaches are central to rehabilitative practice and can inform your practice. Many organisations require regular audits to be completed, then use the results (metrics) to demonstrate success or failure. As you engage with any of these approaches, take time to remember the person who is central and consider the results in context.

Conclusion

Rehabilitation is as much about the way we are with people as it is about a 'thing' that we do; it is more than words and actions. Knowing ourselves and knowing others will enable consideration of the assumptions we make about illness or injury and what people experience. Spending time enabling a person to create their own goals ultimately pays dividends as each person is able to adopt a stepwise approach that resonates with their life experiences, potentials, ambitions, dreams and desires and ultimately helps them to flourish as a person. Human flourishing as a concept is not often associated with rehabilitation, but as we have unpacked in this chapter, positively engaging and involving the person with the opportunities that emerge from illness or injury can create person-centred outcomes. Engaging with the preconditions that influence adjustment and cultivating character strengths in people can create ideal conditions for flourishing in rehabilitation for all involved (Buetow 2019).

Summary

- The constructs of the Person-centred Practice framework and specifically the person-centred processes can be used to frame rehabilitation practice.
- Rehabilitation is a complex process that is most successful when everyone is enabled to be engaged in the process.
- Models, frameworks and assessments are helpful structures to inform goal setting.
- It can take time and requires us to be with a person, using the concepts of engagement to enable rehabilitation and reflexive practice.
- If we notice the opportunities for human flourishing within our rehabilitation practices, there may be more positive outcomes.

References

Bishop, M., Kayes, N., and McPherson, K. (2019). Understanding the therapeutic alliance in stroke rehabilitation. *Disability and Rehabilitation* https://doi.org/10.1080/09638288.2019.1651909.

Buetow, S.A. (2019). Psychological preconditions for flourishing through ultrabilitation: a descriptive framework. *Disability and Rehabilitation* https://doi.org/10.1080/09638288.2018.1550532.

Buetow, S.A., Kapur, N., and Wolbring, G. (2020). From rehabilitation to ultrabilitation: moving forward. *Disability and Rehabilitation* 42: 1487–1489.

Buetow, S.A., Martinez-Martin, P., and McCormack, B. (2019). Ultrabilitation: beyond recovery-oriented rehabilitation. *Disability and Rehabilitation* 41 (6): 740–745.

Dean, S.G., Siegert, R.J., and Taylor, W.J. (eds.) (2012). *Interprofessional Rehabilitation: A Person-Centred Approach*. Chichester: Wiley.

Gracey, J.H., Watson, M., Payne, C. et al. (2016). Translation research: 'Back on Track', a multiprofessional rehabilitation service for cancer-related fatigue. *BMJ Supportive & Palliative Care* 6: 94–96.

McCormack, B. (2001). *Negotiating Partnerships with Older People: A Person-centred Approach*. Oxford: Routledge.

McCormack, B. and McCance, T. (2010). *Person Centred Nursing: Theory and Practice*. Chichester: Wiley.

World Health Organization (2017). *Rehabilitation: key for health in the 21st century*. www.who.int/disabilities/care/KeyForHealth21stCentury.pdf?ua=1

Further reading

www.scope.org.uk

https://journals.sagepub.com/toc/crea/23/4

20

Being person-centred in community and ambulatory services

Caroline Dickson[1] and Lorna Peelo-Kilroe[2]

[1] *Queen Margaret University, Edinburgh, Scotland, UK*
[2] *Health Service Executive, Dublin, Republic of Ireland*

Contents

Fundamentals of Person-Centred Healthcare Practice, First Edition. Edited by Brendan McCormack, Tanya McCance, Cathy Bulley, Donna Brown, Ailsa McMillan and Suzanne Martin.

Learning outcomes

- Recognise the practice contexts within the community as rich learning environments.
- Understand what matters to you as a learner within the community.
- Consider the stepping stones to enable you to be your best self in practice.
- Appreciate community contexts as flourishing workplaces.

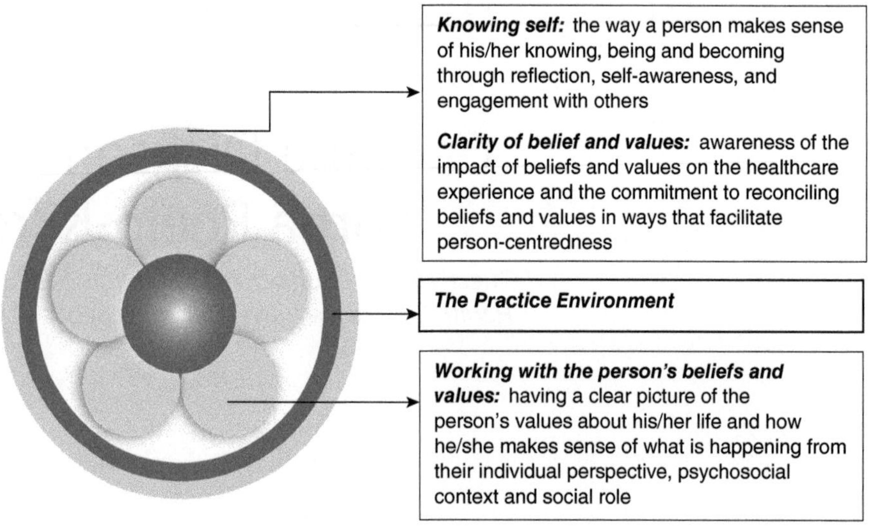

Knowing self: the way a person makes sense of his/her knowing, being and becoming through reflection, self-awareness, and engagement with others
Clarity of belief and values: awareness of the impact of beliefs and values on the healthcare experience and the commitment to reconciling beliefs and values in ways that facilitate person-centredness
The Practice Environment
Working with the person's beliefs and values: having a clear picture of the person's values about his/her life and how he/she makes sense of what is happening from their individual perspective, psychosocial context and social role

Introduction

Community learning contexts are varied across health, social care and the third sector. In the community, you will be part of teams which have an impact on people's lives across the lifespan. Helping people to keep a sense of health and well-being requires autonomous practitioners who can enable people to be the best they can be. To do this, practitioners also have to be the best they can be. The aim of this chapter is to explore how you can use the experience of learning in community contexts to be your best self. This links specifically to the prerequisites in the framework, *knowing self, clarity of beliefs and values* and *the practice environment*. When reading this chapter you may want to also refer to chapter 4 (knowing self), chapter 12 (working with persons' beliefs and values) and chapter 13 (engaging meaningfully and effectively)

Guiding you through some transformative learning processes, and through exploration of community contexts, we encourage you to notice how people engage together and how your values resonate with the public health values that underpin community practices. We hope to inspire you to be the best you can be and consider how you can contribute to flourishing workplaces through a range of activities. Our aim is to help you think about the conditions necessary for you to flourish so that people within the service will flourish also. A healthful culture, the outcome of the Person-centred Practice Framework, is one where everyone experiences human flourishing.

The rich learning environments in community contexts

Inequalities in health are most obvious in community contexts which can provide rich and dynamic learning environments. Taking time to notice determinants of health gives insight into factors influencing people's health across the lifespan. It gives justification for the strengths-based and salutogenic approaches as well as community development activities you may experience and develop. Salutogenesis means health creating (Cowley et al. 2015), whilst strengths based means helping others draw on their existing strengths to promote well-being. Contemporary healthcare is married with social care in the integrated macro context (discussed in more depth in Chapters 3 and 17), providing diverse learning and support opportunities. While your experience in community or ambulatory services may include working alongside community nursing teams such as community mental health or midwifery teams, district nurses, health visitors, school nurses, care home nurses and public health nurses, your practice educator or supervisor and colleagues may be allied health professionals (AHPs). They may be a physiotherapist, occupational therapist or dietician, a social worker or a healthcare worker from a third sector organisation.

The environment of community practice is continuously evolving in response to societal and political needs and expectations. Health policy and professional reforms are having an impact in terms of helping people to stay at home or as near home as possible. The complexity of the community can make it difficult to identify a specific workplace. In reality, many people in ambulatory and community services operate across a multiplicity of workplaces, including clinics, primary care centres, acute units, community hospitals and GP practices, as well as a range of residential settings. Practitioners interact with a diversity of other professionals outside health and social care, for example in third sector organisations, education, voluntary services, police, fire and safety, legal or pharmaceutical services. A move towards advanced practice in the community means you may expect to observe acute care and support in the community as well as supporting people with long-term conditions. This is aimed at keeping people in their own home as far as possible, and avoiding unnecessary hospital admissions. Allied health practitioners, some specialist nurses and community workers have a specific rehabilitation focus in their work. Third sector partners focus on well-being and resilience building, specifically addressing health inequalities. All practitioners have a role in preventing ill health, taking opportunities for early intervention and enabling self-management.

Working in interagency teams may mean practitioners identify with a unidisciplinary core team but work interdependently with a range of other people or professional groups/teams. They are able to do this through communication, shared records, multidisciplinary meetings and case conferences. They are also supported, in some countries like the UK, by joint integrated health and social care organisations. Services are co-located in some areas but quite separate in others. Joint working and integrated organisational systems provide a platform for shared decision making. You may consider how practitioners build working relationships across traditional service boundaries and the effectiveness of such an approach. You may also think about how this context supports the potential for innovation and risk.

Knowing what matters to you being in the community

You have perhaps been asked many times why you have chosen your discipline. The answer may focus on your desire to develop technical skills such as planned interventions, prescribing treatments, giving injections, administering intravenous fluids and drugs or taking blood pressures. Perhaps it is because you like to participate in care or rehabilitation of someone who has experienced trauma. You may know that you are a caring person and want to help people get well. 'Knowing yourself' concerns understanding your values, or what is important to you. This is important because values determine what we feel ought to be done and shape the beliefs we hold and how we express ourselves. They are fundamental to who we are. You will notice that when you encounter something that is at odds with your values, you experience an emotional reaction. This is a trigger to ask questions and engage in reflection and is something you should pay attention to.

One value you hold could be that practitioners are experts and know best. You might think all people have the right to be respected as individuals and are capable of making decisions that are best for them. If your values are the former, then you may believe that 'doing to and for patients' is best. You might also make the assumption that expertise and giving care improve the care experiences and outcomes for people. If you hold the value of respecting people as self-determining individuals, then a belief might be that people should be provided with the opportunity to work in partnership with professionals to make their own choices. The assumption you might therefore make is that people will be active participants in their own care and a professional's role is to engage in shared decision making with the person.

These assumptions of course may or may not be true, and may be a practice that is taken for granted. These are again triggers for you to ask questions. Be mindful, because values and beliefs create culture. Cultures that promote healthfulness prioritise people rather than disease processes or systems. This means that everyone's point of view is valid – practitioners, service users and families.

Shared values can be turned into collective action. In 1998, the World Health Organization made a declaration that globally there should be health for all by 2021. The declaration identified core public health values, upon which each country would build its public health policy (Figure 20.1). These 'healthy public policies' commit to promoting the health of populations through such measures as:

- reducing inequalities in health
- giving children a healthy start in life
- promoting health and well-being across the lifespan
- including mental health
- working with people and communities to build social capital and target groups such as those hard to reach.

The result is a move from treatment and cure, centred around acute hospitals, to helping people stay at home or as close to home as possible, thus avoiding unnecessary hospital admissions.

Public Health Values

- *Equity and social inclusion*
- *Participation, collaboration and community empowerment*
- *Social justice and health as a human right (World Health Organisation 1998)*

Figure 20.1 Public health values.

Activity

To think about what matters to you and how it connects with the team's shared vision, read the WHO European Health Report (2018) Capturing the Health 2020 Core Values: https://www.euro.who.int/en/data-and-evidence/european-health-report/european-health-report-2018/report-by-chapters/chapter-3-capturing-the-health-2020-core-values.

Identify the updated and extended public health values and discuss public health values with your peers and colleagues. Find out what the shared vision of the team is in your practice area. If this is not explicit, ask practitioners about their vision.

Consider how shared values are influencing service user experiences of care. How do they align with public health values? What lessons are you learning about how practitioners are engaging with people within the community and how does that reflect your own values as a practitioner?

The public health ambitions are being tackled in a range of ways. Community practitioners understand the health needs of their populations and know their communities well. They find this out by community profiling. This helps teams respond to health needs, signposting people to appropriate services. This new public health is also achieved by a change in the attitude of professionals and people in society. In the past, professionals were generally viewed as experts and people as passive recipients of care. Today, professionals work with people, enabling them to play their part in their own well-being. They signpost people to resources that lie within communities, encouraging them to be active in contributing to healthy communities. All practitioners working in the community have a role to play in creating a culture of healthfulness with people across the lifespan. This is achieved through:

- resilience building
- promoting healthy lifestyles
- enabling self-care
- building social capital
- ensuring visibility and accessibility of services.

Stepping stones to enable you to be your best self in practice

There are many things to pay attention to whilst working in community and ambulatory services. By focusing on aspects such as working in practice environments that are not clinical settings, establishing clear boundaries with people, working collaboratively and working in person-centred ways, you can be your best self. Non-clinical community settings such as domiciles change practitioners' status from staff to 'guest'. This creates a different power dynamic from other areas, particularly inpatient or clinic settings. You may be used to a workplace where staff in general have control (power) and the people using services have visitor status. Being in someone's home creates a power-sharing dynamic. Being the visitor creates more of a power balance, which is conducive to enabling relationships. Notice how practitioners create this power balance, how they work with people's beliefs and values to understand what is important to them. You may be surprised to discover that what is important to people may be very different from what the practitioner thinks is important. Consider why this might be. Think also about how practitioners identify people's strengths and help them to use these to stay well.

It is important to build mutual trust and promote co-operative and safe relationships with people that enable safe working practice. Establishing clear boundaries is an important aspect of this. Boundary negotiations may include, for example, initial previsit introductory contact, establishing the purpose of visit, negotiation of anticipated outcomes and clarity around responsibilities for equipment, as entry is by invitation and the person always has the right to refuse entry or services whether agreed or not. During the visit/consultation, ensuring there is a shared understanding around expectations helps reduce any differing or unrealistic expectations that could arise. Expectations may already have been negotiated, but it is helpful to be familiar with what is expected of you and what you can expect if you are in learning experience as part of a programme. Your supervisor or assessor will be there to support you during this time and together you can develop a supportive environment where you can safely discuss expectations and share concerns and issues you may have. You will also have support from other members of the team, building a safe supportive learning environment for your placement and your learning goals.

Murphy et al. (2012) suggest that students find it easier to fit into the community than the inpatient practice cultures. This may be because of the collaborative ways of working, not only with other professionals but with service users and their families too. You will find you have a chance to build relationships and get to know people. Notice how these close relationships promote shared decision making, how care is co-produced and how partnerships are developed with people living in the community. As a learner in the community, you will be supported by a practice educator or supervisor and will be expected to seek out learning opportunities that match your intended learning. When you are in the community, arrange to spend time with interagency team members and note their role and responsibilities. Notice their interactions with others and how organisational systems enable these interactions. Think about their approach to care giving.

Working in person-centred ways means working with loving kindness. The aim of any relationship you will have is to be healthful. Healthfulness is a characteristic of person-centred environments and person-centred cultures are collective responsibilities. However, you may observe that not everyone is person-centred and not all workplaces support person-centred practice. Where you notice kindness, think about the impact it has on the quality of relationships as well as care outcomes. If you notice the opposite, how does that impact on healthful relationships? The interactions and relationships that enable flourishing (helping people to be the best they can be) will have a positive effect on workplace cultures. In fact, evidence suggests that enabling people to flourish in their workplaces benefits both individuals and teams. Benefits include improved interpersonal relationships, feelings of self-worth and productivity (Gaffney 2011; Henrekson 2014; McCormack and Titchen 2014; Phelps 2013; Seligman 2011; Titchen 2009; Titchen and McCormack 2010; Yalden and McCormack 2010). Loving kindness can enable human flourishing. This, you will notice, is demonstrated by the value placed on staff relationships, another characteristic of a person-centred practice environment. Loving kindness can be achieved in part by balancing the judgements we make about each other with mercy or kindness so that there is equilibrium between both. Some judgement is always necessary as it is linked to practical wisdom and experience of life. But if it significantly outweighs kindness, judgement becomes autocratic and oppressive. Equally, when kindness is overly dominant in the absence of judgement, practice becomes ineffective.

Community contexts as flourishing workplaces

Consider the Practice Environment domain within the Person-centred Practice Framework. You will see that one characteristic relates to the physical environment and the rest to structures, processes and ways of engagement between staff. Even when we have no control over the physical environment and little control or influence over the quality of staff relationships, we have influence over the choices we make about how we want to 'be' in that environment. That includes our contribution to creating healthful relationships with colleagues and others we work with and our responsibility to our physical and psychological safety. Whilst in community and ambulatory care settings, you are encouraged to think not only about the responsibilities of our employers in creating a healthful workplace, but our own role in relationships and keeping ourselves safe in work. You are encouraged to think about your contribution in creating conditions where all people feel safe, and to be kind to yourself as your role becomes increasingly autonomous.

Regardless of how many different people you work with every day in different locations, these locations are your workplaces. The European Agency for Safety and Health at Work (2013) published a literature review to assess the status of well-being at work across the European Union. The report concluded that well-being at work does not relate only to how the organisation, system structures and jobs are designed, but also includes the quality of work and workplaces. It is not merely about the prevention of harm to someone's health, but the fulfilment of the person's goals as well. This elevates the importance of workplaces for us as persons, as well as employees, beyond a mere physical location with organisational structures. It spreads the responsibility across employers and employees to make sure workplace health, safety and well-being considerations are equally valued.

As you become increasingly autonomous within community and ambulatory services, managing risk is an ever-present consideration. The experience of psychological safety is also a consideration for any team. Brené Brown (2018, p. 36) describes psychological safety as 'feeling safe to take risks and being vulnerable in front of each other'. In psychologically unsafe workplaces, people are reluctant to take risks and admit mistakes for fear of retribution and harsh judgement. This limits opportunities for learning through critical reflection and feedback, which ultimately stifles learning and innovation. Brown and McCormack (2011) identified psychological safety as significant to the development of positive relationships and person-centred practice. If the characteristics within the Practice Environment domain are embedded in teams' ways of working, there is some mitigation against psychologically unsafe workplaces. This is enabled by supporting structures where there is high tolerance and an expectation that mistakes happen when people are being innovative and taking risks with new ideas and learning.

Activity

Linking back to your own values and beliefs that we mentioned earlier, it may be useful for you to stop and think about your own tolerance to risk and mistakes. Take a few minutes to think about the following questions.

- How do you feel about taking risks?
- How critical are you of yourself when you 'slip up'?
- Do you find it annoying when others make mistakes?
- What connection do you see between innovation, risk taking and punishment?
- Do these connections enable or disable you from being innovative?

These questions may help you to better understand your own values and beliefs about risk taking and mistake making and ultimately help you to know yourself better.

Psychological safety is embedded in healthful workplace cultures. Culture creates social norms that are taken for granted and largely go unchallenged in the absence of reflection and detached observation of that workplace (Manley and Jackson 2013). What this means is that the longer a person works in one place, the less likely they are to notice the culture there because they unconsciously accept the social norms that exist. When you are new, you notice the culture straight away; you notice patterns of practice, for example, how decisions are made, who is included, what gets prioritised. You will notice how you are welcomed to the team and how people introduce themselves, show interest in you and your work or placement experience. Do they invite you to accompany them on visits perhaps and ask open questions? You will also notice the interactions between team members and how they talk to and about each other. These experiences are powerful and create an immediate reaction to how safe and open a workplace might be and how psychologically safe you feel.

As you become increasingly autonomous, you will increasingly be working alone. You need to consider this as you plan your learning experience. Perhaps you will be undertaking community profiling or gaining insight into other community roles and services, taking you to a range of settings across the community. A greater degree of autonomy is often very welcome but it does raise issues of safety in community work. Physical safety is served by safety policies, guidelines and technology for good lone working practices. This is coupled with useful insider knowledge often accumulated over time by team members and shared when required. As a learner in the community, your practice educator or supervisor should always know where you are at any time during the day. This should be agreed as your day or week is being planned and there will be an agreed checking-in process used to ensure that you are never vulnerable in any location.

Remember to be kind to yourself. Working in the diversity of workplaces within community and ambulatory services may feel very new and different for you. We hope by using the stepping stones and signposts offered within this chapter, you will access the support and kindness you need to flourish within your workplaces.

Conclusion

On our journey, we have encouraged you to notice how people living in communities connect together and connect with practitioners. We have encouraged you to get to know yourself better and understand what motivates you. We have explored the uniqueness of our values and beliefs and have recognised how they shape the way we view our world and create meaning in our lives. The complexity of person-centredness has emerged, as has the fundamental tenet of the need to be aware of our own values and beliefs, those of the people we work with, as well as people we provide a service to. We know that values affect the quality of our interactions with others and ourselves as human beings. Along our journey, we have signposted healthful relationships aimed at helping people to live, work well and flourish within their communities. Through seeking out learning opportunities in a broad range of experiences in community and ambulatory services, we hope you learn from these healthful relationships. Whilst this can be challenging, we encourage you to keep being curious, asking questions and reflecting on your practice. With growing awareness of what it means to be person-centred, enhanced by the intention to enable human flourishing and loving kindness for all, there is hope for a kinder workplace and more effective outcomes for those using and providing community services.

Summary

- Experiences in community contexts offer opportunities to work with people's beliefs and values.
- Public health values underpin community practice.

- Being in unfamiliar situations and taking time to make your values explicit may challenge your belief systems.
- Knowing yourself is fundamental to being the best you can be.
- Loving kindness is an essential component of human flourishing.
- A healthful culture enables staff and service users to be the best they can be.

References

Brown, B. (2018). *Dare to Lead. Brave Work. Tough Conversations. Whole Hearts.* London: Vermillion.

Brown, D. and McCormack, B. (2011). Developing the practice context to enable more effective pain management with older people: an action research approach. *Implementation Science* 6 (9).

Cowley, S., Whittaker, K., Malone, M. et al. (2015). Why HV? Examining the potential public health benefits from HV practice within a universal service: a narrative review of the literature. *International Journal of Nursing Studies* 52 (1): 465–480.

European Agency for Safety and Health at Work (2013) Wellbeing at work: creating a positive work environment.https://osha.europa.eu/en/publications/literature_reviews/well-being-at-work-creating-a-positive-work-environment

Gaffney, M. (2011). *Flourishing*. London: Penguin Books.

Henrekson, M. (2014). Entrepreneurship, innovation, and human flourishing. *Small Business Economics* 43 (3): 511–528.

Manley, S.A. and Jackson, C. (2013). Working towards a culture of effectiveness in the workplace. In: *Practice Development in Nursing and Healthcare* (eds. B. McCormack, K. Manley and A. Titchen), 146–168. Oxford: Wiley Blackwell.

McCormack, B. and Titchen, A. (2014). No beginning and no end: ecology of human flourishing. *International Practice Development Journal* 4 (2): 1–21.

Murphy, F., Rosser, M., Bevan, R. et al. (2012). Nursing students' experiences and preferences regarding hospital and community placements. *Nurse Education in Practice* 12 (3): 170–175.

Phelps, E. (2013). *Mass Flourishing: How Grassroots Innovation Created Jobs, Challenge, and Change*. Princeton, NJ: Princeton University Press.

Seligman, M. (2011). *Flourish*. Australia: Random House.

Titchen, A. (2009). Developing expertise through nurturing professional artistry in the workplace. In: *Revealing Nursing Expertise Through Practitioner Inquiry* (eds. S. Hardy, A. Titchen, B. Mc Cormack and K. Manley), 219–241. Oxford: Wiley Blackwell.

Titchen, A. and McCormack, B. (2010). Dancing with stones. Critical creativity as methodology for human flourishing. *Educational Action Research* 18 (4): 531–554.

World Health Organization (1998). *Health 21: The health for all policy framework for the WHO European Region*. www.euro.who.int/__data/assets/pdf_file/0010/98398/wa540ga199heeng.pdf

Yalden, B.J. and McCormack, B. (2010). *Constructions of Dignity: A Prerequisite for Flourishing in the Workplace. International Journal of Older People Nursing*, 137–147. Oxford: Blackwell.

Further reading

Edwards, N. (2014). *Community Services – How they Can Transform Care*. London: King's Fund www.kingsfund.org.uk/sites/default/files/field/field_publication_file/community-services-nigel-edwards-feb14.pdf.

Scottish Government (2016). *The Modern Outpatient: A Collaborative Approach 2017–2020*. Edinburgh: Scottish Government www.gov.scot/publications/modern-outpatient-collaborative-approach-2017-2020.

World Health Organization (Europe) (2016). *Integrated Care Models – An Overview*. Copenhagen: World Health Organization.

21

Experiencing person-centredness in long-term care

Kevin Moore[1] and Fiona Kelly[2]

[1] Ulster University, Northern Ireland, UK

[2] Queen Margaret University, Edinburgh, Scotland, UK

Contents

Fundamentals of Person-Centred Healthcare Practice, First Edition. Edited by Brendan McCormack, Tanya McCance, Cathy Bulley, Donna Brown, Ailsa McMillan and Suzanne Martin.

Learning outcomes

- Identify and discuss the complex and multifaceted issues involved in the transition from one's own home to a long-term care setting, from both the person's perspective and that of their family/significant other.
- Discuss the importance of engaging in a person-centred way with a person living in a long-term care setting.
- Explore and explain the critical importance of 'truly knowing the person' as a means of providing compassionate and responsive care to a person within long-term care settings.
- Understand the centrality of effective communication and interpersonal skills in establishing, developing and maintaining a therapeutic relationship.

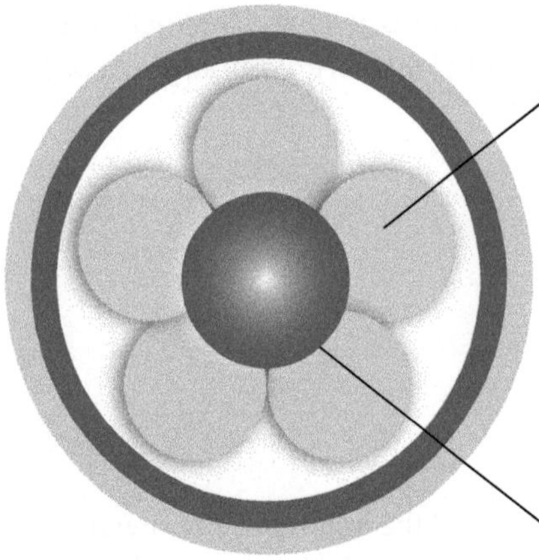

The Practice Environment

Shared Decision-Making Systems + Effective Staff Relationships

A person-centred practitioner through observation, communication, reflection in and on practice, self-awareness, and engagement with the person moving into long-term care and their families, will require sensitivity to the emotions and complexities involved in transitioning from 'home' to 'care home'.

Person-Centred Processes

Engaging Authentically + Shared Decision Making + Working Holistically

The way a person within long-term care settings can experience person-centred care that enables their voice, choice, control and ultimately their quality of life to be enhanced – with reciprocity for staff and the community.

Introduction

As people are living longer, the global population of older people is increasing (World Health Organization [WHO] 2019a). These trends are significant policy drivers throughout Ireland, the United Kingdom (UK) and Europe, consistently recognising the ageing population and the societal challenges that this entails, particularly related to provision of long-term care. As people age, there are many potential issues they may face including chronic ill health, cognitive decline, physical ill health and mental ill health. Moreover, an ageing society provides significant challenges for the provision of effective and responsive health and social care, irrespective of the environment within which it is delivered. This chapter provides an overview and exploration of issues related to the provision of person-centred care in long-term care settings. We will draw on different components of the Person-centred Practice Framework (PcPF), in particular the care environment and person-centred processes (McCance and McCormack 2017) to illustrate the complexities of this type of care and the importance of 'getting it right' for all persons involved.

Residential and long-term care: supporting quality of life

Care homes provide accommodation, with or without nursing care, to people who need extra support in their daily lives. People may move into a care home for various reasons, including a period of rehabilitation following hospital admission, often related to falls at home; to provide some respite for a family carer; following a crisis event such as the death of their main carer; or for longer-term care when their physical care needs can no longer be met at home. Regardless of the reason, the transition from home into a care home can be a stressful and anxiety-provoking time, causing upset for people as there are new sounds, smells, sights, routines and people to get used to and feelings of loss and grief for the life and home they are leaving behind. Person-centred practitioners in care homes can ease this transition by communicating in ways that acknowledge and respect the feelings of new residents and value what is important to them to maintain a good quality of life. Many elements of the PcPF covered in this book in are relevant in this setting.

Activity

Imagine you have just moved to a care home. What might you be feeling? What would you like the care home staff to do to help you to settle in? Listen to the voices of two services users below to help your reflections (Moore and Ryan 2017).

> 'Well they listen to anything I say to them and they treat me like a civil person, which I think I am still, and anything I ask for they do their best, I don't feel I'm being walked over or anything like that. It's all to do with choices and changes in my life' (Mary)
>
> 'Talk about care, you couldn't get that at home as they [staff] understand older people and that's important as is introducing yourself and explanations are essential' (Ann)

The WHO (2019b) defines quality of life as an:

> . . . individual's perception of their position in life in the context of the culture and value systems in which they live and in relation to their goals, expectations, standards, and concerns. It is a broad ranging concept affected in a complex way by the person's physical health, psychological state, personal beliefs, social relationships and their relationship to salient features of their environment.

In the context of care homes, quality of life can be achieved by spending time with family and friends, experiencing pleasure, having autonomy, choice, privacy, security and good relationships with staff and peers.

Murphy et al. (2006) highlighted four broad domains of quality of life in long-term care.

- Independence and autonomy of the resident.
- A resident's ability to maintain his/her personal identity and sense of self.
- A resident's ability to maintain connectedness, social relationships and networks within and outside the care setting.
- A resident's engagement in meaningful activities.

Meyer and Owen (2008) identified eight integrated best practice themes that are important for promoting voice, choice and control and, ultimately, quality of life of residents, staff and the community. They suggested that creating community and optimising relationships within the environment enabled a sense of belonging, purpose and achievement, and promoting a positive culture resulted in moving to a care home being viewed as a positive option. They took a person-centred approach to explore person-centredness in action from the perspectives of those living and working in care homes.

Each care home is unique and those who live and work in or visit a care home are also unique, therefore the elements of best practice will differ from care home to care home. What is important, however, is that care staff work in ways that consider a person's beliefs and values, engagement, sharing decision making, having a sympathetic presence and providing holistic care (McCormack and McCance 2017).

Choosing the right long-term care setting and holding that difficult conversation

Making the decision to move into a care home or move a family member into a care home is influenced by many complex factors. Cole et al. (2018) identified a variety of factors influencing family carers' decisions to move their relative or family member into a care home. These included the person's deteriorating health and the carer's growing recognition that they are no longer able to cope physically or psychologically. Ultimately, carers see a move into a care home as a last resort and want to feel ready to instigate the move, although often this is a process of evaluating and re-evaluating when is the right time to make the move. When choosing a care home, family carers want it to be clean, spacious, with caring friendly staff, a homely environment, with no adverse smells, culturally appropriate and near friends or relatives (Cole et al. 2018).

The range of emotions associated with a move to a care home extend from guilt and shame to feelings of relief, with the 'readiness' of the person moving into the care home an important determining factor in how difficult or easy family carers find the decision-making process. However, some people, particularly those with dementia, may not really be 'ready' or remember the decision to move. Innes et al. (2011) reported that people with dementia described being 'brought in' to the care home, reflecting the lack of choice and control they had over the process. Moore and Ryan (2017) illustrate this lack of choice below.

> My sister shipped me here, I never wanted to come here really. I had been in hospital after a bad fall at home. Was in hospital for months. They wouldn't let me come back to my own home. She [my sister] told me it would only be

> for four weeks. But sure, it has been four weeks, then another four weeks and then another four weeks. I actually don't know really how long I have been here now, over six or eight months. (Mary-Jane)

These findings are similar to a study carried out in Australia with 17 older people in a care home (Vahid et al. 2016), where the decision to move to a care home was made without the involvement of the older person. One way of ensuring that the transition reflects the values of choice and shared decision making is to offer psychological support before a decision has to be made and follow this up with further support if a decision to move to a care home is then made. Ryan et al. (2012) specifically focused on rural family carers' experiences and suggested that older people had a deep attachment to their own homes and entry to care was seen as a last resort. They suggested that family carers had close relationships with health and social care practitioners and felt supported in the decision-making process. The resultant choice of care home was, they asserted, linked to a sense of familiarity that existed in rural communities. Moreover, this sense of familiarity also influenced the timing of the placement and the responses of family carers. Ryan and McKenna (2015) have articulated that it is the 'little things' that matter to people in such circumstances and knowing, appreciating and respecting these things enabled a more effective transition to a long-term care setting. This is a beautiful example of being sympathetically present! (McCance and McCormack 2017).

The transition from 'home' to 'home'

Supporting the person

We have described some of the complexity in discussing and deciding on a move to a care home. Ultimately, it will be the older person who will move and who will have to adapt and settle into this new way of living. Research by Cooney (2012) identified four categories as critical to identifying and 'finding home' in long-term care settings: (i) 'continuity', which helped to create a sense of security, comfort and predictability for the person, (ii) 'preserving a personal identity', which centres around having time on their own, privacy and personal belongings and most importantly feeling known and valued as an individual, (iii) 'belonging', where the resident feels part of a group, has companionship, relaxation and fun, and (iv) 'being active and working', with structured activities within the home to help residents gain a sense of satisfaction within their daily lives. Cooney (2012) concluded that long-term care settings are first and foremost a resident's home and moving beyond the technical and procedural aspects of care enabled staff to meet the holistic needs of the individual. These findings map to the elements of the person-centred outcomes in action within the PcPF.

Creating 'home'

New residents entering a care setting are often encouraged to bring some personal belongings or small pieces of furniture with them to help them 'feel at home' (Lovatt 2018), although for those who are less independent or have few visitors, buying new possessions might not be an option (Paddock et al. 2019). However, 'home' cannot simply be transferred from one place to another with objects, nor does feeling at home necessarily require familiar objects. In her study within residential homes, Lovatt (2018) identified that residents actively turned the spaces of their rooms into places of home, creating an everyday sense of being at home. She emphasised the importance of engaging with objects and space through actions such as cleaning or hosting visitors. She also suggested that imagination in place making can still be possible in residential care, thus contradicting conventional design theory (Dementia Services Development Centre 2001) of the need for design to focus on past aesthetics or what is familiar.

Nordin et al. (2017) identified the role of good environmental design (small scale, logical layout, reference points to support safety and promote independence) in compensating for decreasing function and for enhancing opportunities for well-being. However, as residents plan to 'age in place', consideration also needs to be given to supporting the needs and wishes of those who are no longer able to be independent. Fleming et al. (2015), in their study with people living with dementia, care home staff and recently bereaved family members, identified key components of the physical environment necessary to support those nearing the end of life, particularly those who may not have the capacity or ability to move independently. These include comfort through engagement with the senses, feeling at home, a calm environment, privacy, dignity and use of technology to remain connected.

Thus it is clear that residential settings need to be designed to accommodate a wide variety of abilities, needs and wishes while also supporting an organisational culture that facilitates person-centred care. These findings contribute evidence to the role of the physical environment in facilitating person-centred practice and ensuring person-centred outcomes for everyone.

Supporting relatives

Davies and Nolan (2004) suggested that making the move to long-term care required an exploration of the relatives' experiences as they ultimately were closely linked to the final decision-making process. They identified three phases to the transition from the relatives' perspective: 'making the best of it', 'making the move' and 'making it better'. Lee et al. (2013) suggested that professionals should move away from considering the transition as a stage-based process ending in acceptance. Instead, they should focus on how residents perceive relocation in relation to previous life experiences, unspoken fears evoked by moving and how the environment and relationships with staff may be altered to assist residents in maintaining their identity and sense of control. Davies and Nolan (2004) asserted that health and social care practitioners have enormous potential to influence relatives' experiences of care home entry and that such experiences are enhanced if family carers perceive that they are able to work in partnership with care staff in order to ease the transition for the older person. This research places significant emphasis on the availability, or not, of supportive mechanisms to support families through the adaptation process and on the need for effective communication between the care team and the family.

Activity

Mr Jones is coming to live in your care home. He and his family have just arrived and you are going to be their named person as he settles in. Using the care processes, list the ways in which you will help Mr Jones to feel at home and to create 'home'.

Nursing and caring expertise in residential care settings

Clearly there is a need to provide responsive, compassionate, quality-orientated care within residential and nursing homes. However, ageist attitudes and stigma related to older persons' care can undermine the significance and importance of the quality of care provided to such residents. This may have a demoralising effect on the positive care provided by such dedicated staff. It is now increasingly recognised that providing high-quality care to older people in care homes requires significant skill, underpinned by a person-centred approach. Person-centred care is regarded as an optimum way of delivering healthcare (McCormack and McCance 2010) and has been broadly defined as valuing people as individuals (see Chapter 2 for more information about person-centred care).

McCormack et al. (2012) suggested that staff working with older people need to understand the importance of their role in developing meaningful relationships with older people themselves, families and colleagues to foster a culture of effectiveness. Moore and Ryan (2017) articulated the importance of truly understanding and knowing the person as central to the concept of providing 'homely care' in a nursing home. Taking a more practical approach, the National Institute for Health and Care Excellence (NICE 2015) recommends collaborative care planning, offering individualised information and support, supporting self-management, ensuring continuity of care, socialisation, autonomy, choice, and maintaining respectful and dignified interactions.

Effective leadership and management is also crucial and must underpin all aspects of care provision; it must be clearly accountable and compliant with legislation and professional regulations within the care home's jurisdictions. Transparent and collaborative decision making that acknowledges the prevalence of risk, capacity, resources and person-centred outcomes must underpin the strategic approaches to such care, whilst also acknowledging the ever increasing financial costs for the provision of such care.

Dignity and the importance of effective communication and interpersonal skills

The primacy of the practitioner–resident relationship has been well documented in the literature and many have drawn upon the influence of early scholars in the field of interpersonal relationships (see Rogers 1951). It is likely that, in the absence of a therapeutic relationship or therapeutic alliances within care, mutuality of trust, respect and dignity cannot occur. This means that staff must develop effective communication skills to engage residents and thus to provide significant and meaningful care.

Compassionate care and engagement with a person as they age wisely is a cherished value (Silverman and Siegel 2018). The provision of hope, self-efficacy, well-being and empowerment of the person is viewed as intrinsic to compassionate, dignified person-centred care. There is no denying that dignity and respect are key for effective and compassionate care for all people, not just older people. Indeed, Yalden and McCormack (2010) stated that dignity was a prerequisite for flourishing in the workplace. The vulnerability of many older people with multiple and complex needs, coupled with resource constraints, can make it difficult for staff to deliver care that is person-centred, respectful and courteous.

However, abusive practice and deviation from acceptable standards of care are not acceptable to anyone (Commission on Dignity in Care 2012). The Commission on Dignity in Care (2012) asserts that every staff member is responsible for dignity in care provision and they postulated 'Always' events as the foundation for dignity in care.

- Always treat those in your care as they wish to be treated: with respect, dignity and courtesy.
- Always remember nutrition and hydration needs.
- Always encourage formal and informal feedback from older people and their relatives, carers and advocates to improve practice.
- Always challenge poor practice at the time, and learn as a team from the error.

- Always report poor practice where appropriate; the people in your care have rights and you have professional responsibilities.

(Commission on Dignity in Care 2012, p. 12)

We will conclude with the voice of Jack, reflecting on what it feels like to experience person-centredness within a care home.

> Very happy and content and very secure because times I get pain and be sick, and they're more than attentive, they were there right away, just on the ball. Very generous with their time. They respect me a lot and I respect them and I know they do good work too (Jack). (Moore and Ryan 2017)

Activity

You have just entered a long-term care facility to visit a relative when another female resident, who had been knocking and banging on the exit door, attempts to leave the environment. She grabs you by the arm firmly, she is visibly tearful and upset. She has an outer coat on and has a red handbag on her arm. Take some time to reflect on what is unfolding in this situation and how you can make sense of it. How can you respond in a person-centred way?

Conclusion

In this chapter, we have considered some of the reasons for older people moving into a residential or care setting, some of the challenges with making the decision to move and how a person-centred approach can make the transition easier and more fulfilling. While we have explored these issues using a variety of research evidence, the key uniting principle is person-centred practice. The outcomes of a person-centred approach for people living in care settings include being supported in decision making, feeling valued and respected as a person, experiencing dignified care that respects the person's choice and autonomy and ultimately enables human flourishing. Achieving these outcomes requires care home staff to have sensitivity to the emotions and complexities involved in transitioning from home to care home and to have excellent observational, communication, practice and reflective skills. Moreover, the intrinsic and connected nature of the therapeutic relationship and knowing the person are fundamental to the provision of a 'home from home' experience.

Summary

- With increased numbers of people living into old age, the need for long-term care is clear.
- Person-centred care enables the voice of the person to be heard in decision making, which is important as the transition into long-term care can be stressful.
- Care staff should adopt the PcPF and therefore consider each person's beliefs and values, engagement, sharing decision making, having a sympathetic presence and providing holistic care.

References

Cole, L., Samsi, K., and Manthorpe, J. (2018). Is there an "optimal time" to move to a care home for a person with dementia? A systematic review of the literature. *International Psychogeriatrics* 30 (11): 1649–1670.

Commission on Dignity in Care (2012). *Delivering Dignity: Securing dignity in care for older people in hospitals and care homes.* www.ageuk.org.uk/Global/Delivering%20Dignity%20Report.pdf?dtrk=true

Cooney, A. (2012). 'Finding home': a grounded theory on how older people 'find home' in long-term care settings. *International Journal of Older People Nursing* 7: 188–199.

Davies, S. and Nolan, M. (2004). 'Making the move': relatives' experiences of the transition to a care home. *Health & Social Care in the Community* 12 (6): 517–526.

Dementia Services Development Centre (2001). *Dementia Design Audit Tool.* Stirling: University of Stirling.

Fleming, R., Kelly, F., and Stillfried, G. (2015). 'I want to feel at home': establishing what aspects of environmental design are important to people with dementia nearing the end of life. *BMC Palliative Care* 14: 26.

Innes, A., Kelly, F., and Dincarslan, O. (2011). Care home design for people with dementia: what do people with dementia and their family carers value? *Aging & Mental Health* 15 (5): 548–556.

Lee, V.S.P., Simpson, J., and Froggatt, K. (2013). A narrative exploration of older people's transitions into residential care. *Aging & Mental Health* 17 (1): 48–56.

Lovatt, M. (2018). Becoming at home in residential care for older people: a material culture perspective. *Sociology of Health & Illness* 40 (2): 366–378.

McCance, T. and McCormack, B. (2017). The person-centred practice framework. In: *Person-Centred Practice in Nursing and Healthcare: Theory and Practice*, vol. 2 (eds. B. McCormack and T. McCance), 36–66. Chichester: Wiley Blackwell.

McCormack, B. and McCance, T. (2010). *Person-Centred Nursing. Theory and Practice.* Oxford: Wiley Blackwell.

McCormack, B. and McCance, T. (2017). Underpinning principles of person-centred practice. In: *Person-Centred practice in Nursing and Healthcare: Theory and Practice*, vol. 2 (eds. B. McCormack and T. McCance), 13–35. Chichester: Wiley Blackwell.

McCormack, B., Roberts, T., Meyer, J. et al. (2012). Appreciating the 'person' in long-term care. *International Journal of Older People Nursing* 7: 284–294.

Meyer, J. and Owen, T. (2008). Calling for an international dialogue on quality of life in care homes. *International Journal of Older People Nursing* 3: 291–294.

Moore, K.D. and Ryan, A.A. (2017). *The Lived Experiences of Nursing Home Residents in the Context of the Nursing Home as their 'Home'. A Grounded Theory Study.* Ulster University and Nursing Homes Ireland.

Murphy, K., O'Shea, E., Cooney, A. et al. (2006). Improving Quality of Life for Older People in Long-Stay Care Settings in Ireland. Report No 93. National Council on Ageing and Older People (NCAOP). Dublin.

National Institute for Health and Care Excellence (2015). Older people with social care needs and multiple long-term conditions. www.nice.org.uk/guidance/ng22/chapter/Recommendations

Nordin, S., McKee, K., Wijk, H., and Elf, M. (2017). The association between the physical environment and the well-being of older people in residential care facilities: a multilevel analysis. *Journal of Advanced Nursing* 73: 2942–2952.

Paddock, K., Brown Wilson, C., Walshe, C., and Todd, C. (2019). Care home life and identity: a qualitative case study. *Gerontologist* 59: 655–664.

Rogers, C. (1951). *Client Centred Therapy*. London: Constable.

Ryan, A.A. and McKenna, H. (2015). 'It's the little things that count'. Families' experience of roles, relationships and the quality of care in rural nursing homes. *International Journal of Older People Nursing* 10: 38–45.

Ryan, A.A., McKenna, H., and Slevin, O. (2012). Family care-giving and decisions about entry to care: a rural perspective. *Ageing and Society* 32: 1–18.

Silverman, I.I. and Siegel, E.B. (2018). *Aging Wisely...Wisdom of our Elders.* Burlington, MA: Jones and Bartlett Learning.

Vahid, Z., Vahid, P., Azad, R. et al. (2016). Older people's experiences involving the decision to transition to an aged care home. *International Journal of Medical Research and Health Sciences* 5 (8): 346–355.

World Health Organization (2019a). *Ageing and Life Course*. www.who.int/ageing/en

World Health Organization (2019b). *World Health Organization Quality of Life*. www.who.int/mental_health/publications/whoqol/en

Yalden, B.J. and McCormack, B. (2010). Constructions of dignity: a pre-requisite for flourishing in the workplace? *International Journal of Older People Nursing* 5: 137–147.

Further reading

Age UK. (2019). *Support moving into a care home*. www.ageuk.org.uk/information-advice/care/arranging-care/care-homes/moving-into-care-home

Appleby, J. (2011). *Rapid review of Northern Ireland Health and Social Care funding needs and the productivity challenge: 2011/12–2014/15*. The Appleby Report. Department of Health Social Services Public Safety. www.health-ni.gov.uk/publications/appleby-report

World Health Organization (2019). *Integrated care for older people (ICOPE): guidance for person-centred assessment and pathways in primary care*. www.who.int/ageing/publications/icope-handbook/en

22

Being person-centred in mental health services

David Banks[1], Josianne Scerri[2], and Jessica Davidson[3]

[1] Queen Margaret University, Edinburgh, Scotland, UK
[2] University of Malta and Kingston and St George's Medical School, University of London
[3] NHS Lothian and Queen Margaret University, Edinburgh, Scotland, UK

Contents

Fundamentals of Person-Centred Healthcare Practice, First Edition. Edited by Brendan McCormack, Tanya McCance, Cathy Bulley, Donna Brown, Ailsa McMillan and Suzanne Martin.

Learning outcomes

- Understand the historical and social context of stigmatisation of people, whether experiencing mental distress or recognised forms of mental illness.
- Explore key challenges in supporting people to equitably access person-centred healthcare, specifically in the context of gender violence, rape and mental illness.
- Understand that acute trauma can be considered a mental health emergency.
- Describe how use of the Person-centred Practice Framework can contribute to the development of effective care for persons experiencing acute trauma.
- Understand the importance of the impact of trauma and its contribution to mental illness and the overall well-being of the person in any healthcare context.

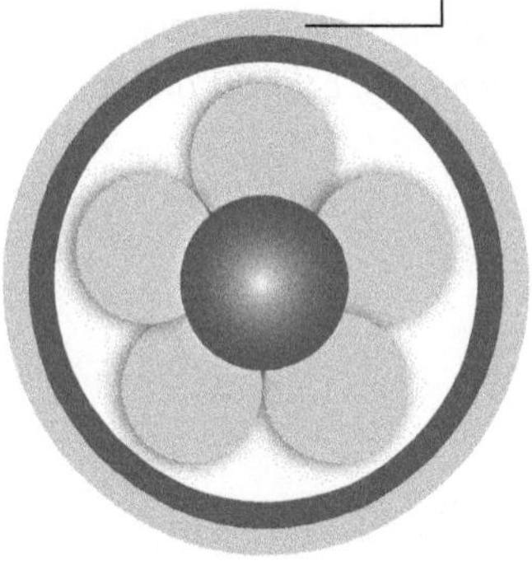

Developed interpersonal skills: the ability of the person to communicate at a variety of levels with others, using effective verbal and non-verbal interactions that show personal concern for their situation and a commitment to finding mutual solutions

Knowing self: the way a person makes sense of his/her knowing, being and becoming through reflection, self-awareness, and engagement with others

Clarity of belief and values: awareness of the impact of beliefs and values on the healthcare experience and the commitment to reconciling beliefs and values in ways that facilitate person-centredness

Introduction

This chapter addresses challenges facing persons with experience of trauma and mental illness. The authors will particularly discuss how working with survivors of rape, from person-centred perspectives, necessarily means tackling societal norms based on patriarchal and other socially excluding assumptions about person, identity and relationships.

How rights-based approaches can inform person-centred care of people experiencing mental distress

Providing person-centred care incorporates a humanistic and holistic approach, one in which the unique life story of the person in a particular context is valued. It is based on a collaborative, inclusive and active participatory partnership between healthcare staff, the person with a mental illness and people significant to them. Such a partnership is underpinned by a shift in emphasis, from focusing solely on symptoms and the prominence of a diagnostic label to one in which the experiences and expectations of people with a mental illness are valued and their dignity and right to self-determination respected.

A gap, however, exists between the rhetoric of person-centred care and the actual reality experienced by people with a mental illness. First-person narratives by people seeking mental health support often emphasise their lack of involvement in decisions relating to their own care, and their experience of continuous scrutiny under the lens of a diagnostic framework by healthcare professionals (Dixon et al. 2016).

The cultural framing of such attitudes from practitioners effectively impedes people in mental distress from properly occupying a collaborative and active role in decisions relating to their own care. The reality of these experiences conflicts too often with professional claims that they are the true protagonists of their own life stories. Furthermore, stigmatising attitudes by professionals may result in diagnostic overshadowing that can negatively influence how persons with a mental illness can access necessary healthcare, thus leading to their potential disempowerment within both general and mental health services.

Professional perceptions and assumptions in socially constructing the meaning of age, gender, social class, sexuality and race are known to be key factors in determining who is considered 'worthy' of access to appropriate care (Brown 1995). This is of major concern, since healthcare services are '. . . the main avenue by which mental health service users are likely to achieve satisfactory integration or re-integration into society' (Carrara et al. 2019, p. 317). Equitable access to appropriate services is key to recovery for such people. Stigmatising attitudes by healthcare professionals have also been identified as exacerbating mental health problems (Sartorius 2007), or influencing decision making by clinicians, based on mistaken assumptions (Shim and Rust 2013).

Stigma and self-stigma are therefore key concepts in understanding how the identities of people are negatively influenced by mental distress and psychological trauma. Goffman argued the former is a key product of social interaction. Goffman (1963, p. 9) classically categorised three forms of social stigma that can be imposed on a person: stigma through negative character traits; physical stigma; and stigma attributable to group identity. Physical stigma would be characterised by perceived physical deformities, whilst stigma by group identity emanates from perceived membership of a particular 'other' race, nation, religion or social group. Consequently, stigma, in any social interaction, is at the foreground of that interaction. This is illustrated, for example, in health professionals changing their behaviour when speaking and listening to someone whom they might construe as socially 'abnormal' and of course different from themselves. The person in such circumstances faces the risk of being dehumanised. On an everyday basis, people react to signs of stigma exhibited by another in various ways, including rejection, excessive acceptance or by plain embarrassment. Their main concern is to manage such an individual's deviance, at the expense of not engaging with the whole of their personality.

There is evidence that such forms of public stigma can lead to the development of self-stigma through a process of internalisation of traumatic events by the victim (Vogel et al. 2013). Consequently, staff from all healthcare settings need to develop an awareness of how their attitudes and discriminatory behaviours may negatively impact on the care experience and feelings of well-being of people for whom they provide services (Caldwell and Jorm 2000).

Another emerging movement within the public health sector has explicitly linked the environment to well-being. The study of 'place' in people's health has a role in connecting communities and providing a sense of belonging. Casey (2013) argues that culture manifestly exists most concretely in places, rather than in minds and signs. Inequalities in environment can create serious disadvantages, with women in deprived areas experiencing 22.6 fewer years of good health (Voluntary Health Scotland 2018). This is also exemplified in African American feminist literature; the matriarchal experience within a harsh and violent patriarchy translates into culture and environment and creates stigma, often somatised into health inequalities for the individuals and groups in the greatest need.

According to Walker (1992), the slave society heritage of poverty, hatred, segregated schools, slum neighbourhoods and the worst of everything constitutes the historical inheritance and material reality of black motherhood. So, if rights are inhibited in such a way as to adversely affect female liberties, experience and the potential for flourishing, then a new imagining for relationships has to begin, and this can find fertile ground within relationships with caregivers that can mimic sisterhood and filial relationships (Hopson 2018). This other way of working is often expressed through the advanced practitioner–patient dyad in person-centred care delivered during times of great crisis. Thus, any claim to the practice of person-centred care should emphasise the humanity of the person in that relationship and the significance of recognising agency on the part of that person in negotiating their own care and treatment.

A vital strand of this evolving public health discourse has now emerged through the voices of service users with mental illness and through social movements campaigning from rights-based political and social agendas, which have been themselves heavily influenced by the postwar African American civil rights movement addressing political and social emancipation in the USA. These health social movements (HSMs) have campaigned for society to reach beyond merely providing a welfare safety net to assisting people at risk of exclusion or marginalisation to self-actualise as citizens, whilst also campaigning for broader social change. HSMs have, therefore, collectively challenged medical policy, public health policy and politics, and belief systems through sponsoring alternative research and practice. They constitute a rich network of formal and informal organisations, supporters, including sympathetic mental health workers, networks of co-operation and media. Gay Pride and Mad Pride are provocative manifestations of these new forms of public engagement, seeking to reframe public perception of other identities (Allan 2006).

Health social movements have consequently made many challenges to political power, professional authority and personal and collective identity. These movements have tackled access to healthcare services, labelling of disease, illness experience, disability, and contested illness, and most importantly they have challenged health inequality and inequity based on race, ethnicity, gender, class and/or sexuality (Brown and Zavestoski 2004). Such rights-based arguments have also helped shape discourses around health education curricula. The concept of person-centred care is increasingly being offered by educators and researchers as necessarily informing the professional values of staff working with people who have been historically stigmatised and marginalised, and indeed excluded from society, such as persons experiencing acute trauma.

Activity

Spend a few minutes reflecting on the word 'stigma'. What does it mean to you? In what ways have you seen stigma being played out in society?

In reflecting on 'stigma' you may have thought about the ways that certain groups of people in society are seen as 'different'. For example, the way in which people who identify as LGBTQ have particular stereotype labels applied to them (such as being camp, liking particular music, being promiscuous etc). You may have considered the way these labels serve to dehumanise such persons and impact on how they live their day to day lives. You might also have thought about people you know who don't fit these labels and thus are somehow 'atypical' of the ascribed stereotype. Such stigma can have profound implications for how we persons are seen by society and accepted into communities.

Implementing the Person-centred Practice Framework in the context of mental distress and trauma informed practice

In modern healthcare systems, mental health practice is too often considered to be a specialist area of work, to be accessed and provided outside the everyday work of mainstream health professionals in major healthcare organisations. Furthermore, in such general acute care settings it is not unusual for the technical and physical aspects of treatment and care to be prioritised at the expense of more holistic practice. Yet if person-centred care is to be achieved, that necessarily must mean the development of new ways of working with people with mental illness, including marginalised members of society, such as victims of abuse, in a manner that will cross traditional team and agency boundaries.

The following section presents a case study of a young woman called Jane (a pseudonym) who experienced the trauma of rape and violence. It highlights various shortcomings in the quality of care that was provided, as a consequence of extant traditional assumptions.

> Jane was a university student in a city centre who was drugged, brutally assaulted and repeatedly raped in a stranger's flat after a night out in the city. She subsequently decided to report this to the police. Her complaint to Police Scotland was upheld on many grounds, not only because of the particular circumstances of her case, but because of inherent structural weaknesses in the provision of care for women, and indeed children and men, who have been raped or sexually assaulted in Scotland.
>
> Jane has described her painful ordeal in detail through various social media and how her medical examination was especially bungled. Her story draws attention to what other women subjected to such attacks have repeatedly reported, regarding the retraumatising effects of attempting to engage with health and welfare professionals and systems, which often appear ignorant and insensitive to the psychological and social effects of rape on the person concerned. Jane not only presents as a survivor of a horrendous assault, but she is also now a significant voice in a health social movement in Scotland seeking to address gender violence through legal and healthcare reform.

The HM Inspectorate Scotland (2017) produced a seminal report recognising that its service to victims of sexual assault and rape was failing the women and children concerned. Its recommendations have heavily influenced current policy to develop person-centred trauma informed services. However, Jane experienced badly mismanaged treatment and care, not only from Police Scotland police officers but also from other significant welfare workers, most importantly, members of the forensic medical service who were tasked to provide her care and treatment and to ensure proper retrieval of evidence.

Jane's case is not a solitary or isolated incident. In fact, sexual assault is far too commonplace as a societal phenomenon, not only in the UK but globally. The World Health Organization produced a unique review of the impact of violence on global public health. This includes a major chapter summarising survey work on the incidence and nature of sexual violence, despite the largely hidden contexts in which it is practised (Krug et al. 2002). The victims are overwhelmingly women and children, with the available data indicating that nearly one in four women may experience sexual violence from an intimate partner in some countries, and nearly a third of girls reported being forced into their first sexual encounter. Such sexual violence has major effects on mental and physical health, where aside from the frequent reporting of physical injuries, it is linked with an increased risk of a range of sexual and reproductive health problems, with short-term and long-term consequences.

The subsequent impact on mental health can be as serious as any physical impact and may be equally long lasting. Common mental effects of sexual assault or rape can be expressed as diagnosable mental disorders, including long-term mental illness. This especially incorporates acute trauma and posttraumatic stress disorder (PTSD); the symptoms include flashbacks, nightmares, severe anxiety and uncontrollable thoughts. Depression is also commonplace amongst survivors of these assaults, who may also experience prolonged sadness, feelings of hopelessness, unexplained crying, weight loss or gain, loss of energy or interest in activities previously enjoyed. Suicidal thoughts or attempts have also been widely reported, as well as murder, the latter occurring either during a sexual assault or subsequently, as a murder of 'honour'. Women have further described how dissociation can also interfere with their everyday lives. These effects include not being able to focus on work, school study, or homework, as well as not feeling present in everyday settings.

It is important to grasp that women may also suffer a range of permanent or temporary physical injuries as a consequence of gender violence, in the form of rape. Some of the most common injuries include bruising, bleeding (vaginal or anal), difficulty in walking and soreness, dislocated or broken bones, sexually transmitted diseases and pregnancy. However, in many cases of rape, contrary to some people's beliefs, vaginal injury is not visible, or absent. But it is thought that the presence of a vaginal injury is more conducive to the survivor being believed and the rapist being successfully prosecuted, such is the layperson's conscious and unconscious bias as to the understanding of the crime of rape (Sawyer Sommers 2007).

For the survivor, there are also powerful emotional effects in terms of the construction of personal identity and relationships with others, including family, friends and co-workers. This can move from initial shock, numbness, disorientation and a sense of loss of control to a sense of helplessness, fear and vulnerability. Feelings can also be affected such as experiencing a sense of anger and blame towards self as well as others for allowing the assault to take place, in addition to changes relating to trusting others. Such feelings may also be self-interpreted by the survivor as a sign of weakness.

Sexual violence can also fundamentally influence the social well-being of victims who may be consequently stigmatised and excluded by family and others. Coerced sex may result in sexual gratification on the part of the perpetrator, though its underlying purpose is frequently the expression of power and dominance over the person assaulted. Often, men who coerce a spouse into a sexual act claim their actions are legitimate since they are married to the woman. In fact, although sexual violence can be directed against both men and women, in the main, women and children are typically targeted by men exercising various forms of formal or informal power (Krug et al. 2002, p. 149).

The raping of women and of men is often deployed as a military tactic to humiliate and intimidate the perceived enemy. Trafficking of women across borders, as a form of sexual commodification, has also been noted as a common global occurrence. Refugees have reported sexual assault being used to punish women within their own communities for transgressing social or moral codes, for instance those prohibiting adultery or drunkenness in public. Women and men have also reported being raped when in police custody or in prison.

A key problem in terms of social justice for people experiencing gender violence has been 'victim blaming'. This gendered response has historically characterised the responses of too many health, police and legal practitioners with regard to the assumed moral careers of the women concerned. Jane has shown undoubted courage in sharing her experiences and making a case for restitution, not only for herself in her own journey of recovery but for thousands of other women who have been similarly assaulted. Jane's personal campaign for better services, in partnership and co-production with Rape Crisis Scotland, has made a significant policy contribution in helping to open up the debate on gender violence and influence current attempts to reform provision of forensic care to people who have shared her experiences in Scotland. It is now clear that the Scottish Government has accepted the need to provide person-centred care that properly addresses issues from a trauma informed action-based perspective. The Scottish Government Taskforce on Sexual Assault and Rape is explicitly focusing on development of better welfare services. It is properly concerned to assist all people who in the past have chosen not to disclose their experiences because they were too intimidated, by fear of adverse public opinion and the potential failure of a prosecution case against offenders.

Secondary analysis of Scottish data from the British National Survey of Sexual Attitudes and Lifestyles identified 19% of women respondents as reporting that someone had attempted to make them have sex against their will. Half of these women went on to report in such cases that a completed rape or assault took place. Women were more likely to report being raped or sexually assaulted than men (Fuller et al. 2015).

To report such attacks to the police and healthcare agencies is in itself a daunting task. Victims of assault commonly make first contact with someone whom they implicitly trust, usually close relatives and friends, rather than directly contacting the police. This is partly about looking for support and seeking advice about reporting the crime and managing the consequences. In 2017–18 it was reported that Scottish court conviction rates were highest for vehicle offences, with 94% of people prosecuted and a 98% conviction rate achieved. Prosecutors achieved a rather lower conviction rate for cases of rape and attempted rape, only 36% of cases being successfully prosecuted in the UK (Office for National Statistics 2018). WHO worldwide data on gender violence, as referenced above, show an even grimmer global picture elsewhere with regard to reporting and prosecuting offenders and care and treatment of survivors of sexual assault, particularly in Latin America, Africa and Asia.

It is important to appreciate that access to appropriate services whilst reporting a serious crime presents a challenge for rape survivors. Healthcare professionals clearly have vital roles to play in enabling appropriate treatment and care to such services. It is well understood that reporting such assaults is unlikely to happen for the majority of victims. This is not only a British welfare issue – similar outcomes can also be shown further afield.

In the longer term, many people who are survivors of sexual assault are likely to seek help from general mental health services, especially in dealing with longer term experiences of anxiety and depression; this may or may not involve initial self-disclosure by the victim. It is also very likely that such self-disclosure may emerge in non-mental healthcare contexts where healthcare workers may also not necessarily anticipate sexual abuse to be an underlying issue for the person seeking help.

The necessity of developing a shared understanding

The Person-centred Practice Framework contributes to the development of effective mental health services by outlining practitioner attributes that are essential in the provision of effective person-centred care. One such attribute outlines the need for practitioners to engage in self-awareness ('knowing self'), which incorporates an ongoing process of self-discovery and self-reflection. This involves making sense of our own belief framework and also that of persons with a mental illness (refer to Chapter 12 for more detail about the importance of beliefs and values in person-centred practice). By engaging in critical reflection (see Chapter 29), we become aware of how our beliefs and values may influence our mode of practice and the way we develop relationships and engage with others (McCance and McCormack 2017), including persons who have experienced abuse.

Reflecting on our practice also incorporates listening to people and exploring their needs, concerns and the perceived barriers encountered, such as the economic, psychosocial, emotional and physical 'costs' of actively engaging in a care plan. This is of particular significance amongst deprived, marginalised and minority communities where issues relating to limited individual resources and the higher levels of stigma aimed at people with mental illness have been identified (Lamb et al. 2012).

Story telling as a means of therapeutic engagement

It is through a narrative approach that people who have experienced mental distress or psychological trauma can share the meaning that they attach to an experience. This meaning furthermore is not contextualised within a vacuum, but rather immersed within their social and cultural background. By exploring these narratives, the professional healthcare practitioner acknowledges any person in mental distress, or with a defined mental illness, as a unique person with a unique perspective to share. Furthermore, by working together with their beliefs and values, the formulation of personalised care plans can be undertaken, as opposed to imposing a 'one size fits all' paradigm of care.

Healthcare workers can also 'know self' by reflecting on the way they communicate both verbally and non-verbally with others. This is of importance as this perspective 'will influence what we say, how we say it, the language used and the use of specific strategies' (McCance and McCormack 2017, p. 44). The communication of stigmatising attitudes may negatively impact on any attempt to foster a therapeutic relationship between the professional and persons experiencing mental distress or illness, leaving them and their families feeling increasingly more vulnerable.

It is through the acquisition of effective communication skills and careful reflection on the potentially implicit meanings conveyed in the language that they use (when referring to the people who use services and the services provided) that practitioners may gain an in-depth insight into what is of importance to the person regarding the potential impact of decisions relating to care and treatment decisions. As Jane's story illustrates, failure by the practitioner to attend to what is of particular significance to the person leads to discordance between the perceptions of the practitioner and the person experiencing mental distress engaged in that dyad. Consequently, the victim of abuse may have concerns regarding any care services being recommended or provided. This in turn may negatively influence their decision to access or continue utilising care services, with a possible impact on their overall quality of life and care experience. Healthcare workers are therefore required to work with a view to 'intentional doing', that is working with the person as an equal partner in planning their care, taking proper account of their opinions and ensuring that they are respected. This requires not only the planning of care with the person but also thinking reflexively about the effect of their interactions on the person as a whole, including the person's potential relationships with others.

Activity

- The '#MeToo' movement is a global movement against sexual violence perpetrated against women in particular. The movement originates to the work of Tarana Burke, sexual violence survivor and activist. Watch Tarana Burke's TED Talk here https://www.ted.com/talks/tarana_burke_me_too_is_a_movement_not_a_moment
- Tarana Burke more recently referred to the movement as "an international movement for justice for marginalized people in marginalized communities"
- What does the #MeToo movement mean to you? Think about your own views of the movement in the context of the Person-centred Practice Framework. Can you use the framework to challenge gender-based aggression in society?

Conclusion

Leaders and service managers need to provide the necessary situational leadership, resources and support to facilitate their colleagues to provide high-quality person-centred services. Healthcare practitioners need to critically recognise that they can influence across all the levels of the Person-centred Practice Framework, being mindful of wider macro influences, joining HSMs to effectively challenge poor-quality service providers claiming to provide high-quality services (Lynch 2015).

Such services should be underpinned by a commitment to people with mental ill health as individual citizens and practitioners, and avoiding the desire to fit people into existing services and 'window dress' this up as person-centred services (Wolfensberger 1991). Leaders and managers should be transparently held to account professionally and, when necessary, legally for how well they do this in their role, alongside direct care practitioners, who should be more openly addressed when their services fail to achieve the required standards. This will include healthcare practitioners collectively campaigning with other stakeholders, including the service user movement, in defence of those values.

Summary

- Understanding mental distress and practising trauma informed care should inform everyone's business.
- Persons accessing both general and mental health services clearly say they are negatively labelled when seen through a diagnostic framework, rather than as unique individuals within a context.
- Stigmatising attitudes towards persons who have experienced traumatic abuse can have a negative impact on the therapeutic alliance between the practitioner abd person within a mental illness dyad.
- The Person-centred Practice Framework highlights that all practitioners must 'know self' when exploring their own beliefs and values towards persons experiencing mental illness or distress.

References

Allan, C. (2006). *Misplaced pride*. www.theguardian.com/commentisfree/2006/sep/27/society.socialcare.

Brown, P. and Zavestoski, S. (2004). Social movements in health: an introduction. *Sociology of Health & Illness* 26 (6): 679–694.

Brown, P. (1995). Naming and framing: the social construction of diagnosis and illness. *Journal of Health and Social Behavior* 35: 34–52.

Caldwell, T.M. and Jorm, A.F. (2000). Mental health nurses' beliefs about interventions for schizophrenia and depression: a comparison with psychiatrists and the public. *Australian and New Zealand Journal of Psychiatry* 34: 602–611.

Carrara, B.S., Aparecida, C., and Ventura, A. (2019). Stigma in health professionals towards people with mental illness: an integrative review. *Archives of Psychiatric Nursing* 33 (4): 311–318.

Casey, E. (2013). *The Fate of Place. A Philosophical History*. Berkeley, CA: University of California Press.

Dixon, L., Holoshitz, Y., and Nossel, I. (2016). Treatment engagement of individuals experiencing mental illness: review and update. *World Psychiatry* 15 (1): 13–20.

Goffman, E. (1963). *Stigma: Notes on the Management of Spoiled Identity*. Harmondsworth: Penguin.

Fuller, E., Clifton, S., Field, N. et al. (2015). *The National Survey of Sexual Attitudes and Lifestyles Natsal-3 Report: Key findings from Scotland*. https://www2.gov.scot/Resource/0047/00474316.pdf

HM Inspectorate of Constabulary in Scotland (2017). Strategic Overview of Provision of Forensic Medical Services to Victims of Sexual Crime. www.hmics.scot/sites/default/files/publications/HMICS%20Strategic%20Overview%20of%20Provision%20of%20Forensic%20Medical%20Services%20to%20Victims%20of%20Sexual%20Crime.pdf

Hopson, C.R. (2018). "Tell nobody but god": reading mothers, sisters, and "the father" in Alice Walker's The Color Purple. *Gender and Women's Studies* 1 (1): 3.

Krug, E., Mercy, J., Dahlberg, L., and Zwi, A. (eds.) (2002). *World Health Organization World Report on Violence and Health*. Geneva: WHO.

Lamb, J., Bower, P., Rogers, A. et al. (2012). Access to mental health in primary care: a qualitative meta-synthesis of evidence from the experience of people in 'hard to reach' groups. *Health* 16 (1): 76–104.

Lynch, B. (2015). Partnering for performance in situational leadership: a person-centred leadership approach. *International Journal of Practice Development* 5 (Suppl): 5.

McCance, T. and McCormack, B. (2017). The person-centred practice framework. In: *Person-Centred Practice in Nursing and Healthcare: Theory and Practice* (eds. B. McCormack and T. McCance), 36–64. Chichester: Wiley Blackwell.

Office for National Statistics (2018). *Sexual Offending: Victimisation and the Path through the Criminal Justice System*. www.ons.gov.uk/peoplepopulationandcommunity/crimeandjustice/articles/sexualoffendingvictimisationandthepaththroughthecriminaljusticesystem/2018-12-13#convictions

Sartorius, N. (2007). Stigma and mental health. *Lancet* 370 (9590): 810–811.

Shim, R. and Rust, G. (2013). Primary care, behavioural health, and public health: partners in reducing mental health stigma. *American Journal of Public Health* 103: 774–776.

Sawyer Sommers, M. (2007). Defining patterns of genital injury from sexual assault. A review. *Trauma Violence Abuse* 8 (3): 270–280.

Voluntary Health Scotland (2018). *The Zubairi Report. The lived experience of loneliness and social isolation in Scotland*. https://vhscotland.org.uk/wp-content/uploads/2018/11/The-Zubairi-Report-VHS-Nov-2018.pdf

Walker, A. (1992). *You Can't Keep a Good Woman Down. Short Stories*. Toronto: Women's Press.

Wolfensberger, W. (1991). Reflections on a lifetime in human services and mental retardation. *Mental Retardation* 29 (1): 1–15.

Vogel, D., Bitman, R., Hammer, J., and Wade, N. (2013). Is stigma internalized? The longitudinal impact of public stigma on self-stigma. *Journal of Counseling Psychology* 60 (2): 311–316.

23

Person-centred support for people with learning disabilities

Owen Barr[1], Martina Conway[2], and Vidar Melby[1]

[1] Ulster University, Northern Ireland, UK
[2] Health Service Executive, Letterkenny, Republic of Ireland

Contents

Fundamentals of Person-Centred Healthcare Practice, First Edition. Edited by Brendan McCormack, Tanya McCance, Cathy Bulley, Donna Brown, Ailsa McMillan and Suzanne Martin.

Learning outcomes

- Define the nature of a person with a learning disability.
- Outline the development of services for people with learning disabilities.
- Explain key challenges in supporting people with learning disabilities to access person-centred health and social care.
- Explain the importance of interpersonal skills, professional competence (and confidence), authentic engagement and sharing decisions to the successful provision of person-centred services to a person with learning disabilities.

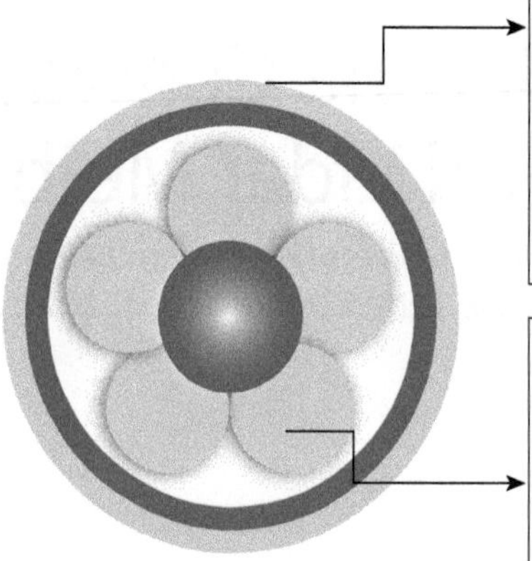

Professionally competent: the knowledge, skills and attitudes of the person to negotiate care options, and effectively provide holistic care

Developed interpersonal skills: the ability of the person to communicate at a variety of levels with others, using effective verbal and non-verbal interactions that show personal concern for their situation and a commitment to finding mutual solutions

Working with the person's beliefs and values: having a clear picture of the person's values about his/her life and how he/she makes sense of what is happening from their individual perspective, psychosocial context and social role

Sharing decision making: engaging persons in decision making by considering values, experiences, concerns and future aspirations

Engaging authentically: the connectedness between people, determined by knowledge of the person, clarity of beliefs and values, knowledge of self and professional expertise

Being sympathetically present: an engagement that recognises the uniqueness and value of the person, by appropriately responding to cues that maximise coping resources through the recognition of important agendas in their life

Introduction

This chapter presents an overview of the importance of citizenship as a service principle in policies guiding services for people with learning disabilities and the definition of a person with learning disabilities. The use of the Person-centred Practice Framework to guide the use of effective interpersonal skills, being professionally competent and confident, engaging on a person to person level and supporting shared decision making is explored as a way of overcoming some of the key challenges in providing person-centred services for people with learning disabilities.

The majority of people with learning disabilities live with their families and/or in community-based facilities, with a small minority of people living in larger congregated settings, such as hospitals or village communities. Therefore, you can expect to come in contact with people with learning disabilities across a wide range of services. These include primary care services, such as local health centres, secondary care, including hospitals as people attending for planned or emergency treatment, and tertiary care services, including specialist continuing care and end of life services. More effective health and social care for people has supported more children to live into adulthood and adults to live into older age, often into their 70s. These developments have resulted in many people with increasingly complex health and social care needs that require the knowledge and skills of interdisciplinary and interagency team members to design, plan and deliver services.

Definition of a person with a learning disability

The language used when talking to and about people can convey the values we hold about people. The term 'learning disabilities' is widely used in the United Kingdom within conversation, policy and legislation. Internationally, the term 'intellectual disabilities' is more widely used across Europe and Australia, with the term 'intellectual and developmental disabilities' (which also includes some people with non-progressive physical disabilities such as cerebral palsy) also being used in some countries, including the United States of America. Although these terms are widely used in health and social care policy or legislation, there continues to be confusion about the meaning, definition and boundaries of these terms in practice settings.

Activity

In your own words, write your definition of people with learning disabilities. Discuss your definition with colleagues and reflect on the meanings they have taken from your definition and the words you have used.

Consider what your definition is based upon; have you started your definition with 'a person with' or have you sought to define learning disability without reference to a person? What does your definition say about a person's ability to learn new skills or to successfully live in and contribute to society?

How is the 'person with learning disabilities' being communicated about in your definition? What other labels or abbreviations have you heard used or personally used when referring to a person with learning disabilities (for example, LD, the learning disabled, or related to physical or behavioural characteristics, wheelchair user, epileptic, etc.)? How do you feel these terms reflect the valuing of personhood of the person with learning disabilities?

In the UK, a person with a learning disability is defined as a person with:

> a significantly reduced ability to understand new or complex information or to learn new skills (impaired intelligence), with a reduced ability to cope independently (impaired social functioning), which started before adulthood with a lasting effect on development. (DHSSPS 2005, p. 18)

The World Health Organization (WHO) uses the same definition for the term 'intellectual disability' (www.euro.who.int/en/health-topics/noncommunicable-diseases/mental-health/news/news/2010/15/childrens-right-to-family-life/definition-intellectual-disability).

These definitions of learning disability emphasise the importance of recognising the personhood of people with learning disabilities and their ability to continue learning, and the need for these opportunities to be provided. The definitions also consider a person's ability to cope independently. This is an important revision of earlier definitions which had been based only on intelligence quotient (IQ). Alongside this revised definition, the previous categories of profound, severe, moderate and mild learning disabilities and the use of the concept of 'mental age' as criteria to make generalisations about a person's ability and potential future achievements are called into question.

Person-centred principles that have underpinned services for people with learning disabilities

The importance of recognising and valuing the uniqueness, abilities, needs and aspirations of people with learning disabilities has been an integral part of service policies that developed from the theory of 'normalisation' since the 1970s. In 1983, Wolfensberger developed the earlier theory of normalisation to one more focused on the importance of attaching social value to the role of people with learning disabilities in society, which he called social role valorisation (SRV). SRV was defined as 'the enablement, establishment, enhancement, maintenance, and/or defence of valued social roles for people, particularly for people at value-risk by using, as much as possible, culturally valued means' (Wolfensberger 1983, p. 235).

This approach to service provision advocated increased choice and control for people with learning disabilities over decisions that affected their lives. These values were actioned in approaches such as Individual Programme Planning and Shared Action Planning which sought to support and actively find out about a person's aspiration and to involve people with learning disabilities in decisions that affected their lives. O'Brien and Lyle-O'Brien (1987) put forward five accomplishments that services should provide for people with learning disabilities that should result in the five valued experiences of:

- belonging
- being respected
- sharing ordinary places
- contributing to others and society
- choosing.

However, there were key limitations of these previous approaches to Individual Programme Planning and Shared Action Planning. These principle-based approaches had very broad objectives and were largely focused on the processes to be followed rather than the outcomes to be achieved for people with learning disabilities (Mansell and Beadle-Brown 2004). The degree to which a person with a learning disability was actively involved in the discussions and decisions about his/her care could have been limited, with an overemphasis on the needs and limitations of the person, rather than focusing on their aspirations for their future (Greasley 1995). In contrast, in the Person-centred Practice Framework, staff are actively challenged 'to think about the person first and then the disease or disability' (McCance and McCormack 2019, p. 305).

It is clear that these previous person-centred models did not adequately acknowledge the complexity and influence of service cultures, as articulated in the macro context, prerequisites and aspects of the care environment now integrated into the Person-centred Practice Framework. It is important for staff to be aware of the service principles in national and local policy documents, and how these influence or can be used to influence workforce development, strategic leadership of services and the priorities of service managers. This awareness is necessary for staff to be able to engage in innovative practice and lead the development of services, within their sphere of influence.

Health and social care staff also need to consider how these service principles stated at a macro level are evident in their practice. This includes the need for people with learning disabilities to be treated as full citizens of the country in which they live and the role of staff in maximising the opportunities for the person with learning disabilities to be involved as fully as possible in making decisions that affect him or her (Scottish Executive: Same as You 2000; Department of Health: Valuing People 2001; Department of Health, Social Services and Public Safety: Equal Lives 2005).

Activity

Service Principles in Your Practice

Familiarise yourself with the stated services principles within the national policy documents that guide services for people with learning disabilities in the country in which you are working. Thinking about your experience of meeting/supporting people with learning disabilities, consider these principles and provide a practical example of how these evidenced the services you have worked in or have contact with. Reflecting on your own practice, which service principles are evident in your professional practice, noting if any of these are not clearly evident?

Based on your reflections, identify three actions you can take to further enhance the embedding of these service principles in your practice.

The ongoing need for a person-centred framework that is evidenced in practice

In 1991, Wolfensberger, a prominent advocate for people with learning disabilities, reflected on his lifetime work in services and concluded that he had seen substantial progress in the development of SRV in services for people with learning disabilities during his career. At the same time, he urged caution that this progress should not be used as 'window dressing' that will hide what he referred to as the 'larger dismay realities' (p. 14) of limited rights, citizenship and inclusion for many people with learning disabilities.

This cautionary view is still relevant in current services. There has been the development of less congregated models of residential accommodation and increased support for people living at home. These have included an emphasis on providing services built on a recognition of citizenship, individual support and interdisciplinary working. However, the person-centred outcomes, for example in relation to involvement in decision making and exercising choice achieved for people with learning disabilities, have been variable across services and are not significantly associated with smaller purpose-built services (Ratti et al. 2016). There is also clear evidence from recent research that people with learning disabilities are normally not actively involved in the care planning process relating to their care (Doody et al. 2019).

There are persistent and growing concerns about access to primary care, general hospital care and mental health care for people with learning disabilities. This is evidenced in the fact that the median age of death for men with learning disabilities is 60 years and for women 59 years, which is 23 years and 27 years younger, respectively, than members of the general population. Concerns have been highlighted about the failure of general health services to undertake effective assessments of a person's abilities and needs, to actively involve people in decisions that affect them and to make reasonable adjustments that facilitate a person to make effective use of the services available. These factors often result in the presence of a person's learning disability and associated stereotypical views of health and social care professionals about people with learning disabilities, resulting in 'diagnostic overshadowing' (Barr and Gates 2019). This occurs when the presence of learning disabilities is incorrectly used to explain changes in a person's physical and mental abilities that are in fact due to changes in a person's health. Diagnostic overshadowing has been as a factor contributing to preventable and premature deaths of people with learning disabilities (Heslop et al. 2013; LeDeR 2020).

The development of community-based services for people with learning disabilities has been focused on supporting people to live fulfilling lives with their families or in their own homes and there has been a major move away from the previous model of large congregated services. However, in the last decade there have been five major inquires into care services in the UK and Ireland. These inquiries all happened in apparently new community-based services, that were described as person-centred, purpose-built specialist assessment and treatment services, including Winterbourne View (2011), Ralphs Close (2012), Veilstone (2011), Aras Attracta (2016), and Muckamore Abbey Hospital (2019). The lessons from these inquires for individual staff and service managers, in respect of development of services for people with learning disabilities, need to be learnt and action taken to truly deliver person-centred services in practice for people with learning disabilities.

Delivering person-centred health and social care services for people with learning disabilities

Reflecting on the successful progress made towards more person-centred services for people with learning disabilities alongside the limitations of current services, it is argued that two key areas require renewed attention to provide more person-centred services for people with learning disabilities.

- Interpersonal skills, professional competence (and confidence) (prerequisites).
- Engaging authentically, being sympathetically present, sharing decision making (person-centred processes).

Interpersonal skills

Effective communication is one of the 'four Cs' identified by Marsden and Giles (2017) and colleagues as necessary to provide effective reasonable adjustments in healthcare. The starting point for effective communication is the firm belief that *all* people can communicate, maybe not verbally or even vocally, but perhaps by the use of gestures, facial expressions and sounds. From this starting point, an assessment of how a person with a learning disability communicates should only need the answer to one question: 'How does (person's name) communicate?' and your assessment should answer this question, explaining how the person conveys their message and how best to share information with them. There is no need for further 'tick boxes' (such as verbal, non-verbal, hearing, vision) to explain how a person communicates.

Staff need to be accurate and honest in their assessment of their own communication abilities. Therefore, if the person with learning disabilities is able to communicate effectively with other people who know them well and you are unable to understand them, then this identifies a learning need for you and should increase your self-awareness of your abilities and limitations (see more about identifying learning needs in Chapter 33). It is not professionally acceptable to 'blame' the person with a learning disability for your difficulties in understanding their means of communication to others. The majority of people with learning disabilities will try to find ways to make their communication clearer to you, if you continue to show your commitment to listen, engaging authentically with them as a person and trying to hear their message. Equally, many people with learning disabilities will also know when you are trying to pretend you understood or 'fobbing them off' as if you understand them. Such action is unprofessional, devalues the person with a learning disability and can have a lasting negative effect on your relationship with the person.

Professional competence and confidence

Many staff unfamiliar with working with people with learning disabilities can often feel awkward and lack confidence in their interactions with people with learning disabilities, which can leave them feeling professionally inadequate and not focused on listening to the person. Bear in mind that the person with learning disabilities is first and foremost a person and is likely to be accessing services for largely the same reasons as people who do not have a learning disability, for example feeling unwell, in pain, distressed. Draw confidence from your previous learning and do not let your actions become overwhelmed by the person having learning disabilities. In your role, you possibly know most of what you need to do so the key to doing this successfully is your ability to make reasonable adjustments that may be necessary at that time. Work hard to avoid the pitfall of 'diagnostic overshadowing' and in the first instance, consider what you would do if the person did not have a learning disability (as that is probably a lot of what needs done). Then, through your interacting with, listening to and observing people with learning disabilities and speaking to people who know them, consider what adjustments to your usual practice you need to make. Most reasonable adjustments are not major changes to your practice (for example, speaking more slowly; using more clear language supported by gestures; allowing more time for appointments; using accessible information to explain). Such apparently small changes can have a major impact on your ability to provide services and should enhance your confidence in working with people with learning disabilities.

Activity

A large amount of accessible resources about healthcare have been developed to explain many aspects of care to people with learning disabilities. In discussion with colleagues, obtain copies of accessible resources that are available in your service. If no local resources exist, visit http://easyhealth.org.uk and select two resources that are relevant to your practice. Select one resource designed to provide information to people with learning disabilities (e.g. leaflet or video) and another resource designed to provide you with information about the person with learning disabilities (e.g. pain or distress assessment). Read over the resources and make notes on how you feel these could be of use in providing clearer explanations to or receiving clearer information from people with learning disabilities using the services you provide.

Engaging authentically and being sympathetically present with a person with learning disabilities and colleagues

Developing an ability to effectively communicate with (in particular, listen to) people with learning disabilities is critical to you being able to provide person-centred services. Integral to this is your willingness and ability to engage authentically on a person-to-person level and being open to learning from the person with learning disabilities. One of the key areas identified in limiting the provision of person-centred services and access to healthcare is a focus on assessing the needs of a person with learning disabilities without seeking to learn about their abilities and aspirations (Heslop et al. 2013). This can require you to spend more time with the person with learning disabilities than you may with another person in your services. You need to look beyond a person with apparent limited abilities and on occasions set aside your preconceived ideas and maybe those of colleagues that have been communicated to you, in order to see and hear the person more clearly. At the end of your assessment with a person with learning disabilities, you should be able to explain your understanding of their abilities, aspirations and needs. From that position, it is possible to agree objectives for your engagement that will build on their abilities to respond to their needs and move them closer to their aspirations in life. When an assessment is problem focused and seeks only to establish a person's needs, there is often a large amount of missed information about the 'person' and their potential to be actively involved in decision making is not fully appreciated.

A similar level of engagement should also be offered to colleagues, as the need for respect and working collaboratively is key to the Person-centred Practice Framework. Therefore you need to be willing on occasions to ask colleagues who you feel may be having difficulties in their work environment how they are (not 'Are you ok?') and provide encouragement and feedback to them. It is clear from several of the major inquiries noted earlier that colleagues and managers were aware of difficulties staff were experiencing, including problems in their workplace culture, but often failed to acknowledge this and act. These reports from inquiries have documented the limitations of support provided to people with learning disabilities, but are rather more silent about the negative impact on individual health and social care staff who have worked in these environments.

Shared decision making

Sharing decision making has an impact on all the person-centred outcomes and is an aspect of the care experience which is a problem encountered by many people with learning disabilities. Often there is confusion about the relationship between consent and capacity to make a decision. The policy guidance on consent to examination, treatment and care across the UK and internationally (for example, DHSSPS 2003; HSE 2019) is clearly based on the view that all people, including people with learning disabilities, must be given the opportunity to make informed decisions about things that will affect them. The provision of informed consent is a process and is not reliant on a signed form. The process of obtaining consent starts from the position that consent is decision and person specific. It recognises that while a person may be able to consent to one decision, they may not be able to provide informed consent in another decision. However, the presence of learning disabilities should never be taken to equate to a person not being able to give informed consent.

Informed consent requires that information be provided in a format that is accessible and understandable to the person with learning disabilities. People with learning disabilities should feel they can make their decisions free from duress (including time pressure) and know they may withhold or withdraw consent without the need to provide a reason. These principles apply to all decisions, including some decisions that you may feel uncomfortable discussing with a person with learning disabilities, such as end of life care. Recent research has shown that in a UK-wide retrospective study of end of life care of people with learning disabilities, 22% of people with learning disabilities, compared to 51% of the general population, 'certainly' or 'probably knew' they were going to die before they were dying (Hunt et al. 2019). In the same study, it was reported that 46% of people with learning disabilities, compared to 86% of people in the general population, were involved in decisions about their care as much as they may have wanted.

It is not acceptable to overturn a decision made by a person with learning disabilities on the grounds that you feel it is irrational or unreasonable if the person made an informed decision, unless you have reason to question the person's capacity to make that specific decision. A person's capacity to make a decision should only be considered when reasonable attempts have been made to seek informed consent and there is reason to believe that the person with learning disabilities does not have the capacity to make that decision at that time. If this is the view, then guidance should be sought about the capacity legislation within the jurisdiction in which you are working as the specific details can differ across the devolved countries of the UK and internationally.

It is critical to remember that if a person over the age of 18 years is unable to give consent, no one can give consent on their behalf, including family members. In these circumstances, discussion should include the person with learning disabilities, carers (including relevant family members) and health and social care professionals who will undertake the examination, treatment or care for which the consent is being sought. Discussions should be focused on making a decision in the person's (not the service's) 'best interests', following the process required in the respective country's legislation.

Conclusion

Providing person-centred services for people with learning disabilities continues to present many challenges despite the apparent commitment to this philosophy across national and international service policies (Barr and Gates 2019). To move forward, it is essential that staff in all settings recognise the centrality of their values, commitment and continuing professional development. The primacy of the person with learning disabilities and their citizenship must underpin all actions by staff.

Practitioners need to recognise the need to develop services that fulfil all the levels of the Person-centred Practice Framework. Leaders and service managers also need to provide the necessary leadership, resources and support to facilitate staff to provide high-quality person-centred services. Such services should be underpinned by a commitment from staff and managers within a collective leadership approach to working collaboratively with people with learning disabilities as individual citizens. This also includes effectively addressing any pressure (real or perceived) to fit people into existing services and 'window dress' this as a person-centred service. This will involve leaders and managers, alongside direct care workers, being transparently held to account professionally, and when necessary legally, for how well they do.

Summary

- The need to recognise the citizenship and personal abilities, aspirations and needs of people with learning disabilities is a national and international service principle.
- Many people with learning disabilities experience difficulties in accessing and using general health and social care services.

- The Person-centred Practice Framework provides a structured approach to delivering person-centred services for people with learning disabilities in practical and visible ways.
- People with learning disabilities can be actively involved in shared decision making about decisions that may affect their lives.
- Health and social care professionals need to become confident and competent in communicating and engaging authentically with people with learning disabilities.

References

Barr, O. and Gates, B. (eds.) (2019). *Oxford Handbook of Learning and Intellectual Disability Nursing*. Oxford: Oxford University Press.

Department of Health (2001). *Valuing People. A New Strategy for Learning Disability for the 21st Century*. London: Department of Health.

Department of Health, Social Services and Public Safety (2003). *Reference Guide to Consent for Examination, Treatment or Care*. Belfast: DHSSPS.

Department of Health, Social Services and Public Safety (2005). *Equal Lives. A review of policy and services for people with a learning disability in Northern Ireland*. Belfast: DHSSPS.

Doody, O., Lyons, R., and Ryan, R. (2019). The experiences of adults with intellectual disability in the involvement of nursing care planning in health services. *British Journal of Learning Disabilities* 47: 233–240.

Health Service Executive (2019). *National Consent Policy*. Dublin: HSE.

Heslop, P., Blair, P., Fleming, P. et al. (2013). Confidential Inquiry into premature deaths of people with learning disabilities. www.bristol.ac.uk/media-library/sites/cipold/migrated/documents/fullfinalreport.pdf

Hunt, K., Bernal, J., Worth, R. et al. (2019). End-of-life care in intellectual disability: a retrospective cross-sectional study. *BMJ Supportive and Palliative Care* https://doi.org/10.1136/bmjspcare-2019-001985.

LeDeR (Learning Disabilities Mortality Review Programme) (2020). *Annual Report 2019*. Bristol: University of Bristol.

Mansell, J. and Beadle-Brown, J. (2004). Person-centred planning or person-centred action. A response to the commentaries. *Journal of Applied Research in Intellectual Disabilities*. 17 (1): 31–35.

Marsden, D. and Giles, R. (2017). The 4C framework for making reasonable adjustments for people with learning disabilities. *Nursing Standard* 31 (21): 45–53.

McCance, T. and McCormack, B. (2019). Person-centred practice framework. In: *Oxford Handbook of Learning and Intellectual Disability Nursing* (eds. O. Barr and B. Gates), 305–306. Oxford: Oxford University Press.

O'Brien, J. and Lyle-O'Brien, C. (1987). *A Framework for Accomplishments*. Lithonia, Georgia: Responsive Systems Associates.

Ratti, V., Hassiotis, A., Crabtree, J. et al. (2016). The effectiveness of person-centred planning for people with intellectual disabilities: a systematic review. *Research in Developmental Disabilities* 57: 63–84.

Scottish Executive (2000). *Same as You. A review of services for people with learning disabilities*. Edinburgh: HMSO.

Wolfensberger, W. (1983). Social role valorization: a proposed new term for the principle of normalization. *Mental Retardation* 21 (6): 234–239.

Wolfensberger, W. (1991). Reflections on a lifetime in human services and mental retardation. *Mental Retardation* 29 (1): 1–15.

Further reading

Barr, O. and Gates, B. (eds.) (2019). *Oxford Handbook of Learning and Intellectual Disability Nursing*. Oxford: Oxford University Press.

LeDeR (Learning Disabilities Mortality Review Programme) (2020). *Annual Report 2018*. Bristol: University of Bristol.

RQIA. (2018). *Guidelines for caring for people with learning disabilities in general hospital settings*. www.rqia.org.uk/RQIA/files/41/41a812c6-fee8-45ba-81b8-9ed4106cf49a.pdf

24

Being person-centred in maternity services

Honor MacGregor[1] and Patricia Gillen[2]

[1] *NHS Tayside and Queen Margaret University, Edinburgh, Scotland, UK*
[2] *Southern Health and Social Care Trust and Ulster University, Northern Ireland, UK*

Contents

Fundamentals of Person-Centred Healthcare Practice, First Edition. Edited by Brendan McCormack, Tanya McCance, Cathy Bulley, Donna Brown, Ailsa McMillan and Suzanne Martin.

Learning outcomes

- Acquire a deeper understanding of what it means to provide person-centred maternity care.
- Consider how the concept of power sharing impacts on the maternity practice environment and person-centred care provision.
- Be able to reflect on how the person-centred processes enable and support the provision of person-centred maternity care.

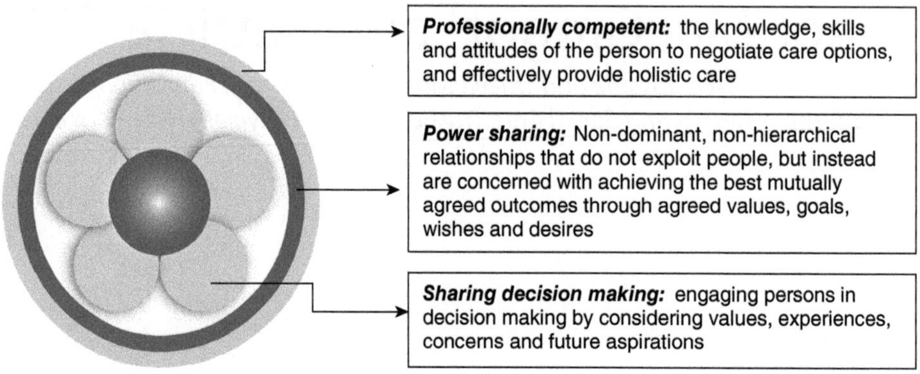

Professionally competent: the knowledge, skills and attitudes of the person to negotiate care options, and effectively provide holistic care
Power sharing: Non-dominant, non-hierarchical relationships that do not exploit people, but instead are concerned with achieving the best mutually agreed outcomes through agreed values, goals, wishes and desires
Sharing decision making: engaging persons in decision making by considering values, experiences, concerns and future aspirations

Introduction

This chapter focuses on how the Person-centred Practice Framework can assist us to develop as a member of a person-centred team in a maternity care setting. In particular, we will consider the prerequisite of being *professionally competent*; the practice environment characteristic of *power sharing*; and the person-centred process of *shared decision making*. We will explore the meaning of person-centred care to women, their babies and families, taking account of the context of the maternity care practice environment and how this helps or hinders person-centredness. We will also reflect on how person-centred processes enable us to offer person-centred modern maternity care that meets the needs of women and their babies, while recognising and accommodating the diversity and needs of the contemporary families to which women belong. In Chapter 3 you were introduced to the Person-centred Practice Framework. This chapter offers you the opportunity to consider your actions and intentions that immediately surround the central aspiration of a healthful culture for all in maternity services.

Contemporary maternity care

Care received during pregnancy and birth influences not only the current physical and psychosocial health and well-being of women, families and communities, but may also contribute to the health of future generations (Renfrew et al. 2014). The House of Commons Health and Social Care Committee (2019) and the World Health Organization (2018) also highlight how profound the health, development, social and economic consequences of childbirth and the early weeks of life are. Contemporary care from a midwife must therefore be person-centred to meet the current and future needs of women, babies and families.

Women and their families should have a positive experience of maternity care that places them at the centre of all care decisions, taking account of their preferences and individual needs. Midwives therefore have a key role to play, alongside other maternity care providers, in ensuring this happens for all women (Scottish Government 2010; DHSSPSNI 2012). Midwives are required to meet the often straightforward but sometimes complex needs of a woman, her baby and family through pregnancy, childbirth and the postpartum period. Some women may need or choose to access care from an obstetrician, while all women regardless of their care needs and preferences will benefit from the expertise of a midwife (Sandall 2012). Modern maternity care can be offered at home, in an alongside or free-standing midwifery unit or birth centre and in an obstetric hospital setting. However, while the role of the midwife may differ across these contexts, the expectation is that maternity care is person-centred regardless of where it takes place.

Being professionally competent as a midwife

Professional competence as one of the defining prerequisites of the Person-centred Practice Framework is key in ensuring a person-centred response to the needs and wishes of women and their families within the maternity care setting. Midwives are ideally placed, as their name suggests, in being 'with woman' to respond to the needs and wishes of a woman at a defining moment in that woman's and her family's life. They bring their professional competence which is derived from a unique mix of knowledge, skill and attitudes to facilitate women to make individualised yet flexible care plans that optimise the experience and outcome for the woman, her baby and her family. The midwifery workforce are increasingly working within models of care that provide continuity of care and carer for women during pregnancy, birth and for up to 10 days following birth, in line with recent strategic policy changes and a growing evidence base.

The fundamental concept of midwifery care is based around the relationships that midwives develop with individual women. This relationship is quite unique in healthcare and is a demonstration of human caring and kindness that is established early in pregnancy and develops during the year that includes pregnancy and the early postnatal period. The woman relies on the professional competence of the midwife to understand and discuss pertinent evidence, in order to assist her in making pregnancy and childbirth choices. Care provided by a midwife working in a continuity model has been proven to reduce harm to babies. Women being cared for by a midwife known to them are less likely to give birth to a preterm baby, the baby is less likely to require admission to the neonatal unit and the baby is less likely to be born with a low birthweight (Dahlen 2016). Sandall et al. (2016) also found that women who have care in a model that values continuity of carer were less likely to experience preterm birth and their babies were less likely to die, when compared to other models of care. Women being cared for by a midwife known to them are also less likely to experience intervention during labour. These are significant physical outcomes for women and babies; additionally, care delivered where continuity of carer is valued is also associated with the woman feeling more satisfied with the quality of care received.

Activity

Can you identify the benefits and challenges of continuity of care models from the perspective of the woman and the midwife? You could perhaps use this as a focus for a supervision session.

The key to enabling holistic and person-centred care for women is the ability to develop a meaningful, compassionate and respectful relationship with the woman and her family that reflects a partnership approach to care. However, the midwife works as a member of the maternity care team and in order to be an effective part of that team, midwives must be professionally competent and have the ability to communicate appropriately with all members of the maternity team, other professionals, women receiving care and their family members (Royal College of Midwives 2016). This is also further supported by the Nursing and Midwifery Council (2018) and Royal College of Obstetricians and Gynaecologists (2019), who state that communication is an essential aspect of person-centred care in maternity services.

Often the way that teams communicate among themselves and with others is recognised as having the most powerful impact on outcomes for women and babies and not always in a positive way (Kirkup 2015; The Shrewsbury and Telford Hospital NHS Trust 2017). Indeed, West and Lyubovnikova (2013) highlight the *illusions* (p. 134) of working in teams in healthcare, stating that few teams actually have shared objectives, work closely and interdependently or assess their effectiveness on care provision and outcomes. Within the maternity care context, in order to be professionally competent, the midwife must work collaboratively with a range of colleagues and maintain effective working relationships. This competence is vital in order to respond to the individualised and personalised care of women and their families.

Power sharing in person-centred maternity care

As mentioned earlier, the context of maternity care could be an obstetric hospital, a midwifery unit (birthing centre) or a woman's home. Each of these contexts provides different challenges and opportunities for the maternity care team and for the women and babies receiving care. It is important that wherever possible, continuity of care and carer is maintained. This is particularly challenging for those women who require a consultation with others, such as our obstetric colleagues. A woman who has care that crosses the boundaries of midwifery and obstetric care often relies on a midwife to act as her advocate to support and enable her to remain active in decision making about her care. Effective communication between the midwife and obstetrician is invaluable so that where possible, the woman transfers back into the care of the same midwives if the reason for obstetric input resolves. This is an example of power sharing that places the woman at the centre of care and optimises outcomes for the woman and her baby.

In particular, continuity of carer facilitates a relationship to build between the woman and the midwife that enables power sharing which respects each individual woman's wishes and desires for her pregnancy and childbirth. This includes decisions about place of birth that may be informed by the woman's life or previous childbirth experiences. A mutually trusting and respectful relationship with care providers is required to promote honest conversations and power sharing that is reflected in midwives being supportive of the woman's informed choices, even when they are not aligned with local policy and practice guidelines.

Increasingly, power sharing between professionals is being extended to women and their families within the context of maternity care. The principles of co-production are being used with women to co-design and provide services and resources that meet women's needs (Department of Health 2018). Examples of co-produced evidence-based maternity care practice guidelines and resources designed with and for multidisciplinary colleagues and women are available at www.rqia.org.uk/what-we-do/rqia-s-funding-programme/guidelines.

Enabling person-centred maternity care through shared decision making

Midwives often describe the privilege afforded to them of being 'with woman'. Earlier in this chapter we explored how professional competence and power sharing are key to the provision of safe and effective person-centred care, but it is also important to consider how person-centred processes such as shared decision making enable person-centred care.

The World Health Organization standards and guidelines focus on various aspects of care during pregnancy and childbirth. The recent guidelines on intrapartum care (World Health Organization 2018) highlight the need for person-centred care in labour and childbirth in order to optimise experiences and outcomes for women and babies. This includes the recognition that every person has the human right to be treated with respect and dignity. The WHO expects that its guidelines will be used as the basis for the development of national and local guidelines and protocols that will assist maternity care providers, including midwives, to optimise the provision of person-centred care. In addition, national policy guides how we organise and deliver maternity services locally. Policy often provides a vision that states clearly how care should be delivered, where care should be delivered and who is the most appropriate person to be the lead care provider. This ensures that services are of high quality, safe and effective for all. In recent years, each of the four countries in the UK has developed strategies and policies to provide a framework for how maternity care will be delivered in the future. Their intention is to ensure that all women and babies are offered a truly person- and family-centred, safe and compassionate approach to care.

An example of this is in The Best Start (Scottish Government 2017) which highlights the importance of ensuring that families are actively encouraged and supported to become an integral part of all aspects of care. It promotes the need for all women to experience continuity of care and carer from a multiprofessional team who have an open and honest team culture where everyone's contribution is equally valued. One of the core recommendations across these documents is that maternity care should be personalised and co-designed with each woman and her family. From the first time they meet, the woman should be provided with information and evidence to enable her to make informed decisions in partnership with her family, her midwife and the wider care team when required. The woman and her family are always at the centre of a service that is safe, effective and person-centred, with shared decision making and collaboration being the foundations of safe, effective, person-centred maternity care (Department of Health 2010). This is also supported by guidance from the National Institute for Health and Care Excellence (NICE) (2012) which makes it clear that a woman's decisions should be respected, even when they are contrary to the views of the healthcare professional. This is more likely to be realised where women experience continuity of care and carer.

Continuity of carer is a key focus in current UK maternity care policy (DHSSPSNI 2012). There are many examples of teams across the UK where service redesign is ensuring that women will have continuity of care from one midwife. As mentioned earlier, women having care offered in this way have been shown to have better outcomes than those who had care from different midwives. This trusting relationship and shared decision making are key in reducing harm and ensuring the provision of safe and effective care.

The National Institute for Health and Care Excellence (2019) guidelines recommend that women, their families and partners should all be treated with dignity, respect and kindness. These guidelines also recommend that professionals offering care should not make assumptions about what matters to women and their families during pregnancy and in the postnatal period. The views, values and beliefs of not only the woman who is pregnant but also those people important to the pregnant woman should be sought and respected. Building healthful relationships and effective communication are essential if we are to be truly person-centred in providing care.

Activity

When reading this scenario, think about what you have read in this chapter so far and whether or not the power-sharing aspect of the care environment and the person-centred process of shared decision making are evident.

When Jane and I met, she spoke of a previous experience with her first baby that left her with a distrust of health professionals. She was in the first trimester; she wanted to discuss how she arranged a water birth at home. Jane was pregnant with triplets; she lived an hour away from the hospital in a remote setting. Jane was really practical, I admired her need for information and knowledge, she wanted the very best for these babies, she needed to be in control of this pregnancy. We talked about many different pregnancy outcomes at different gestations. Jane was well supported by her husband. Jane managed and co-ordinated her own pregnancy with help and support and chose a semi-elective caesarean section when labour started at 28 weeks gestation. she gave birth to three identical girls.

What elements of person-centred care have you been able to identify? How, for example, did Jane know that she was being heard, and that shared decision making was being facilitated? Is this different to how you have either witnessed or undertaken care in the maternity setting? How can you further develop person-centredness as a way of being?

There is increasing evidence to support the importance of the first 1000 days in life (House of Commons Health and Social Care Committee 2019) and indeed recognition of the importance of the in utero environment to which the baby is exposed prior to birth. Therefore, it is vital that maternity services offer women individualised, personalised care that not only meets the specific care needs of the woman during and after her pregnancy, but also respects her values, experiences, concerns and future aspirations. Maternity care, if provided well, will not only enable and support women and their families during pregnancy and birth but has the potential to improve the woman's ability to provide the best care for her baby (WHO 2017, 2018).

Conclusion

It is important that women have the opportunity and are supported to make informed decisions about their care during pregnancy, birth and in the postnatal period. Women should always be equal partners in any decisions relating to them; they should be supported to disagree with care options that are being suggested to them if they do not align with their beliefs and values. Members of the team delivering maternity care are accountable for ensuring the woman and her family are always at the centre of care, are actively involved in decision making and are provided with information in an unbiased way. While the Person-centred Practice Framework in its totality is helpful in encouraging us to challenge our ways of thinking and working, this chapter has explored elements of the Person-centred Practice Framework that are of most relevance to maternity care.

Summary

- Being professionally competent is an essential prerequisite for safe and effective person-centred maternity care.
- Power sharing is an important aspect of the maternity care practice environment, both between professionals but also with women and families who are accessing maternity care.
- Shared decision making that respects the underpinning values and beliefs of the woman is one of the cornerstones of contemporary midwifery care.

References

Dahlen, H. (2016). *Continuity of midwifery care models improve outcomes for young women and babies.* https://ebn.bmj.com/content/ebnurs/19/3/72.full.pdf

Department of Health (2010). *Midwifery 2020: Delivering expectations.* https://assets.publishing.service.gov.uk/government/uploads/system/uploads/attachment_data/file/216029/dh_119470.pdf

Department of Health (2018). *Co-Production Guide: Connecting and Realising Value Through People.* Belfast: Department of Health.

DHSSPSNI (2012). *Northern Ireland: A Strategy for Maternity Care in Northern Ireland 2012–18.* Belfast: DHSSPS.

House of Commons Health and Social Care Committee (2019). *First 1000 Days of Life.* Thirteenth Report of Session 2017–19. London: Stationery Office.

Kirkup, B. (2015). *The Report of the Morecambe Bay Investigation.* www.gov.uk/government/uploads/system/uploads/attachment_data/file/408480/47487_MBI_Accessible_v0.1.pdf

National Institute for Health and Care Excellence (2019). *Antenatal care for uncomplicated pregnancies: Clinical Guideline 62.* www.nice.org.uk/guidance/cg62/chapter/Woman-centred-care

National Institute for Health and Care Excellence (2012). *Patient experience in adult NHS services: improving the experience of care for people using adult NHS services Clinical Guideline 138.* www.nice.org.uk/guidance/cg138

Nursing and Midwifery Council (2018). *The Code. Professional standards of practice and behaviour for nurses, midwives and nursing associates.* www.nmc.org.uk/standards/code

Renfrew, M.J., McFadden, A., Bastos, M.H. et al. (2014). Midwifery and quality care: findings from a new evidence-informed framework for maternal and newborn care. *Lancet* 384 (9948): 1129–1145.

Royal College of Midwives (2016). *The RCM standards for midwifery services in the UK.* www.rcm.org.uk/media/2283/rcm-standards-midwifery-services-uk.pdf

Royal College of Obstetricians and Gynaecologists (2019). *Departmental and team interventions.* www.rcog.org.uk/en/careers-training/workplace-workforce-issues/improving-workplace-behaviours-dealing-with-undermining/undermining-toolkit/departmental-and-team-interventions/

Sandall, J. (2012). *Every woman needs a midwife, and some women need a doctor too.* www.ncbi.nlm.nih.gov/pubmed/23281954

Sandall, J., Soltani, H., Gates, S. et al. (2016). Midwife-led continuity models versus other models of care for childbearing women. *Cochrane Database of Systematic Reviews* (4): CD004667.

Scottish Government (2010). *Midwifery 2020: delivering expectations.* https://assets.publishing.service.gov.uk/government/uploads/system/uploads/attachment_data/file/216029/dh_119470.pdf

Scottish Government (2017). *The best start – a five-year plan for maternity and neonatal care.* www.gov.scot/publications/best-start-five-year-forward-plan-maternity-neonatal-care-scotland

The Shrewsbury and Telford Hospital NHS Trust (2017). *The Royal College of Obstetrics and Gynaecology Reports*. www.sath.nhs.uk/wp-content/uploads/2018/07/12-RCOG-Report.pdf

West, M.A. and Lyubovnikova, J. (2013). Illusions of team working in health care. *Journal of Health, Organisation and Management* 27 (1): 134–142.

World Health Organization (2017). *WHO Recommendations on Antenatal Care for a Positive Pregnancy Experience*. Geneva: WHO.

World Health Organization (2018). *WHO recommendations: intrapartum care for a positive childbirth experience*. www.who.int/publications/i/item/9789241550215

Further reading

Afulani, P.A., Phillips, B., Aborigo, R.A., and Moyer, C.A. (2019). Person-centred maternity care in low-income and middle-income countries: analysis of data from Kenya, Ghana, and India. *Lancet Global Health* 7: e96–e109.

Downe, S. (2019). Focusing on what works for person-centred maternity care. *Lancet Global Health* 7: e10–e11. www.thelancet.com/action/showPdf?pii=S2214-109X%2818%2930544-8.

Sudhinaraset, M., Giessler, K., Golub, G. et al. (2019). Providers' and women's perspectives on person-centered maternity care: a mixed methods study in Kenya. *International Journal for Equity in Health* 18: 83.

25

Being person-centred in children's services

Ruth Magowan[1] and Brian McGowan[2]

[1] Queen Margaret University, Edinburgh, Scotland, UK

[2] Ulster University, Northern Ireland, UK

Contents

Fundamentals of Person-Centred Healthcare Practice, First Edition. Edited by Brendan McCormack, Tanya McCance, Cathy Bulley, Donna Brown, Ailsa McMillan and Suzanne Martin.

Learning outcomes

- Reflect on your current practice and think about how person-centred you are.
- Develop your knowledge about person-centredness and person-centred processes in children's services.
- Enhance your practice with children and their families using person-centred practice processes.

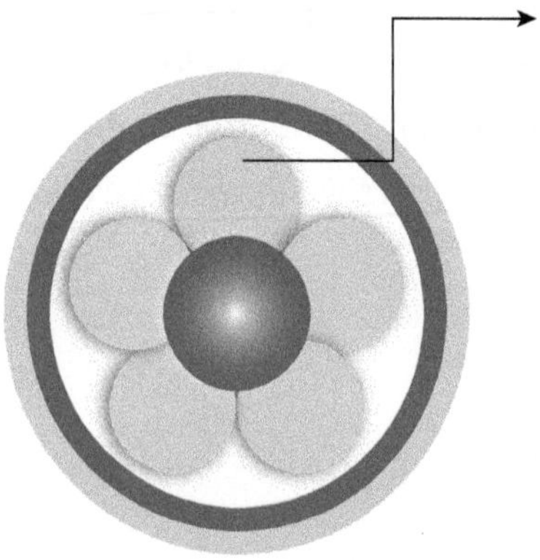

Person-centred processes:

Working with the person's beliefs and values: having a clear picture of the person's values about his/her life and how he/she makes sense of what is happening from their individual perspective, psychosocial context and social role

Sharing decision making: engaging persons in decision making by considering values, experiences, concerns and future aspirations

Engaging authentically: the connectedness between people, determined by knowledge of the person, clarity of beliefs and values, knowledge of self and professional expertise

Being sympathetically present: an engagement that recognises the uniqueness and value of the person, by appropriately responding to cues that maximise coping resources through the recognition of important agendas in their life

Working holistically: ways of connecting that pay attention to the whole person through the integration of physiological, psychological, sociocultural, developmental and spiritual dimensions of persons

Introduction

Working in children's services for all health professionals is an exciting and challenging field of practice. It could be argued that being person-centred in children's services adds another layer of complexity to an already complicated picture. By and large, we think of being person-centred as something that is relational, that happens between adults where the interpersonal connection is immediate and direct. We work with children, however, and whilst we still enjoy a direct connection that respects the child's personhood, we must consider the significant others who will be (and must be) involved. When we consider person-centred practice as outlined in Chapter 3, we will focus on the person-centred processes important to professionals working in children's services. Person-centred relationships must be developed with children, young people, their families and all included in and connected to the care situation. An example of this is a teenager who is living with a lifelong condition such as diabetes. Health professionals require a participative, collaborative and inclusive approach, and the work of educating others about the young person's condition will extend in a wide circle. This will include peers, sports coaches, teachers and anyone else whose understanding and support will help the young person live with the condition and not be limited by it.

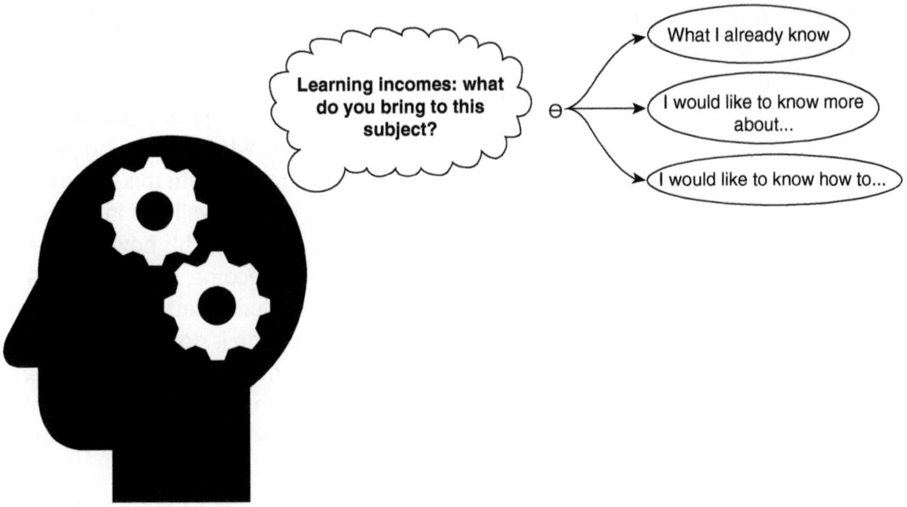

Figure 25.1 Learning incomes. Source: From Race P. (2014).

Children's services currently take the position that they practise family-centred care and whilst we recognise that this is a good thing, we argue that sometimes it does not have the same underpinning ideas that truly empower individuals. For example, a study by Stuart and Melling (2014) found that definitions of family-centred care were still very much underpinned by what people did (tasks), as opposed to how they felt or who they were. According to Ford et al. (2018), this approach tends to sideline children and downplay their needs in favour of parents; it is therefore parent-centred. In addition, Smith (2018) argues that family-centred care is an abstract concept and that nurses have trouble putting it into practice. Over the course of this chapter, we invite (or challenge) you to question your assumptions about what you mean when you say family-centred. We expand on the ways in which person-centred processes can be enacted when working in children's services.

Activity

You have read the learning outcomes above that state what we think you may get out of reading this chapter, but what do you think? Learning incomes are those things that you bring to the subject when beginning to engage with it (Race 2014). Spend a little time thinking about what you know and what you would like to know. Figure 25.1 explains this.

Person-Centred Processes

Working in children's services is different from caring for people in adulthood (whilst appearing remarkably similar). That is, we are still striving for the same person-centred outcomes and these will be facilitated in the same type of care environments and have the same organisational requirements and prerequisites, discussed in Chapter 3. To that end, we have focused on the person-centred processes and considered how they would be enacted in the context of working with children and their families.

We start from a belief that the professional person in children's services has an honorary position in a family (although we accept that sometimes this doesn't happen for a variety of reasons). We are invited to join in with the family and are afforded the opportunity to walk beside them. This may only be for a short time, such as at a time of crisis or for a planned short-term intervention. It could also be over a longer period when the young person is living with a long-term condition. Part of the professionalism associated with this is knowing, accepting and respecting that this is a position of power. Doing our job well and in a person-centred manner means that we are able to behave appropriately and share this power with the person and family in order to make sure that they do not feel, or become, subordinate. As a young person moves towards transition to adult services, this includes 'letting go' and supporting increased autonomy of the person and family unit. Once our job is done, we need to recognise that there is a right time to respectfully step away. In this chapter, we are not suggesting that person-centredness is *different* for children; rather that when you work in children's services, you must be adept at being person-centred for adults and for children too. For more detail on person-centredness see Chapter 2.

It is natural to come to a subject such as this with 'baggage' or assumptions that underpin your practice (Brookfield 1995). Some of your assumptions may be around definitions of person-centred practice for children's services. Historically, professionals who work with children thought of themselves as being 'child-centred' and/or 'family-centred'. Take time to challenge these assumptions because as O'Connor (2019) argued, they may not be truly person-centred and can often be more about service provision and delivery than the individual people we are connecting with.

Working with the person's beliefs and values

As we mentioned above, working with children adds some extra factors that need to be considered when working on a day-to-day basis. In our context we are not only working with the child's beliefs and values but also those of their primary carer, significant others or those with parental responsibility. When it comes to the child themselves, we need to think about the child's stage of development and capacity for understanding their current circumstances. Depending on their cognitive ability, a child's capacity to understand consequences may be limited, (Berk 2013), and we need to make sure that we are (where possible) reducing anxiety. The innocuous phrase of 'we need to take your blood' can, in a child's mind, become a horrific proposition. It may sound like you wish to remove all of their blood. Therefore, you need to be clear, for example 'we need to take *some* blood' and show the child that you will not take a lot. Such a routine procedure is probably normal to you by now, but it could be very daunting for someone on the receiving end for the first time. Try to make sure that your reassurance doesn't seem indifferent or careless; instead try to engage authentically.

Engaging authentically

When working with children and their families, you will have learnt about stages of cognitive, social, emotional, language and physical development and their implications for your practice in terms of communication, (Bornstein and Lambe 2011). Essentially, this is a reductionist approach that disassembles the person into component parts to better understand how they work. But this approach has a fundamental flaw and could even be labelled as antiholistic. In your practice, you need to be able to bring all the components back together and address not only the whole child but the whole family unit.

George Bernard Shaw pointed out, 'The single biggest problem in communication is the illusion that it has taken place'. Whilst he wasn't thinking about children when he said that, it has implications for practice. So now might be a good time to revise your communication skills. A formal approach to communication and development will act as a useful knowledge base but when engaging with children, think about what they like to do and hear and what are the things that interest them and bore them.

An active approach is always recommended when working with children. Expecting them to sit passively whilst information is being thrown at them is a likely way of losing their attention and invites chaos. Think about how you can engage children when talking with them on a daily basis. Most people love a story, (Smidt 2011), and according to Bruner (1966) stories form the basis of how we live our lives and interpret the world around us. It is a process of sense making and Bruner and Haste (1987) wisely point out that 'making sense is a social process'. Telling a story may be a useful approach when explaining what is going to happen whilst in hospital. You could also encourage children to tell their own stories.

Hearing the child's story can help us to be authentic in our response and ways of engaging. Authentic means being genuine and going beyond merely stating our values, to trying to live them. We want our values to be visible in our practice and ways of working. Being authentic can be a challenge, however. Authenticity can go unchallenged when things are going well but can be more troublesome when times are tough or when we are called to account.

Sharing decision making

Sharing decision making can be something that a lot of us have some trouble with. When people agree with what we say, sharing can be easy. In contrast, when it seems that someone is rejecting something we believe is in their best interests, it can be hard to live up to the idea of sharing decision making. Some of your assumptions around definitions of person-centred practice for children's services might be interfering with your efforts to be person-centred.

Sharing decision making is additionally complicated by the developing intellectual capacity of children, affecting their ability to understand complex information and fully understand the consequences of their actions. Communication is key, along with involvement. Children are curious and want to know why things are the way they are. Ostroff (2012) pointed out that over 70% of 2–4-year-old children's questions are about human motivation. This is where we rely upon parents or those with parental responsibility to work with us. The sharing of decision making goes beyond a one-to-one interaction to one that has multiple actors contributing in a variety of ways. Legal and/or technical guidance exists that can assist with understanding this; however, in the moment we must engage with children and their families and try to understand the shape and dynamics of their family. We then need to seek admission to that dynamic and find our own place where we can contribute and help. All too often, we can insert ourselves into the mix in a brusque fashion and over time can do more harm than good.

We need to be careful that our shared decision making is genuine and authentic. As technical authorities, we have 'a pass' into the family dynamic and this must be used wisely. Family members may ask you 'What would you do?'. Although it is tempting and easy to answer this question, this is not shared decision making. We need to provide the impartial information and evidence that they need to come to a decision together, and then support them in their chosen path. Once a decision has been reached, our role may be to support parents when they discuss this with the child. This too has its pitfalls, because parents themselves have different views about how much involvement their children have in day-to-day decision making. Suddenly being asked to be involved in decision making in healthcare may impact negatively on a child.

This means that getting to know the family as individuals as well as a unit is of vital importance. As McCormack and McCance (2017) point out, this will enable true collaboration, participation and negotiation. There are resources available to help you with decision making, such as NICE guidelines available from its website and useful documents from the King's Fund.

- www.nice.org.uk/about/what-we-do/our-programmes/nice-guidance/nice-guidelines/shared-decision-making
- www.kingsfund.org.uk/sites/default/files/Making-shared-decision-making-a-reality-paper-Angela-Coulter-Alf-Collins-July-2011_0.pdf

Being sympathetically present

Being sympathetically present has additional layers when working with children and their families. Being sympathetically present is explored in depth in Chapter 15. When considering sympathetic presence with adults, there is a focus on accepting the other person's beliefs, values and priorities and attending to their feelings and identity in the moment (McCormack and McCance, 2017). Being sympathetically present for a child also requires the health professional to try to understand, or remember, what it is like to see the world through a child's eyes. Running concurrently with this is the need to alter one's focus and imagine what it must be like for a parent.

It is now well recognised that children's and parents' needs and emotions in a health crisis are very different, for example, during a hospital admission or diagnosis. In two studies by Coyne (2015) and Magowan et al. (2017), children described needing appropriate explanations and space to ask questions, to be prepared for events, and to have enough information to understand their care. It may surprise many health professionals that parents' needs are usually much more on an emotional level. When listening to their stories, even when parents seemed outwardly to be coping with their child's illness, often this did not reflect their feelings. They talk of the time of diagnosis as feeling that the 'bottom had fallen out of their world' and that 'their family would never experience normal again' (Magowan et al. 2017). Clearly health professionals need to be able to meet the needs of both children and parents.

On a day-to-day basis we need to be aware of our language; we often use terms that to us seem to be normal or even common sense; for service users coming into hospital or any healthcare environment, however, that language can be impenetrable or frightening. For example, we tend to refer to all things child-orientated as paediatric. This is a common enough word, but not one that everyone understands. We must be sympathetic to what people know and what they don't, rather than making assumptions.

Working holistically

Normally the provision of holistic care hinges upon us understanding that people are more than the sum of their parts and not treating them as biological systems that need fixing. In the case of children, this also holds true but adds a new perspective – of the family in whatever shape or configuration it comes in. Each family is unique and has its own shape, dynamic and history. Traditional notions of a nuclear family are less dominant than they were and increasingly families are blended and have parents with myriad roles that need to be understood. Therefore, the first step to the provision of holistic care is to understand the family in front of you.

Activity

Take a few moments to think about your family. What shape is it and who occupies which roles? Placing yourself at the centre of your family map, what does it look like? Who are the really significant people in your life? What is a 'normal' family? Where do your views about what is normal come from?

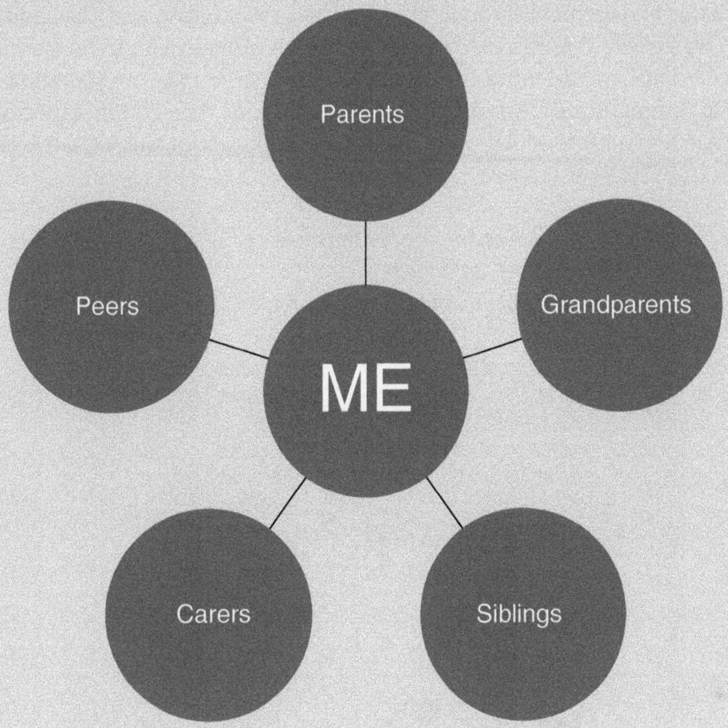

In all these person-centred processes, it is important to consider carefully how we make sure that children feel involved in their care. The key language in which you need to become fluent is play. All children play (and all people should play). Play could be the key to accessing the child's inner life world and acts like a carrier wave for information and things you need to do. Its also a two-way communication system whereby the children get to know you and establish a trusting therapeutic relationship. Once that trust has been gained, it needs to be handled with care and treated with respect.

Provision of care is still dominated by a discourse of doing things *to* children. Definitions of family-centred care moved the agenda somewhat by including parents in that equation, but they are still essentially doing things *to* as opposed to *with*. The challenge is to move your care towards working with the child and family and doing this in the context of an interprofessional approach to care. A uniprofessional development of holistic care delivery is probably doomed to failure. We don't work in isolation; each of our actions is informed and contextualised by the people we work with and we must strive to ensure that the child and family are included in that team as full members.

Conclusion

In conclusion, we wish to point out that we do not believe this chapter to be definitive. Indeed, it is the very act of questioning that defines our practice and we urge you to do this. Working with children and their families has different layers of complexity when compared to working with adults and it is important to consider how person-centred processes can be enacted when working in this context. Respecting children's personhood can be a challenge in practice but with authentic engagement through creativity (e.g. story telling and play) and a sympathetic presence, we believe that this can be facilitated. This requires you to be alert and mindful of your surroundings and attentive to what children are saying to you. Sometimes, children can be trying to communicate ideas or feelings that are beyond their current capacity and this leads to frustration and misinterpretation or misunderstanding. Engaging with this is best summed up by Mackesy (2019) as follows;

I'm so small", said the mole
"Yes", said the boy.
"But you make a huge difference".

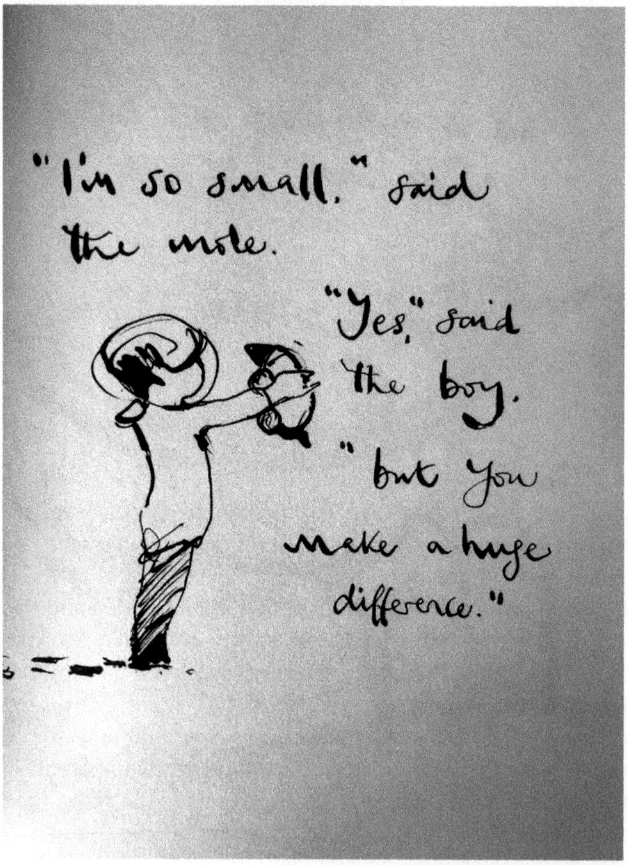

Read widely and think deeply. Many activities that run as a thread throughout this book depend on your ability to reflect. However, according to Boud (1985), in order to reflect we must first *notice*. To illustrate this, we leave you with some words from Seamus Heaney (2010) who points out the importance of being able to notice things.

Had I not been awake
Had I not been awake I would have missed it,
A wind that rose and whirled until the roof
Pattered with quick leaves off the sycamore
And got me up, the whole of me a-patter,
Alive and ticking like an electric fence:
Had I not been awake I would have missed it,
It came and went so unexpectedly
And almost it seemed dangerously,
Returning like an animal to the house,
A courier blast that there and then
Lapsed ordinary. But not ever
After. And not now.

Summary

- Working with children's and families' values and beliefs is complicated and relies on listening and finding out what is important to each person.
- Families come in all shapes and sizes. Spending time mapping out a family's shape, dynamic and history will be time well spent to help you explore the best way of being in partnership and providing a sympathetic presence.
- Communicate clearly and authentically with children and their families as equal partners in the decision-making process
- Be creative, tell stories, listen to stories and make stories together
- Reflect on your culture and care environments and challenge ways of working that are not healthful and person-centred. Above all, when working with children, don't forget to play

References

Berk, L. (2013). *Child Development*, 9e. London: Pearson.

Bornstein, M.H. and Lamb, M.E. (2011). *Cognitive Development: An Advanced Textbook*. New York: Taylor and Francis.

Boud, D., Keogh, R., and Walker, D. (1985). *Reflection: Turning Experience into Learning*. Abingdon: Routledge.

Brookfield, S.D. (1995). *Becoming a Critically Reflective Teacher*. San Francisco: Jossey-Bass.

Bruner, J.S. (1966). *Toward a Theory of Instruction*. London: Belknap Press.

Bruner, J.S. and Haste, H. (1987). *Making Sense: The Child's Construction of the World*. London: Methuen.

Coyne, I. (2015). *Child and family-centred care: promotion of person-centred care*. National Association of Children's Nurses 40th Jubilee Conference, Stockholm, 5th November.

Ford, K., Dickinson, A., Water, T. et al. (2018). Child centred care: challenging assumptions and repositioning children. *Journal of Pediatric Nursing* 43: e39–e43.

Heaney, S. (2010). *Human Chain*. London: Faber and Faber.

Magowan, R., Chalmers, A., Millin, T. (2017) Person-centred paediatric care: capturing the experience and collaborating for the future. www.fons.org/Resources/Documents/Project%20Reports/Person-Centred-Paediatric-Care---Capturing-the-Experience-and-Collaborating-for-the-Future.pdf

Mackesy, C. (2019). *The Boy, the mole, the fox and the Horse*. London: Ebury Press.
McCormack, B. and McCance, T. (eds.) (2017). *Person Centred Practice in Nursing and Healthcare: Theory and Practice*, 2e. Chichester: Wiley Blackwell.
O'Connor, S., Brenner, M., and Coyne, I. (2019). Family-centred care of children and young people in the acute hospital setting: a concept analysis. *Journal of Clinical Nursing* 28: 3353–3367.
Ostroff, W.L. (2012). *Understanding How Young Children Learn. Bringing the Science of Child Development to the Classroom*. Alexandria: ASCD.
Race, P. (2014). *Making Learning Happen. A Guide for Post-Compulsory Education*, 3e. London: Sage.
Smidt, S. (2011). *Introducing Bruner: A Guide for Practitioners and Students in Early Years Education*. New York: Routledge.
Smith, W. (2018). Concept analysis of family-centred care of hospitalized pediatric patients. *Journal of Pediatric Nursing* 42: 57–64.
Stuart, M. and Melling, S. (2014). Understanding nurses' and parents' perceptions of family-centred care. *Nursing Children and Young People* 26 (7): 16–20.

Further Reading

www.nice.org.uk/about/what-we-do/our-programmes/nice-guidance/nice-guidelines/shared-decision-making
www.kingsfund.org.uk/sites/default/files/Making-shared-decision-making-a-reality-paper-Angela-Coulter-Alf-Collins-July-2011_0.pdf
https://phil-race.co.uk

26

Being person-centred when working with people living with long-term conditions

Anne Williams[1], Suzanne Martin[2], and Vivien Coates[2]

[1] Queen Margaret University, Edinburgh, Scotland, UK

[2] Ulster University, Northern Ireland, UK and Western Health and Social Care Trust, Londonderry, Northern Ireland, UK

Contents

Fundamentals of Person-Centred Healthcare Practice, First Edition. Edited by Brendan McCormack, Tanya McCance, Cathy Bulley, Donna Brown, Ailsa McMillan and Suzanne Martin.

Learning outcomes

- Critically reflect on current approaches to delivering person-centred care for people with long-term conditions.
- Develop an understanding of the barriers and facilitators of self-management for adults with a long-term condition.
- Apply models of care that support self-management for people living with long-term conditions and their families.

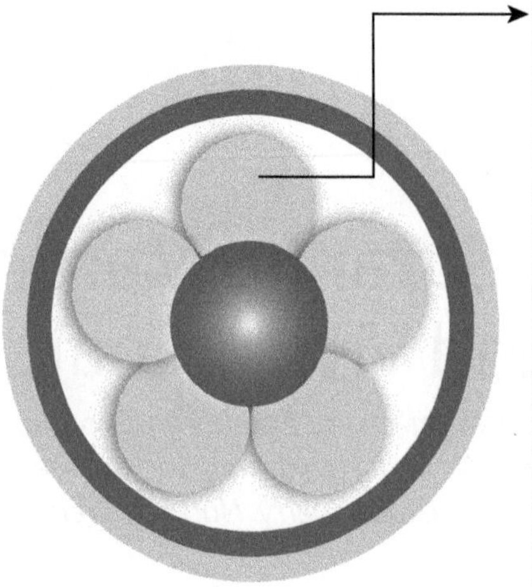

Working with the person's beliefs and values: having a clear picture of the person's values about his/her life and how he/she makes sense of what is happening from their individual perspective, psychosocial context and social role

Sharing decision making: engaging persons in decision making by considering values, experiences, concerns and future aspirations

Engaging authentically: the connectedness between people, determined by knowledge of the person, clarity of beliefs and values, knowledge of self and professional expertise

Being sympathetically present: an engagement that recognises the uniqueness and value of the person, by appropriately responding to cues that maximise coping resources through the recognition of important agendas in their life

Working holistically: *ways of connecting that pay attention to the whole person through the integration of physiological, psychological, sociocultural, developmental and spiritual dimensions of persons*

Introduction

In this chapter we will critically explore the opportunities and challenges that arise when working with people living with long-term conditions, and how this relates to the *processes* domain of the Person-centred Practice Framework.

The context and challenges of living with a long-term condition

A long-term condition is defined as 'a condition that cannot, at present, be cured but is controlled by medication and/or other treatment/therapies' (Department of Health 2012, p. 3). As a health professional, it is highly likely you will work with people living with one or more physical long-term conditions such as diabetes, arthritis, respiratory or coronary heart disease, cancer, obesity, dementia or AIDS. It will be important for you to recognise the different challenges that arise for individuals such as physical symptoms, the demands of navigating healthcare systems, managing polypharmacy (more than one medication), and balancing social roles and responsibilities (Gallacher et al. 2014).

It is estimated that one in three adults in the United Kingdom (UK) lives with a long-term condition (Department of Health 2012), often leading to premature death, disability and significant costs to the healthcare system. Advances in healthcare are more likely to control than cure, so people may live longer, while dealing with complex problems and treatments (Nolte and McKee 2008). In a study of 314 medical practices in Scotland, Barnett et al. (2012) reported that 23.2% of people lived with multi-morbidities related to several co-existing physical and mental health conditions, with the prevalence much higher in those over 65 years and in areas of socioeconomic deprivation. Therefore, significant personal, social and economic burdens are often associated with long-term conditions, which vary widely depending on individual circumstances, stage of the condition, the need for lifestyle and specialist interventions, and the individual capacity to self-manage (Eaton et al. 2015).

The World Health Organization takes a human rights perspective on long-term conditions, recognising the need to empower people and their communities, focus on international co-operation, evidence-based approaches to prevention, and multisector action in addressing lifestyle and wider determinants of health such as poverty (WHO 2013). The Person-centred Practice Framework is aligned to this as it encourages us to think holistically about the person and what matters to them (see Chapter 16), within this global and developing context of humanising healthcare systems that support dignity, equity and partnership as universal principles (McCormack and McCance 2017, Chapter 1).

Activity

Think about a person you know or someone that you cared for, perhaps in hospital, community or a care home setting, who has one or more physical long-term condition. Make a note of the main difficulties or challenges they experience. In what ways does the care environment influence your ability to provide person-centred care?

Healthcare system design

Healthcare systems such as the National Health Service (NHS) have traditionally followed a medical model, with acute services often organised within medical specialties and single-condition services, for example coronary care. These do not reflect the needs of those living with multi-morbidities. For people living with more than one condition, care becomes fragmented and poorly co-ordinated (NHS England 2019), and the scope for person-centred practice is limited.

Over several decades, care of people with long-term conditions has become a key priority within health policy (Barclay and Lawson 2016), shifting the care from acute services into community-based integrated, interprofessional health and social care services (Scottish Government 2016). New approaches to healthcare delivery seek to place the person at the centre of services and dismantle the traditional barriers between health, social care and third sector providers to ensure genuine partnerships are developed between service users and providers (www.england.nhs.uk/ourwork/clinical-policy/ltc/our-work-on-long-

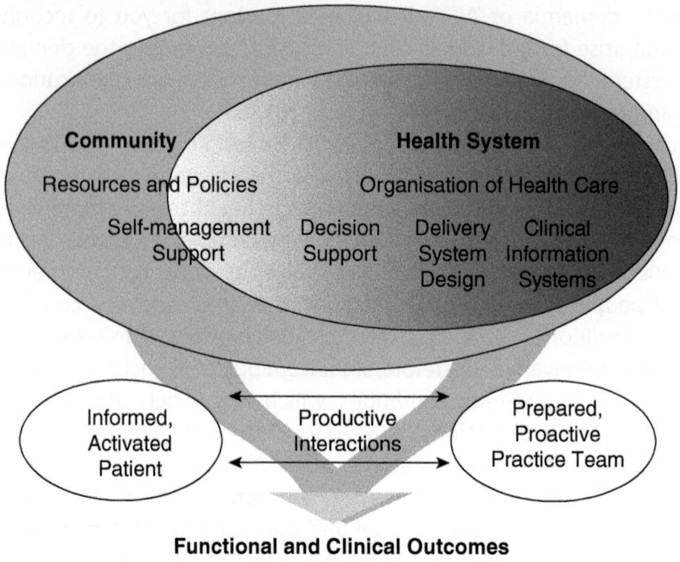

Figure 26.1 Chronic Care Model. Source: Wagner, E.H. et al. (2005).

term-conditions/). This quote from National Voices, a coalition of health and care organisations, emphasises a key focus for services (National Voices 2019):

> We want person-centred care: people having as much control and influence over their care as possible – as patient, carers and members of communities.

Service models

There are numerous models of care underpinning service delivery. Here we will outline two models that have been developed to address the challenges of long-term conditions: the Chronic Care Model and the House of Care.

The Chronic Care Model

The Chronic Care Model (Wagner et al. 2005) recognises that chronic conditions place a different set of demands on people than acute conditions, requiring continual decision making and adjustments to changing circumstances. The model focuses on linking informed and active people with long-term conditions with proactive teams of professionals. Wagner and colleagues acknowledge that when you live with a long-term condition, a significant proportion of the care takes place outside traditional healthcare settings and they identify six elements of importance to improve outcomes. These elements are shown in Figure 26.1.

The House of Care

Coulter et al. (2016) described the development of a co-ordinated service delivery model in the UK, incorporating collaborative personalised care planning, enabling clinicians and patients to work together in a collaborative process of shared decision making. The metaphor of a House

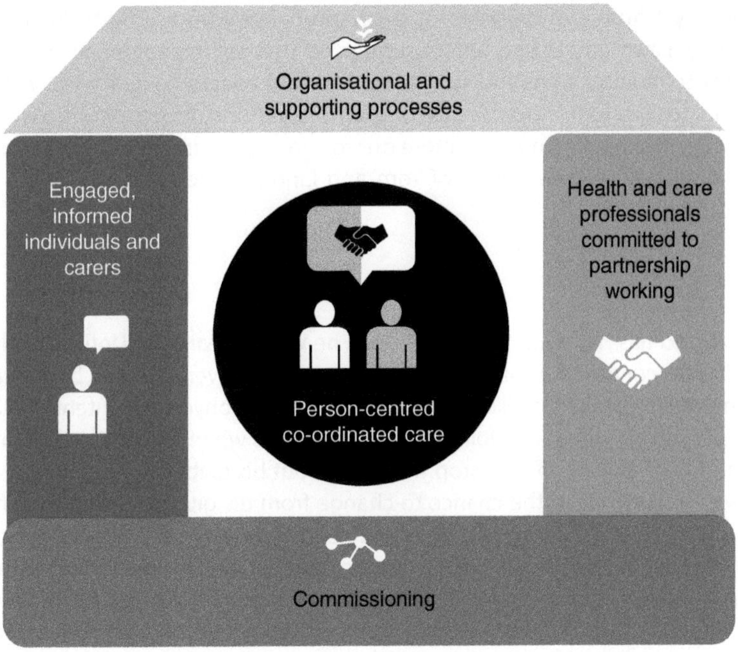

Figure 26.2 House of Care Model. Source: Modified from Taylor, A (2015).

of Care reflects a whole-system approach and the interdependency of each component part in meeting the needs of people with long-term conditions (Figure 26.2). The model fits the commissioning context of the NHS in parts of the UK, but further evaluation is required (Taylor 2015).

Supporting people with long-term conditions

Here we will explore in more detail the opportunities person-centred healthcare staff have to support people with long-term conditions, using the Person-centred Practice Framework within the models of care outlined above. Long-term conditions are complex and management requires commitment and adherence to treatment by the person who has the condition. This is generally referred to as self-management. Supporting self-management has been a central focus for policy and strategic development, with self-management being described as:

> The successful outcome of the person and all appropriate individuals and services working together to support [a person] to deal with the very real implications of living the rest of their life with one or more long-term condition. (LTCAS 2008, p. 5)

We are all involved in the everyday work of self-managing our health through attending to what we eat, taking exercise, caring for our bodies. 'Illness work', such as taking regular medications, monitoring blood glucose or blood pressure, and managing symptoms often become key features of daily life of a person living with a long-term condition (Vassilev et al. 2013). Lawn and Schoo (2010) suggested that self-management requires knowledge, the ability to monitor signs and symptoms and the capacity to deal with emotional, physical, social and occupational impacts of a long-term condition. As people who work in healthcare, we must therefore take time to explore our role in supporting people with self-management. We are going to use the stories of Tom and Linda in the scenarios below to deepen our understanding.

Scenario 1: Tom's story

Tom is 25 and has had type 1 diabetes since he was 11 years old. Until recently he found self-managing his condition a challenge. He frequently felt overwhelmed by the need to monitor his blood glucose, take his insulin, be aware of the carbohydrate content of all he ate and the impact of days when he was doing nothing and days when he was 'on the go' all the time. At times he would 'switch off' and stop thinking about his diabetes.

He was recently given the chance to change from his glucose monitoring meter to having a flash glucose sensor so that he does not need to do so much finger pricking. He likes this device as he feels it is easier to check his glucose levels and his diabetes control has improved. He has now been offered an insulin pump and has been told that many young people find these preferable to having insulin injections. Before he can have a pump, he needs to complete a five-day course about diabetes self-management; he does not want to miss work at the moment but realises that this course could help him.

However, the change that he thinks is helping him the most is that the diabetes team have a different approach to managing diabetes. At the clinic, less time is spent talking about targets, hypoglycaemia and bloods and he is encouraged to explore issues that are important to him. These are rarely about blood sugars. He feels the team have a better understanding of him as a person and his own goals in life. They understand that he can't take on the diabetes education course now due to his job but will offer him another chance next time the course runs. He feels more able to open up about how tedious life with diabetes can be, that he is not judged when expressing negative views and that staff are keen to explore ways of supporting him to manage his diabetes without it dominating his life or his lifestyle.

Activity

Barriers and facilitators to self-management

With Tom's story in mind, make notes on the most useful ways in which members of the diabetes team can support him. More broadly than just the diabetes team, what will help Tom (facilitators) and what are the barriers to him managing his diabetes? You may wish to consider how the prerequisites of healthcare workers, their knowledge of self, their professional competence, interpersonal skills and commitment to the job enable them to effectively apply person-centred processes. These processes may include working with Tom's beliefs and values, and sharing decision making, enabling him to have a good care experience. The environmental context of care and the way in which the service is delivered are also important. An outpatient clinic in which staff appeared harried and with a waiting room full of patients is unlikely to be conducive to a young person engaging in meaningful discussion about a complex condition that can affect all elements of their life.

In the next section we will use Linda's story to explore our work in undertaking assessment to provide holistic care.

Assessment in the context of providing holistic care

Scenario 2: Linda's story

Linda is the 59-year-old mother of Jade and Ellen. Linda has lipoedema, a poorly recognised fat disorder affecting women, which leads to disproportionate enlargement of her legs and buttocks, bruising and pain on pressure to the tissues (Williams 2019). Linda now has secondary lymphoedema and was recently admitted to hospital with recurrent cellulitis of the leg. Her mobility is significantly worse than last year due to the leg swelling; she also has plantar fasciitis, making walking more challenging. The lipoedema first began when she was 14 years old, when she noticed changes in her leg shape. Linda remembers being called 'thunder thighs' at school. She tried to lose weight by dieting for several decades, without success. She has also had depression for many years.

Linda is a member of a closed Facebook peer support group, run by a third sector organisation that supports women with lipoedema. Linda has shared with other women the difficulties she had with staff at the GP surgery, who have constantly chastised her for being 'obese', due to her BMI of 36; she has often left the surgery in tears. She has recently attended a self-management group run by a third sector organisation, over five weeks. Linda feels her self-esteem has improved and she is more confident to self-manage her lipoedema, making changes to her diet, taking appropriate exercise in water, wearing compression garments and taking antibiotics.

You will see from the complex problems experienced by Linda that she is likely to meet a range of healthcare professionals over the years including nurses, midwives, physiotherapists, occupational therapists, dieticians and podiatrists. Each professional has their own scope of practice, but consistent to all is the need to undertake a comprehensive assessment in order to work with Linda and support her to make decisions about her care. Linda also provides us with a context of living with a poorly recognised long-term condition where women are faced with stigma and judgemental comments from those around them, often from an early age (Williams 2019). The current focus on 'obesity' as a key health issue and the power dynamics related to this (Knutsen et al. 2011) also mean that Linda has experienced many health professionals labelling her as 'obese' and suggesting that lifestyle changes are the only solution.

Activity

Person-centred assessment

Drawing on your knowledge of the Person-centred Practice Framework, make notes on how you would work with Linda to undertake an assessment, taking into account the person-centred processes:

- being sympathetically present
- engaging authentically.

Consider here how authentic engagement with a person as part of your assessment might enable you to develop a trusting, healthful relationship with people such as Linda, in order to provide holistic person-centred care.

You will have noted that Linda experiences several physical symptoms, bringing her to an embodied knowledge of her lipoedema. She talks of feeling that her body 'has become out of control' (Williams 2019). Bodily changes in physical long-term conditions are often unpredictable and challenging. In Linda's situation, leg swelling, acute cellulitis and pain challenge the everyday silence of her body, and in a sociological sense, Linda views her body as betraying her; to her it has become an alien, changing body in which she must negotiate her relationship with the world (Williams 1996). Merleau-Ponty argues that the body is both a physical presence/object but also mediated through perceptual meaning (Crossley 1995) (see Chapter 1). Engaging authentically (see Chapter 13) as we make an assessment, touch and palpate the tissues, examining and measuring also requires us to recognise that embodied experience and the distress that may be associated with living in a body that is changed. As such there are some considerations for how we work with people.

- Take time to listen to their story.
- Reflect the contrasting approaches to using measurement and examination to objectify or medicalise the body versus using touch and interpersonal communication in a way that enhances the embodied, holistic care experience.
- Draw attention to physical changes in the body that enable people to understand their condition, rationale for self-management, and notice positive changes.
- Consider using a consultation model that helps us to be systematic but also holistic in our approach.

Source: Adapted from Barclay & Lawson (2016).

Critical perspectives

Entwistle et al. (2018) provided an important critique of the philosophical perspectives underpinning self-management. They recognised that policies on long-term condition care have often viewed self-management as a means to reduce demands on health services, by ensuring people change their health behaviours to meet biomedical health targets. For example, in Tom's story, you will see that although he had a blood glucose meter and he had information about his condition to ensure his glucose levels were maintained within 'normal limits', he struggled to do so during his teenage years. Entwistle et al. (2018) argue that this approach may set up ambitious targets for behaviour change, encourage authoritarian behaviours by health practitioners, disempower the person, and underestimate their self-knowledge and ability to make decisions. Entwistle et al. (2018) challenge us to consider whether the aim of self-management for Tom is to biomedically manage his condition well, monitoring the condition and adapt his behaviour, or is it about how we can support Tom to manage better with his diabetes?

Morgan et al. (2017) point out the difference between helping people to manage a condition well (interpreted as achieving clinical targets) and helping people to manage well while living with their health condition (more about quality of life overall). This is a subtle but important change in perspective as we work in a more person-centred way, enabling us to engage authentically and be sympathetically present. Bossy et al. (2019) also identify the potential dichotomy between a medical perspective on self-management and the reality of social and political dimensions of Tom's health-related experiences. This is where a partnership approach takes account of physical, socio-economic and psychological barriers to self-management that may exist, recognising ways in which healthcare practitioners can support and facilitate someone to make significant life changes towards longer term health and well-being. Linda's story also highlights how third sector groups and social media such as Facebook provide additional opportunities for person-centred self-management support (McGowan et al. 2013).

Conclusion

Fiscal challenges and policy drive supported self-management/care as a viable and appropriate mode of healthcare for those people living with long-term conditions. Within this paradigm, the context of care shifts primarily to the home space, and the expectation on people living with a long-term condition to step up within a self-management construct is fairly significant. Ideally, the aim is to support individuals, families and carers to understand fully and manage their health and well-being, with a sharper focus on prevention, rehabilitation and independence, allowing them to flourish and for healthcare staff to flourish (Scottish Government 2016). However, with this fundamental shift in approach to healthcare for long-term conditions, a key task for us is how to ensure that contemporary holistic healthcare, possibly delivered remotely, potentially using technology, does indeed remain person-centred.

Summary

- People living with long-term conditions face many challenges.
- Genuine partnership working can empower people living with long-term conditions.
- The Person-centred Practice Framework encourages us to identify what is important to the person living with their long-term condition to help them manage their condition well beyond the hospital.
- Using a consultation model helps us to be systematic and person-centred in our approach.

References

Barclay, E. and Lawson, V. (2016). Health psychology: supporting the self-management of long term conditions. *British Journal of Nursing* 25 (20): 1102–1107.

Barnett, K., Mercer, S.W., Norbury, M. et al. (2012). Epidemiology of multimorbidity and implications for health care, research, and medical education: a cross-sectional study. *Lancet* 380: 37–43.

Bossy, D., Knutsen, I.R., and Rogers, A. (2019). Moving between ideologies in self-management support – a qualitative study. *Health Expectations* 22: 83–92.

Coulter, A., Kramer, G., Warren, T., and Salisbury, C. (2016). Building the house of care for people with long-term conditions: the foundation of the house of care framework. *British Journal of General Practice* 66 (645): e288–e290.

Crossley, N. (1995). Merleau-Ponty, the elusive body and carnal sociology. *Body & Society* 1 (1): 43–63.

Department of Health (2012). *Long Term Conditions: Compendium of Information*, 3e. Leeds: Department of Health.

Eaton, S., Roberts, S., and Turner, B. (2015). Delivering person centred care in long term conditions. *BMJ* 350: h181.

Entwistle, V., Cribb, A., and Owens, J. (2018). Why health and social care support for people with long-term conditions should be oriented towards enabling them to live well. *Health Care Analysis* 26: 48–65.

Gallacher, K.I., Batty, G.D., McLean, G. et al. (2014). Stroke, multimorbidity and polypharmacy in a nationally representative sample of 1,424,378 patients in Scotland: implications for treatment burden. *BMC Medicine* 12 (1): 151–151.

Knutsen, I.R., Terragni, L., and Foss, C. (2011). Morbidly obese patients and lifestyle change: constructing ethical selves. *Nursing Inquiry* 18: 348–358.

Lawn, S. and Schoo, A. (2010). Supporting self-management of chronic health conditions. Common approaches. *Patient Education and Counselling* 80: 205–211.

Long Term Conditions Alliance Scotland/Scottish Government (LTCAS) (2008). *Gaun Yersel'. The self-management strategy for long term conditions in Scotland* www2.gov.scot/Publications/2008/10/GaunYersel.

McCormack, B. and McCance, T. (eds.) (2017). *Person-Centred Practice in Nursing and Healthcare: Theory and Practice*, 2e. Chichester: Wiley Blackwell.

McGowan, A., Williams, A., Davidson, F., and Williams, J. (2013). A self-management group programme for people with lymphoedema: experience from a third-sector project. *British Journal of Community Nursing* 18: S6–S12.

Morgan, H.M., Entwistle, V.A., Cribb, A. et al. (2017). We need to talk about purpose: a critical interpretive synthesis of health and social care professionals' approaches to self-management support for people with long-term conditions. *Health Expectations* 20 (2): 243–259.

National Voices (2019). www.nationalvoices.org.uk

NHS England (2019). *NHS Long Term Plan*. www.longtermplan.nhs.uk

Nolte, E. and McKee, M. (eds.) (2008). *Caring for People with Chronic Conditions. A Health System Perspective. European Observatory on Health Systems and Policies Series*. Maidenhead: Open University Press/McGraw-Hill.

Scottish Government (2016). *Health and Social Care Delivery Plan*. Edinburgh: Scottish Government.

Taylor, A. (2015). *Building the House of Care; How Health Economies in Leeds and Somerset Are Implementing a Coordinated Approach for People with Long-Term Conditions*. London: The Health Foundation.

Vassilev, I., Rogers, A., Blickem, C. et al. (2013). Social networks, the 'work' and work force of chronic illness self-management: a survey analysis of personal communities. *PLoS One* 8 (4): e59723.

Wagner, E.H., Bennett, S.M., Austin, B.T. et al. (2005). Finding common ground: patient-centeredness and evidence-based chronic illness care. *Journal of Alternative and Complementary Medicine* 11 (Supplement 1): S-7–S-15.

Williams, A. (2019). *A study of the experiences of women living with lipoedema in Scotland*. Oral presentation to the International Lymphoedema Framework Conference, Chicago, 13–16th June.

Williams, S. (1996). The vicissitudes of embodiment across the chronic illness trajectory. *Body & Society* 2 (2): 23–47.

World Health Organization (2013). *Global Action Plan for the Prevention of Noncommunicable Diseases 2013–2020*. Geneva: World Health Organization.

Further reading

Genova, L. (2012). *Still Alice*. London: Simon & Schuster.

Nolte, E., Knai, C., and McKee, M. (2008) *Managing chronic conditions. Experience in eight countries*. WHO, Copenhagen.

Reynolds, R., Dennis, S., Hasan, I. et al. (2018). A systematic review of chronic disease management interventions in primary care. *BMC Family Practice* 19: 11.

Sontag, S. (2009). *Illness as Metaphor and AIDS and Its Metaphors*. London: Penguin.

Woolf, V. (2012). *On Being Ill: With Notes from Sick Rooms by Julia Stephen*. Middletown, CT: Wesleyan University Press.

27

Palliative and end of life care services

Antonia Lannie[1], Erna Haraldsdottir[2], and Juliet Spiller[3]

[1] University of Dundee, Dundee, Scotland, UK
[2] Queen Margaret University, Edinburgh, Scotland, UK and St Columba's Hospice, Edinburgh, Scotland, UK
[3] Marie Curie Hospice, Edinburgh, Scotland, UK

Contents

Fundamentals of Person-Centred Healthcare Practice, First Edition. Edited by Brendan McCormack, Tanya McCance, Cathy Bulley, Donna Brown, Ailsa McMillan and Suzanne Martin.

Learning outcomes

- Understand the overlapping contexts of palliative care ethos and person-centred practice.
- Appreciate the key elements of person-centredness in palliative care
- Understand how a person-centred approach can be made to different contexts and different client groups in palliative and end of life care services.
- Recognise the potential barriers and challenges to person-centred practice within palliative care.

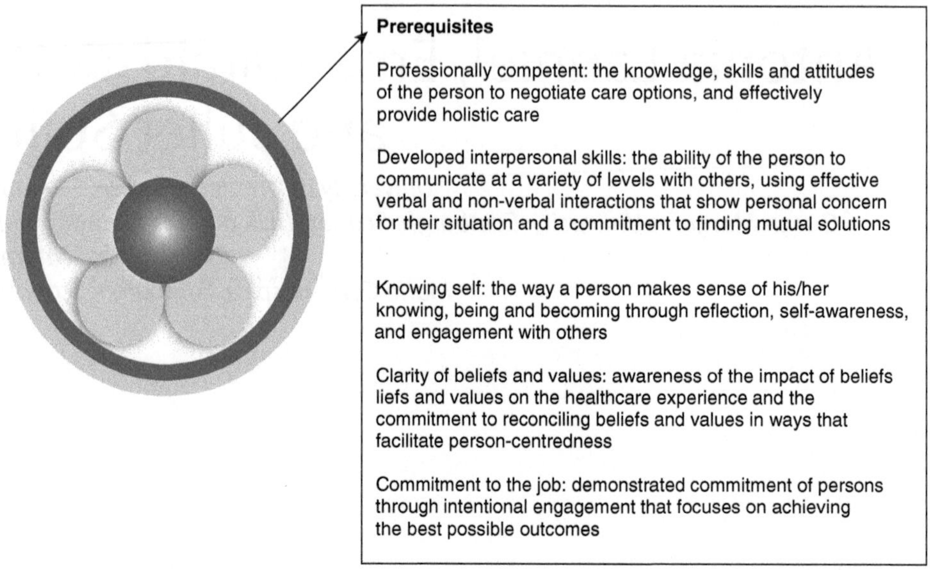
Prerequisites
Professionally competent: the knowledge, skills and attitudes of the person to negotiate care options, and effectively provide holistic care
Developed interpersonal skills: the ability of the person to communicate at a variety of levels with others, using effective verbal and non-verbal interactions that show personal concern for their situation and a commitment to finding mutual solutions
Knowing self: the way a person makes sense of his/her knowing, being and becoming through reflection, self-awareness, and engagement with others
Clarity of beliefs and values: awareness of the impact of beliefs liefs and values on the healthcare experience and the commitment to reconciling beliefs and values in ways that facilitate person-centredness
Commitment to the job: demonstrated commitment of persons through intentional engagement that focuses on achieving the best possible outcomes

Introduction

> You matter because you are you, and you matter to the end of your life. We will do all we can not only to help you die peacefully, but also to live until you die.

These words of Cicely Saunders encapsulate the importance of person-centred care in palliative care (Saunders and Clark 2006). As the founder of the modern hospice movement, Cicely Saunders challenged the culture (or 'the way things were done') around care of the dying. She developed a new system with a strong focus on care, but less so on cure. She highlighted the traditional healthcare service model as inadequate for people who were dying (Saunders and Clark 2006). Saunders knew that her ideas were too radical to be accepted within the established culture of healthcare and therefore created a hospice as a new environment for dying people. Through sophisticated writings based on her practice, she established a new approach that formed the key elements of palliative care, which is now well established within healthcare systems across the world. It has been defined as a person-centred holistic approach to caring for people with progressive and life-limiting illness, which has physical, psychological, social and spiritual dimensions (WHO 2017). From its origins, palliative care has always had person-centred practice (see Chapter 3) at its core. This chapter will illustrate how the key principles of palliative care align with the Person-centred Practice Framework (McCormack and McCance 2017).

Key strategic drivers reflecting the person-centred macro context of palliative care

A person-centred approach in healthcare is advocated internationally by the World Health Organization (2011) and is embedded in national and international palliative and end of life care policy and direction (e.g. Department of Health 2011; Scottish Government 2011). Strategic key drivers in palliative care are influenced by national policy and these will vary between different countries according to how the work of palliative care services relates to each country's healthcare burden generally (WHO 2017). For example, in Western countries, the greatest public health burden is the care of people with non-communicable diseases whereas in sub-Saharan Africa, overwhelmingly, the public health burden is communicable diseases such as HIV/AIDS (Harding et al. 2012). In the past, the strategic direction of palliative care service development has been heavily influenced by cancer. Recently, however, non-cancer diagnoses, including frailty and dementia, have become more influential in driving policy direction (Scottish Government 2018; WHO 2014). There is evidence that recognising and addressing palliative care needs early in a person's illness journey is of benefit to all. Understanding the different illness trajectories of different conditions helps in the identification of early palliative care needs. The differences between the illness trajectories of advanced cancer, organ failure and dementia/frailty were crystallised in 2005 and this differentiation has been at the core of early identification strategies in the UK and worldwide (Figure 27.1).

The benefit of palliative care is well established. It is now well recognised that an increasing number of people require palliative care input prior to death, but we also know that few countries are able to invest further in specialist palliative care services. This has meant a sharpened focus upon 'generalist palliative care provision' (https://hospicecare.com/what-we-do/projects/consensus-based-definition-of-palliative-care/definition). The majority of palliative care is provided by generalist providers, i.e. primary care teams, hospital teams and other healthcare and social care providers within a variety of settings (Scottish Government 2011). Only a small percentage of people will require the input from teams who focus exclusively on the delivery of comprehensive specialist palliative care (Seymour et al. 2010).

Prerequisites: being a person-centred practitioner in palliative care

Vital in palliative care is the ability to 'engage authentically' by developing an open and honest relationship with people who are living with incurable illness, and with their families. There may be significant levels of distress, including anxiety and depression, that need to be addressed (Aktas et al. 2010). The ability to listen with full attention and the intent to gain insight into the feelings, thoughts and values of the other person are essential. Effective communication is crucial in identifying and assessing needs, providing information and enabling shared decision making (Chochinov 2002). The way in which we relate to and communicate with people is underpinned by our attitudes, beliefs and behaviours, and necessary attributes to develop a therapeutic relationship. Furthermore, in palliative care, the concept of dignity-conserving care (Chochinov 2002) has received increasing attention in the literature. The A, B, C and D of dignity-conserving care describes how attitudes, behaviour, compassion and dialogue underpin interactions and how we should ensure the person is valued and respected (Chochinov 2002).

Person-centred practice requires a certain flexibility, whereby the practitioner can deviate from already set routines, priorities and tasks to be available in a moment of person-centred

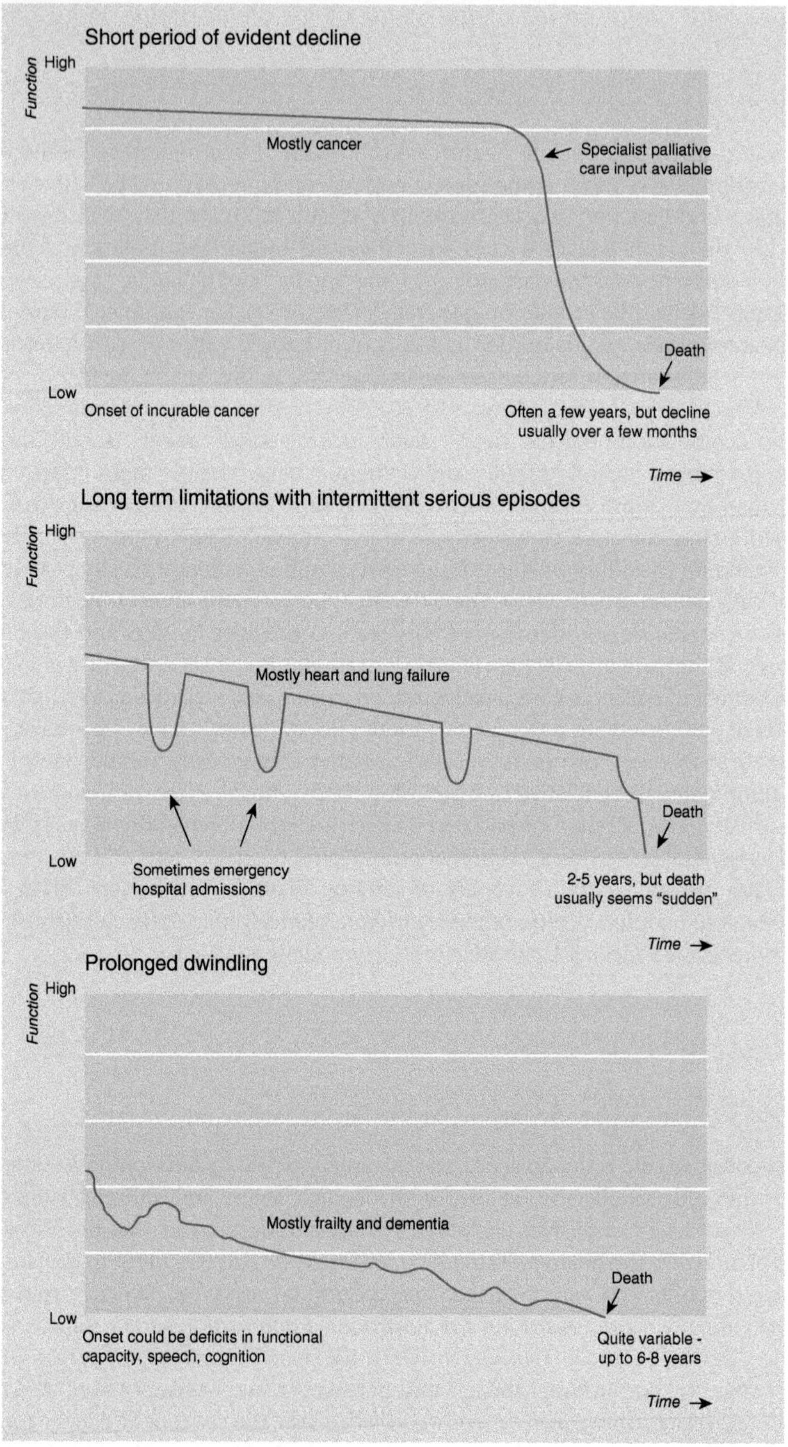

Figure 27.1 Trajectories graphic. Source: Murray et al. (2005).

engagement as the opportunity or need arises. Whilst this flexibility can be incorporated into everyday care, engaging in this way often uncovers issues that need addressing. This can be challenging for various reasons. It may be that it is not perceived as acceptable for the practitioner to prioritise this engagement as there are other system priorities that seem more important. The practitioner may also not feel confident or competent enough to deal effectively with the identified needs. To be available for person-centred moments in care, practitioners must be able adjust to the rhythm of each individual person and their particular needs, and be able to change gear from 'doing' to 'being' (Haraldsdottir 2011). This leads to person-centred outcomes, good care experience and flourishing for both the practitioner and the ill person.

Saunders (Saunders and Clark 2006) developed a new model of care based on her thoughts, values and beliefs, creating new assumptions underpinning healthcare for those with palliative care needs. Her legacy has been integrated into the practice environments of traditional healthcare systems. As palliative care has moved into and become part of mainstream healthcare, professionals are challenged to stay true to their roots, vision and core principles. Working in a culture which is highly influenced by technical systems and task-focused care can push practitioners into focusing on systematised tasks and process-driven routine. This impedes their ability to notice opportunities to provide person-centred and values-based care. Therefore, a key prerequisite in palliative care is the practitioner's clarity of beliefs and values, as described by Cicely Saunders and mirroring person-centred care as we understand it today.

Working with loss, dealing with strong emotion and being open about death and dying can be challenging. Therefore, knowing oneself is a vital part of interpersonal skills in palliative care, as is being able to reflect on one's own feelings, thoughts and core values, and to critically evaluate these.

According to Higginson and Evans (2010), working in teams has been an integral part of the practice of palliative care since its early days. The multiprofessional team varies, but in most cases involves medical practitioners, nurses, allied health professionals, social workers and spiritual carers (WHO 2017). Each professional has their own perspective on palliative care, hence the importance of shared team working

The context of palliative care and person-centred practice

A person's experience of life-limiting illness is unique to them and so a person-centred approach is essential to enable the needs of the individual to be identified and met. Understanding of and insight into people's specific conditions and situations are important. People living with serious chronic and life-limiting diseases face a wide range of problems and each illness brings specific physical symptoms (Aktas et al. 2010). For example, ischaemic heart disease may cause the chest pain of angina, breathlessness or fatigue (WHO 2017); a person with cerebrovascular disease may have difficulty in moving or communicating; while chronic obstructive pulmonary disease may restrict activity because of breathlessness (Edmonds et al. 2006). Chronic diseases often accumulate to create escalating co-morbidity which can further affect an individual's perception of the quality of their life (Davies 2003).

Age and life stage also have an impact on individuals' psychosocial adaptation to illness as well as on the clinical manifestations of their illness (Hubbard et al. 2010). Studies related to psychosocial adaptation have demonstrated that older people have distinct coping processes related to their individual life courses and these processes make them unique individuals who, at the same time, exhibit societal representations of being old (Kagan 2008). Similarly, younger people also display coping adaptations related to their shorter life experience and life stage (Kelly et al. 2004). Thus, the interlinking of a diagnosis with past experience, gender and social ageing brings an interplay of factors to strengthen the argument that caring for a person should be person-centred (Lannie 2014).

Person-centred processes in palliative care

Central to palliative care has been an unwavering focus on what really matters to the individual and to those close to that individual. Realistic care and treatment choices must be tailored to that individual's preferences and to their view of what 'quality of life' is for them. Doing this requires supporting that individual to identify their core values so that goals of care can be aligned with those values.

In the following example we demonstrate the importance of working with people's beliefs and values.

Olivia is 32 years old and has lived with ovarian cancer for two years. She is married, with two children aged 11 and 8, and being a good mum is the thing that matters most. She is distressed and frustrated now that she has advanced ovarian cancer and no longer has the energy 'to be a good mum'. She can't get out of bed and is unable to do any of the things she used to do for her children. Supporting her to identify what her core values are in being a good mum enables her to share that these are being loving and caring. When asked if her kids know that she loves them, she says yes. With everything she is able to do and not do at the moment, will they always know that she loves them? She agrees that they will and is able to see that despite being very weak, she is still able to stay true to her values of being a good mum. Over her last days, she is supported by the health and social care team to focus on 'being with' rather than 'doing for' her children; she is able to spend less time being angry and distressed at her frailty and more time noticing her children as they continue to live their lives with her and alongside her in their home.

Within the palliative care context, the core values which come from personal beliefs can be identified and used to guide a person's goals, choices, decisions and actions. The physical and psychosocial losses that are inevitably associated with a life-limiting illness often obscure core values. This can make it challenging to provide person-centred care, as enabling a person to identify their realistic care goals depends on establishing what really matters to that person (Boa et al. 2014). It is generally accepted that being in touch with one's own core values is essential to enable and support other people to do the same. It is also important to recognise when one's own core values are at odds with those of another person. Person-centred practice relies on that recognition and the willingness to respect the person's values and wishes even when that is not what we would choose for ourselves.

Activity

Think about what your core values might be for the different aspects of your life. What kind of a person do you want to be? What strengths or qualities do you want to develop?

- Relationships
- Work/education
- Personal growth/health
- Leisure

How could you use this awareness of personal values to frame conversations around goals of care in different care settings and with different people? Do you think values identification is a helpful concept to clarify goals of care with people who may not want to think of themselves as 'palliative'.

Source: Harris (2009) https://thehappinesstrap.com/free-resources

To enable the provision of holistic care throughout the person's illness, their needs and concerns should be continuously assessed (Seymour et al. 2010). An individual should be supported to identify and review their goals of care and what matters to them as their illness progresses. The choice of an appropriate assessment tool or questionnaire may depend on the clinical situation or issue, the cognitive and functional ability of the person and the purpose for which it is being used (Sheehan 2012). The Palliative care Outcome Scale (POS) (https://pos-pal.org) measures are a 'family of tools' used to assess people's physical symptoms, psychological symptoms, emotional and spiritual needs and information and support needs. The POS is a validated instrument that can be used in clinical care, audit, research and training. The POS measures are specifically developed for use among people with any chronic and life-limiting illness and enable professionals to be 'working holistically'.

Effective shared decision making is integral to any person-centred care process. It has been established that shared decision making leads to improvements in people's knowledge and their understanding of risk, and to a greater likelihood of getting care aligned with their values. Various models of shared decision making can be helpful in integrating this approach into palliative care in any care setting. Elwyn et al. (2012) propose a three-step model.

Step 1 – Choice Talk

- Explaining that choice exists
- 'Let's work out which choice is right for you'

Step 2 – Option Talk

- Specific details about the options
- Potential risks and benefits outlined for the individual in concrete terms

Step 3 – Decision Talk

- Help the person identify outcomes that matter most
- Explore preferences in the context of what is clinically and practically viable
- Arrive at a shared decision when the person is ready

Activity

Reflect on a person you have recently looked after who has had to make a decision about treatment or care (e.g. antibiotics for an infection, an operation, going to a care home, etc.). For each step of the shared decision-making process, write out a question that you could imagine yourself asking, which would support the person to reach the right decision for them. Reflect on some of the enabling and disabling factors for shared decision making in different care environments you have experienced.

Challenges to person-centred outcomes in palliative care

In this chapter we have discussed the synergy between person-centred practice and palliative care. The assumption is often made that palliative care practice is, in its essence, person-centred. People assume that since person-centredness is inherent to the philosophy of palliative care, it is embedded in day-to-day practice. However, there are challenges to this. The current healthcare system is driven by a strong curative focus. The palliative care approach focuses mainly on care, alongside an acceptance that cure is not possible.

One of the core principles of palliative care is openness towards death and dying. This can be challenging for practitioners and, as discussed earlier in this chapter, requires specific interpersonal skills. The opportunity for deep emotional engagement needs to be accepted and valued within the culture of an organisation, which would include time and support for practitioners to put this into practice. Culture embraces social context that influences the way people behave and talk, and the social norms that are accepted and expected (McCormack and McCance 2017). To transform culture and shift how things are done at practice level requires fundamental changes in mindset, language and behaviour (McCormack and McCance 2017). In order to enable truly person-centred palliative practice, organisations need to pay attention to their own organisational culture, and specifically to how much the traditional biomedical model may negatively influence a person-centred culture.

The Person-centred Practice Framework can be used to guide palliative care practice to enable individuals and organisations to become more person-centred. The framework can provide a starting point for assessing current culture and to inform development of person-centred palliative care practice.

Activity

Reflect on what person-centredness in palliative care means to you and what attributes you have observed in practice that are important to person-centred palliative practice.

Summary

- Person-centred practice within palliative care requires a mindset shift towards shared decision making irrespective of the care setting or illness trajectory.
- Reflection, flexibility and openness to opportunities for core values identification enable person-centred practice to be prioritised within palliative care.
- From its inception, palliative care has evolved with an ethos which overlaps significantly with that of person-centred practice.
- However, attempting to truly integrate person-centred practice into palliative care uncovers many challenges.
- The tension between cure-based care and palliative care is as great as the tension between task-based practice and person-centred practice.

References

Aktas, A., Walsh, D., and Rybicki, I. (2010). Review: symptom clusters: myth or reality? *Palliative Medicine* 24: 373–385.

Boa, S., Duncan, E., Haraldsdottir, E., and Wyke, S. (2014). Goal setting in palliative care: a structured review. *Progress Palliative Care* 22 (6): 326–333.

Chochinov, H.M. (2002). Dignity-conserving care – a new model for palliative care: helping the patient feel valued. *AMA* 287 (17): 2253–2260.

Davies, E. (2003). *What Are the Appropriate Services and Support to Address the Palliative Care Needs of Older People? Report to the Health Evidence Network*. Copenhagen: WHO Regional Office for Europe.

Department of Health (2011). *Holistic Needs Assessment for People with Cancer: A Practical Guide for Healthcare Professionals*. London: Department of Health.

Edmonds, P., Burman, R., Silber, E. et al. (2006). Evaluation of a novel palliative care service for patients severely affected by multiple sclerosis. *Palliative Medicine* 20: 245.

Elwyn, G., Frosch, D., Thomson, R. et al. (2012). Shared decision making: a model for clinical practice. *Journal of General Internal Medicine* 357: 1361–1367.

Haraldsdottir, E. (2011). The constraint of the ordinary 'being with' in the context of end of life nursing care. *International Journal of Palliative Care Nursing* 17 (5): 245–250.

Harding, R., Selman, L., Agupio, G. et al. (2012). Intensity and correlates of multidimensional problems in HIV patients receiving integrated palliative care in sub-Saharan Africa. *BMJ Sexually Transmitted Infections* 88 (8): 607–611.

Harris, R. (2009). *ACT Made Simple; An Easy Read Primer on Acceptance and Commitment Therapy*. Oakland, CA: New Harbinger Publications.

Higginson, I. and Evans, C. (2010). What is the evidence that palliative care teams improve outcomes for cancer patients and their families? *Cancer Journal* 16 (5): 423–435.

Hubbard, G., Kidd, L., and Kearney, N. (2010). Disrupted lives and threats to identity: the experiences of people with colorectal cancer within the first year following diagnosis. *Health* 14 (2): 131–146.

Kagan, S.H. (2008). Ageism in cancer care. *Seminars in Oncology Nursing* 24 (4): 246–253.

Kelly, D., Pearce, S., and Mulhall, A. (2004). Being in the same boat: ethnographic insights into an adolescent cancer unit. *International Journal of Nursing Studies* 41 (8): 847–857.

Lannie, A. (2014). *Experiences of the Older Person with Cancer: A qualitative study of medical and specialist ward settings*. Unpublished thesis, University of Dundee.

McCormack, B. and McCance, T. (2017). *Person-Centred Practice in Nursing and Healthcare: Theory and Practice*. Chichester: Wiley Blackwell.

Murray, S., Kendall, M., Boyd, K., and Shekh, A. (2005). Illness trajectories and palliative care. *BMJ* 330: 1007.

Saunders, C. and Clark, D. (2006). *Cicely Saunders Selected Writing 1958–2004*. Oxford: Oxford University Press.

Scottish Government (2011). *Living and Dying Well: Building on Progress*. Edinburgh: Scottish Government.

Scottish Government (2018). *Long Term Monitoring of Health Inequalities: Dec 2018 Report*. Edinburgh: Scottish Government.

Seymour, J.E., French, J., and Richardson, E. (2010). Dying matters: let's talk about it. *BMJ* 341: c4860.

Sheehan, B. (2012). Assessment scales in dementia. *Therapeutic Advances in Neurological Disorders* 5 (6): 349–358.

WHO (2011). *Palliative Care for Older People: Better Practice*. London: King's College.

WHO (2014). *Global Atlas of Palliative Care at End of Life*. London: Worldwide Palliative Care Alliance.

WHO (2017). *WHO Definition of Palliative Care*. www.who.int/cancer/palliative/definition/en

Further reading and resources

Good Life Good Death Good Grief: www.goodlifedeathgrief.org.uk

PCC4U: www.pcc4u.org

SECTION 4

Approaches to Learning and Development for Person-Centred Practice

The final section of this book builds on the previous chapters that explored what person-centred practice is, how to be person-centred, and how to enact aspects of the Person-centred Practice Framework in different health and social care systems. In this section we focus on how we learn and develop over time. The sections have titles that will be familiar to you, for example, 'reflective learning' and 'critical thinking'. The chapters explore how we embed our person-centred values within these familiar processes and how engaging in this ongoing development is a necessity to being person-centred in our practice.

In Chapter 28, we explore how to be an active learner, and engage all our senses and intelligences in transformative learning that helps us grow as person-centred practitioners. Chapter 29 focuses on the role of reflection within this journey and how to use it in helping us learn from ongoing professional and personal challenges. To develop, we also need to cultivate our ability to think critically in practice, as discussed in Chapter 30, which interlinks with active learning and reflection. Chapter 31 explores how to develop and support practice educators, while Chapter 32 focuses on ways of starting and progressing research and knowledge exchange journeys when embodying person-centered principles and values. Finally, Chapter 33 reinforces the importance of person-centred learning as a lifelong process that includes both 'being' and 'becoming'.

Fundamentals of Person-Centred Healthcare Practice, First Edition. Edited by Brendan McCormack, Tanya McCance, Cathy Bulley, Donna Brown, Ailsa McMillan and Suzanne Martin.

28

Being an active learner

Jan Dewing[1] and Brighide Lynch[2]

[1] Queen Margaret University, Edinburgh, Scotland, UK
[2] Ulster University, Northern Ireland, UK

Contents

Fundamentals of Person-Centred Healthcare Practice, First Edition. Edited by Brendan McCormack, Tanya McCance, Cathy Bulley, Donna Brown, Ailsa McMillan and Suzanne Martin.

Learning outcomes

- Acquire an understanding of the principles of active learning and how they connect to your learning and transformative growth as a person.
- Reflect on the connections between active learning and the prerequisites domain in the PcPF.
- Identify and describe active learning methods that you can use in the classroom setting and the workplace setting

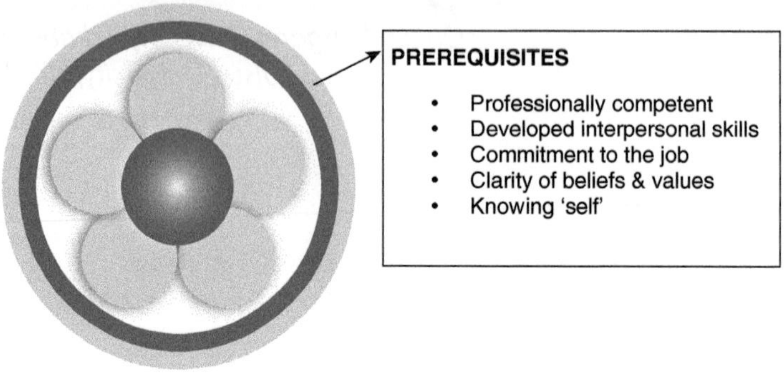

Introduction

In this chapter we invite you to explore the principles of active learning, what they mean to you and how you can work with them as you progress to becoming a person-centred practitioner and working with the Person-centred Practice Framework (PcPF). Active learning is an approach that, in addition to being essential for personal and professional purposes, offers you a structure to help you feel more confident that you are evolving as a person-centred practitioner.

What is active learning?

Broadly speaking, active learning is a methodology or approach that sets out six principles (see Box 28.1) which act as a guide to selecting, using and evaluating active learning methods. These principles are not fixed and can be revised or have other secondary principles added to them. Where this is done, it is important that all the principles are complementary to each other and don't 'argue' against each other. The original principles developed by Dewing (2008, 2010) have been updated and are presented here.

Box 28.1 Active learning: revised principles

- In-depth drawing on the primary senses (including seeing, noticing and observing), and multiple social intelligences.
- Critical dialogue with me and then with other(s) drawing in elements of past, present and future and space/place.
- Intentional action or doing (as part of practice/work); ultimately doing things differently and feeling differently about it.
- Integration of learning into the body/personhood to achieve reflexivity and flow.
- Knowing how to repeat this process consistently over time, so that it contributes to flourishing.
- Enabling or facilitating similar learning experiences with others in the workplace.

Activity

Having viewed Box 28.1, you might like to consider if there are any other principles you would want to add to personalise active learning to you.

What do they say about your values and ideas on (i) persons and personhood and (ii) human flourishing?

Our primary senses as the foundation for learning

According to the philosopher Merleau-Ponty (1945), the world is a canvas for perception. In turn, perception is the background of all our experience, which guides every conscious action and the meaning we give to everything in the world. We cannot separate ourselves from our perceptions of the world. We pull in sensory data or material from all around us into our consciousness and it is, in effect, given a 'make-over' so that it becomes something other than and more than it started out as. Our core sensory perceptions are transformed by different layers of cognitive knowledge. It is therefore helpful to be able to draw on a wide range of ways of knowing – sometimes known as multiple intelligences.

Multiple intelligences

We require a dynamic and 'open' concept of intelligence to enable us to learn as widely as possible. The theory put forward by Gardner (1983) suggests that the traditional theory of a general IQ is too limited. Instead, Gardner initially proposed seven intelligences, then increased this as seen in Table 28.1. Although his theory suffers from a lack of empirical research at present, there is plenty of supporting evidence that there are many different ways of knowing something. It is useful for us to draw on these when considering the range of intelligences we have and from this, to consider how we nurture them through active learning in the classroom and in the practice workplace.

Table 28.1 Gardner's multiple intelligences

Intelligence type	Capability
Linguistic	Words and language
Logical/mathematical	Logic and numbers
Musical	Music, sound, rhythm
Bodily/kinaesthetic	Body movement control
Spatial/visual	Images and space
Interpersonal	Other people's feelings
Intrapersonal	Self-awareness
Naturalist	Natural environment
Spiritual/existential	Religion and 'ultimate issues'
Moral	Ethics, humanity

Activity

Find out more about your own multiple intelligences by (i) noting in order (strongest first) which intelligences you subjectively feel you are best at using in your learning, (ii) entering the term multiple intelligences into a search engine and exploring the content. Try out a free online multiple intelligence assessment to see where your strengths are and the areas you can spend time strengthening. Compare the similarities and differences between your ordering and the test findings. One you have some results or findings, how might you make use of them to help you flourish as a person-centred learner?

What makes active learning necessary for human flourishing?

Being a person is a lifelong process of becoming; a person is never a fully completed entity. Because it is always ongoing and evolving, this implies that different types and levels of change, including transformation, are going on. It is learning that lies at the heart of transformation and growth as a person. Thus, learning that contributes to transformation is of interest in person-centred practice. However, not all learning or the emergent difference is transformational. Belenky and Stanton (2000) suggest that transformational learning theory is too 'narrow' because it tends to focus on the endpoint of development and does not track the many steps people take before they know how they know. While there is no general agreement about what is and what is not transformative learning, or the difference between transformative and other learning, there is agreement that it requires that persons know how they know. For example, how do I know I am tired or angry, and how do I know another person is in pain or scared?

Briefly, transformation in persons comes about by experiencing and learning through a deep, structural shift in the fundamental processes of our thought, feelings and actions. Illeris (2018, p. 5) cites Piaget who proposed that learning takes place in the body and not just the brain. It is a shift in different elements of consciousness that dramatically and irreversibly alters our bodies and our way of being in the world. We know that how we know something is different and can sense, explain the differences and most importantly, say how and why it 'matters'. A key point to pay attention to is that learners need to have an emotional connection to the learning content and learning process to construct meaning and the incentive to direct energies into the learning and into its use in practical terms (Illeris 2018). You can strengthen your learning in the classroom and in practice settings by asking 'What does this mean to me (emotionally) and why does this matter to me?'.

These examples illustrate how the overall experience, and even the physical environment, can be complex yet it is our core senses that have been involved and that will evoke emotions. Learning only becomes transformative when we see a big shift in how we see the real 'me' and/or the world around us and then choose or decide to act on the revised perspective (Cranton 2011, p. 53). What comprises a deep shift varies between persons. Transformational learning can be a sudden disorientating dilemma or a series of related, accumulated experiences over time. This is sometimes referred to as an evolving meaning-schema.

Examples

- In the clinic room, the person is undressing ready for a physical examination with a consultant practitioner. The sight of their significantly altered/adapted body from their health condition, and from what you imagine is the consequences of self-harm, comes as a shock and makes you feel incredibly uncomfortable.
- It's time for the wound dressing to be changed again. No matter that this is the fourth time you've assisted with this dressing change, you still feel butterflies in your stomach. You try to prepare for the smell from the fungating wound, although it never seems to work. The practitioner you work with has not raised the issue with you and you feel unsure whether it's OK for you to do so or not.
- You're in the bedroom with a family when a person in that family dies. The care leading to the death and the support for the family has all gone as planned. The lead practitioners describe the planning as 'textbook'. Then comes a sound from one of the family that you've never heard before and you hadn't expected – the sound of raw grief.
- You overhear your mentor talking about you with their colleague. Your mentor seems to accept the criticism being made of you and even laughs about it. You recognise that you feel hurt and vulnerable. How can you trust your mentor after this?

> Transformative learning may be defined as learning that transforms problematic frames of reference to make them more inclusive, discriminating, reflective, open, and emotionally able to change. (Mezirow 2009, p. 22)

Transformative learning is usually slow and needs to be facilitated by the person and/or by others who are skilled in the facilitation of active learning. Even then, time for processing is a necessary factor in the transformation process. Active learning enhances the probability of life experiences becoming the material for transformation and thus evolvement as a person. It can, to a certain degree, accelerate our rate of transformation.

Activity

From your reading of the examples above, how might you feel in those situations? What would you need to attend to in relation to your learning? How would you know if any transformational learning was taking place?

Active learning and the Person-centred Practice Framework

Active learning can enable more and deeper attention to be given to the PcPF (McCormack and McCance 2017). In this chapter we are focusing on enhancing your attributes within the prerequisites construct in the framework.

Learning more deeply about who you are as a person and a healthcare practitioner is central to developing your own perceptions, emotions, values and beliefs and interpersonal skills; in turn, these are cornerstones of being professionally competent and growing your commitment to the job. It is a life-long habit to acquire and keep refreshing. Given that we are in an age of rapidly expanding technology seen in progress with digital technologies and immersive, augmented and virtual realities, there are exciting times ahead. We can make use of technologies in active learning and to support practitioners in developing professional competence. It's worthwhile considering how ready you feel for these developments.

Activity

To help you consider the connections between active learning and the prerequisites in more depth, look through the contents of Table 28.2.

Active learning in class-based learning

Class-based learning opportunities are rehearsal spaces for the main elements of active learning that take place in care environments. Active learning is not complete until it has been used and evaluated in the workplace (Dewing 2010). Educators and lecturers need to be facilitators of your learning, creating the best conditions in the space/place rather than simply teaching content. Drawing on the principles of active learning shown in Box 28.1, there are a number of 'indicators' of active learning in class-based learning you can look out for (Table 28.3).

Active learning in the workplace

Health practitioners are found in many workplaces, most of which are also care environments. Care environments and workplaces are also places of learning (Hardiman 2017, p. 30). Rycroft-Malone (2004, p. 127) suggests that the learning of new skills in isolation from the workplace may lead to difficulties with application back in the 'hot action' of the care environment. In the everyday work of healthcare, potentially, all aspects of practice allow opportunities for learning and for transformation of our being. The workplace is therefore the primary space in which active learning can occur. Whilst everyday practice has this potential, these opportunities may not be recognised, sometimes because habits and practices are taken for granted and not usually questioned or examined, or because of general busyness.

The ultimate aims of active learning are, first, transforming the workplace to become more person-centred and, second, acting as a catalyst for personal transformation (Dewing 2010). This would mean that person-centred practice and the framework are evident in various ways. Whether learning does or does not take place is in part influenced by the culture in the workplace and the macro level culture in the organisation – the Person-centred Framework sets this out clearly. For example, if organisation A always provides short bursts of mandatory training for teams and organisation B offers facilitated workplace learning sessions, there will be differences in what their employees believe about what learning is and what its purpose is.

Table 28.2 Active learning principles and prerequisites

Central principles of active learning	Connection with the prerequisites
In-depth drawing on the senses (including seeing, noticing and observing) and multiple social intelligences	*Knowing self/me* is the development of our self-awareness through reflection and is fundamental to active learning. It is how we learn every day in relation with others and how we construct our world using our senses and multiple intelligences. Through active learning, we enhance the possibility of integrating what we learn from our life experiences with what we are experiencing in the present moment
My critical dialogue and with other(s) drawing in elements of past, present and future and place	In active learning the practitioner uses a range of *developed interpersonal skills* that originate from engaging all their senses in order to interact with others and experience a specific practice activity. Through critical dialogue with self and others, the practitioner develops a better understanding of the assumptions they hold and their reasons for intentionally adopting a particular practice approach. Active learning can enable the practitioner to gain *clarity about their beliefs and values,* feelings and emotions about a particular experience. Others, skilled in the facilitation of active learning, can support the practitioner in this process. The practitioner needs to be given time to reflect and refine their values so that their true intentions are uncovered naturally. As a result, new approaches open up for the practitioner in the 'doing' of their practice and 'being' in their practice, thereby deepening their understanding and self-awareness
Intentional action or doing (as part of practice/work); ultimately doing things differently and feeling differently about it	The practitioner's intentional action or doing in practice is manifested in their *commitment to the job* and is intrinsically connected to the beliefs and values on which the practitioner acts. When practitioners engage in active learning with the intention of transforming their team culture and/or care, they not only bring about a change in the practice itself but also a change in the consciousness of their own practice and in their feelings about their practice – ultimately a positive difference in *professional competence*
Integration into the body/person to achieve reflexivity and flow	Reflexivity requires a deeper level of *knowing self* and is where you can place yourself in the picture or situation, and appreciate how you and your 'drives' influence action, and where you bring into the world actions that you reflect on further. Active learning is not complete until you have used the learning practically in some way
Enabling or facilitating the same or similar learning experiences with others in the workplace	Being facilitative with others is evidence of *commitment to the job and developed interpersonal skills.* It is an act of social commitment and shows responsibility for the larger community

Table 28.3 Active learning principles and indicators in class-based learning opportunities

Active learning principle	Indicators
In-depth drawing on the primary senses (including seeing, noticing and observing); and multiple social intelligences	Learning begins with tuning into and paying attention to our sensory perception and intelligences. Mindfulness, contemplation, imagination, day dreaming, music, poetry, storytelling and authentic movement are some examples of how this can be facilitated
Critical dialogue with me and then with other(s) drawing in elements of past, present and future and space/place	A critical, creative reflection and drawing on our multiple intelligences and experiences and sharing with others. Introduction of new knowledge and processes by self and/or others
Intentional action or doing (as part of practice/work); ultimately doing things differently and feeling differently about it	Rehearsing how new knowledge can be used in the care environment/workplace and how practitioners can absorb and embody it
Integration of learning into the body/personhood to achieve reflexivity and flow	Helping practitioners be aware of and prepare for the complexity of moving from novice to expertise
Knowing how to repeat this process consistently over time, so that it contributes to flourishing	Helping practitioners be aware of and prepare for knowing how they learn and how this connects with energy, vitality and flow
Enabling or facilitating similar learning experiences with others in the workplace	Enabling practitioners to be open and inclusive of others to assist with knowledge exchange and translation

Actively learning in the workplace with others is a social learning process and our being and practice are changed. However, in order to maximise the impact of active learning and ensure sustainable practice evolves, other person-centred methods and processes must be used as part of active learning. Crucially, person-centred facilitators are pivotal to helping practitioners learn in and from everyday practice and discover and embody new ways of knowing and being. More senior learners can often take on facilitation skills or a role to enable newer learners to actively learn from what is going on around them. Facilitators use a wide range of skills, methods and processes that are aligned to the development level of learners and the context in which they are working. A practitioner's stage of learning may be such that they are unaware of care practices that are routinised, repetitive and less than person-centred; the facilitator is key to helping the practitioner recognise such limitations and get beyond them.

Active learning activities can commence with uncomplicated activities that are challenging and yet relatively unthreatening, such as by observing others who have healthcare expertise, setting one's own goals and objectives, and reflecting and learning from one's own practice experience. More complex learning activities include asking questions, observations of the environment, observations of practice, narratives with persons about their care experience and generally using active learning methods as part of person-centred elevation of practice.

Conclusion

As a developing healthcare practitioner, you will take responsibility for and become the authority over your personal and professional identity, values, actions and feelings. Thus you will need to gradually take on more ownership of how you learn as well as what you learn. There is a challenge with transformational learning as it is 'unbounded' and there are infinite active learning possibilities in workplaces and classrooms. You will need a willingness to stay with uncertainty and unpredictability, to doubt and to have an ability for gracious questioning. Is this you, or can it be you?

> Paradoxically, despite all that we know and all that we have learned, we will spend the remainder of our lives learning to be . . . persons in society. (Jarvis 2018, p. 27)

Summary

- Active learning draws on multiple intelligences to help us make sense of our perceptions of the world around us.
- Being a person is a lifelong process of becoming and transformative learning helps us grow as person-centred practitioners.
- Different types of facilitated class-based learning experience, with time for processing, can enable active learning; it is not complete, however, until used and evaluated in the workplace.
- As well as enabling personal transformation, active learning can enable workplace transformation in ways that enact person-centred principles and support more healthful cultures.

References

Belenky, M. and Stanton, A. (2000). Inequality, development, and connected knowing. In: *Learning as Transformation: Critical Perspectives on a Theory in Progress* (eds. J. Mezirow and Associates), 71–102. San Francisco, CA: Jossey-Bass.

Cranton, P. (2011). Adult learning and instruction: transformative-learning perspectives. In: *Adult Learning and Education* (ed. K. Rubenson), 53–59. Oxford: Academic Press.

Dewing, J. (2008). Becoming and being active learners and creating active learning workplaces: the value of active learning. In: *International Practice Development in Nursing and Healthcare* (eds. K. Manley, B. McCormack and V. Wilson), 273–294. Oxford: Blackwell.

Dewing, J. (2010). Moments of movement: active learning and practice development. *Nurse Education in Practice* 10 (1): 22–26.

Gardner, H. (1983). *Frames of Mind: The Theory of Multiple Intelligences*. Boston, MA: Ingram Publishers.

Hardiman, M. (2017). *Using two models of work-place facilitation to create conditions for development of a person-centred culture: a par study*. Unpublished PhD Thesis, Queen Margaret University, Edinburgh.

Illeris, K. (ed.) (2018). *Contemporary Theories of Learning: Learning Theorists in their Own Words*, 2e. Abingdon: Routledge.

Jarvis, P. (2018). Learning to be a person in society: learning to be me. In: *Contemporary Theories of Learning: Learning Theorists in their Own Words*, 2e (ed. K. Illeris), 15–28. Abingdon: Routledge.

McCormack, B. and McCance, T. (2017). *Person-Centred Practice in Nursing and Healthcare: Theory and Practice*, 2e. Chichester: Wiley Blackwell.

Merleau-Ponty, M. (1945). *The Phenomenology of Perception*. London: Routledge.

Mezirow, J. (2009). Transformative learning theory. In: *Transformative Learning in Practise: Insights from Community, Workplace, and Higher Education* (eds. J. Mezirow and E.W. Taylor), 18–32. San Francisco, CA: Jossey-Bass.

Rycroft-Malone, J. (2004). The PARIHS framework: a framework for guiding the implementation of evidence-based practice. *Journal of Nursing Care Quality* 19: 297–304.

Further reading

Find out more about your multiple intelligences by taking a free assessment on line. Type in multiple intelligences test to your search engine and choose which one you want to do. Examples include: www.literacynet.org/mi/assessment/findyourstrengths.html

The digital age has made it very easy to visit some of the world's most famous museums from wherever you can connect to wifi. Try a visit and find a piece of art that helps you reflect http://mentalfloss.com/article/75809/12-world-class-museums-you-can-visit-online

Get comfortable with being uncomfortable by Luvvie Ajayi (2018). 'Your silence serves no one,' says the writer, activist and self-proclaimed professional troublemaker. Ajayi shares three questions to ask yourself if you're teetering on the edge of speaking up or quieting down – and encourages all of us to get a little more comfortable with being uncomfortable. www.youtube.com/watch?v=QijH4UAqGD8

Theory of Creativity: Duncan Wardle talks about the importance of creativity and why it will be the one core human element to compete in a world that is becoming automated faster than we can think. www.youtube.com/watch?v=_8MwiGYzlyg

29

Knowing and becoming through reflective learning

Donna Brown[1] and Kristina Mountain[2]

[1] Ulster University, Northern Ireland, UK
[2] Queen Margaret University, Edinburgh, Scotland, UK

Contents

Fundamentals of Person-Centred Healthcare Practice, First Edition. Edited by Brendan McCormack, Tanya McCance, Cathy Bulley, Donna Brown, Ailsa McMillan and Suzanne Martin.

Learning outcomes

- Engage in discussions about the nature of knowing and becoming.
- Make sense of how reflection on knowing and becoming can assist you to develop shared understandings for person-centred practice.
- Openly embrace changes in your learning and thinking about knowing and becoming person-centred in your practice.

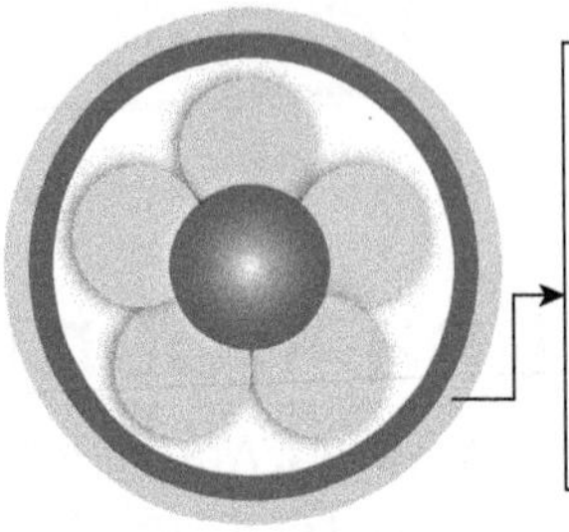

Knowing self: the way a person makes sense of his/her knowing, being and becoming through reflection, self-awareness, and engagement with others

Clarity of beliefs and values: awareness of the impact of beliefs and values on the healthcare experience and the commitment to reconciling beliefs and values in ways that facilitate person-centredness

Introduction

This chapter will primarily focus on the 'knowing self' and 'clarity of beliefs and values' prerequisites of the Person-centred Practice Framework. It will consider how knowing and becoming through reflective learning can help learners achieve a better understanding of the professional and personal challenges that they encounter in practice. It will look at ways of using reflection to help work with the uncertainty of knowing and becoming more person-centred in practice. We need to remember, though, that developing some sense of who we are requires a lifelong commitment to learning about ourselves and our practice. In the context of knowing and becoming person-centred, if you look back and reflect meaningfully on your experiences, you will already have a story that has resulted in your current way of being.

In the Person-centred Practice Framework, prerequisites are deemed to be the essential building blocks that develop and enable people to work in person-centred ways. In the prerequisites, 'clarity of beliefs and values' and 'knowing self' can be found (see Chapter 4). These are key areas for development if we are to understand who we are and why we practise and react in the ways we do (see Chapters 1, 10 and 13). This necessitates us taking responsibility for and entering positively into all learning opportunities, by seeking guidance, feedback and support. Critical reflection offers a medium to grow as we learn about ourselves and others, explore the professional, political and social influences in our professional lives and find new ways to overcome the challenges we may face (Rolfe et al. 2011).

Reflection for person-centred practice

There are many theories and models of reflection that have been adapted in a variety of areas of practice. At its simplest, reflection enables persons to focus on their individual experiences and learn from them (Bolton 2014). Critical reflective practice offers a structured way in which people who provide care can question and appraise the challenges they face in practice and develop new insights into knowing and becoming more person-centred. However, as people in healthcare settings work in complex and messy environments, in which they are frequently challenged to consider their personal and professional values, purposes and interests, there is no single approach to reflection that will work every time. Evaluating your progress, learning through and from experience and considering different ways to enrich your practice are dynamic processes that require the use of different approaches and ways of reflecting, to gain a deeper learning about experiences and why you respond in the ways you do. To learn more about reflective practice and tools see; www.open.edu/openlearn/ocw/mod/oucontent/view.php?id=51386&section=4

In pursuit of knowing and becoming

When we start the process of learning and exploring that sense of knowing and becoming, we take an individual and collective leap into a new reality, with our fellow learners. Each new experience generates moments of learning that have the potential to connect to new ways of knowing, being and becoming (Denzin 2014). We are leaping from a place we know into a new place, new experiences and new relationships. For example, think about your first day in university or a new area of practice; doubtless you experienced feelings of excitement, and also feelings of uncertainty and disorientation (Mezirow 2012). As we adjust in these new situations, we spend time reacting, noticing and then thinking through the experience, to make sense of our new encounters and develop new understandings.

To guide your thinking in this chapter, we will use Mezirow's seven-stage sequence (1994). Mezirow encourages us to reflect critically and in depth as we try to make sense of and cope with changes in our world. He would see this deep critical reflection as a transformative experience, with the initial 'disorientating dilemma' acting as a trigger for learning. Disorientating dilemmas occur when we experience something that does not make sense to us or an experience that does not 'fit' with our expectations. Often, as we think about the experience, we become aware that we will be required to change our view of the world, in some way, to make sense of the situation. This requires examining our 'self' and considering why we have responded in a particular way (Mezirow 1994). As you pause for a moment and 'step back', you might ask why you are feeling like this. It could be that your established beliefs and assumptions are being questioned and you could see this 'pause' as a means of making sense of how you feel and how that builds on your previous experiences, which is reflective learning (Merriam and Bierema 2014). Consciously working through these moments 'with yourself' and talking with others provides opportunities to understand the relevance and significance of the experience in terms of your learning.

Activity

Think about a situation in practice when you have felt really out of your comfort zone. Why was this?

> In this first question you are being guided by the elements of disorientation and self-examination. In order for an experience to encourage learning, a person needs to be faced with a thought-provoking dilemma (disorientation). This can be something that challenges our thinking and we have to mull it over to find a solution, or it could be a sudden 'ah ha' moment. Regardless of how it is experienced, we are required to consider our previous beliefs and values by questioning how we are feeling (self-examination).

Do you think you made assumptions about the people, places and experiences you have just encountered; if so what were these?

Here you are exploring what your intentions may have been, what influenced you and what internal dialogue you are having with yourself. This aspect helps us develop insight into our self and our practice (critical assessment of assumptions).

How can you connect this experience to your values and beliefs as a person (prerequisites)?

Reflecting on our experience through a person-centred lens requires careful consideration of what we believe and value and how this is upheld, or is at odds with the behaviours we witness in others' practice. Consider here what impact your behaviour may have had on others and vice versa. This connects with the idea of 'human agency' discussed in Chapter 13.

Bolton (2014) proposes that it is not sufficient just to think about the decisions we make; it is essential to write down our thoughts. Writing is the key to successful reflection, knowing and becoming. Writing (and telling) our stories of learning can provide a means to make connections between the experience, and all that goes with that, including the mix of emotions, what we are going to do with those moments of learning, and how we understand and link this to theories and research we have encountered (Tyler and Swartz 2012). These stories provide a degree of structure as well as a sense of freedom, as we gather up how we are thinking and feeling about an experience in practice, and what we want to do with that. We are forming a frame of reference, a way to illuminate and make meaning of an experience or situation (Mezirow 2012). This story can be for our 'self' or we can share the story with others.

Activity

Thinking about your story in relation to the first learning activity, start jotting down a few sentences or mapping your thoughts on the questions in a diagram (e.g. concept mapping, Figure 29.1). You are encouraged to share this with a colleague or small group of your fellow learners and discuss these points together. A reflective discussion with peers, an experienced clinical colleague or team members enables you to share your experience with supportive individuals who actively listen and encourage your thinking by asking questions to help you think critically, developing your story. Questioning your assumptions and seeking common understandings opens you up to rich learning opportunities and creates a communicative space (Habermas 1987).

Creating communicative spaces

Creating a communicative space to reflect on learning experiences and develop ways of knowing sits within Habermas' philosophical frame and a constructivist paradigm. It encompasses reflexivity (i.e. standing back from a situation and considering the impact your values, beliefs and actions may have on a given situation) and the development of knowledge through communicative action (Habermas 1987). The act of sharing and talking through our reflections on learning can connect us with others, opening up the discussion

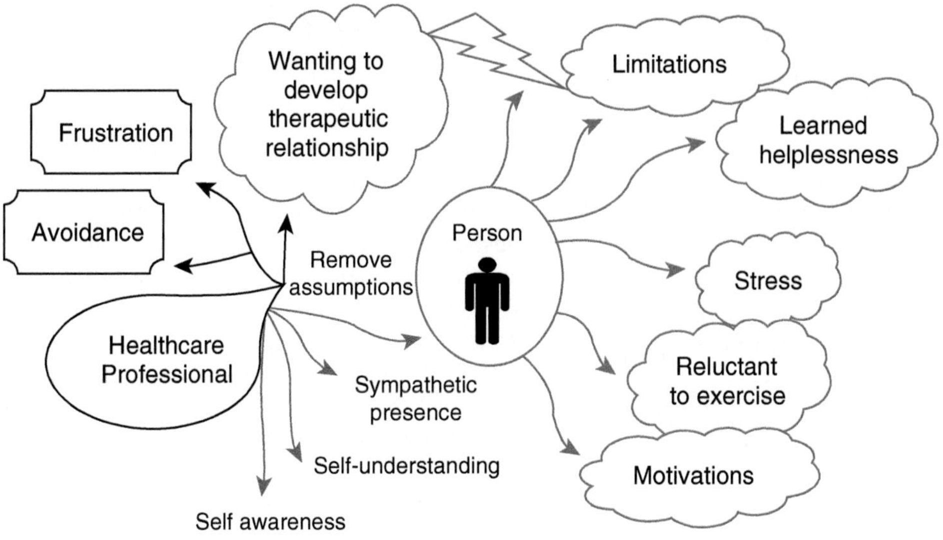

Figure 29.1 Using a concept map. Source: Adapted dimensions of being (McCormack 2004; Dewing 2007).

and introducing different viewpoints and perspectives. This becomes a shared narrative of knowing and a means to interpret our responses to the situation. We are being curious and open to the experience (and the learning from this), with support from each other (Clandinin 2013). This then connects to the concept of us as persons and our personhood; being with self, in place, in relation and in the social world (McCormack 2004). Bringing in the dimension of 'time' places the experience, and the moment of learning, at a specific point in your story of 'becoming' (Dewing 2007).

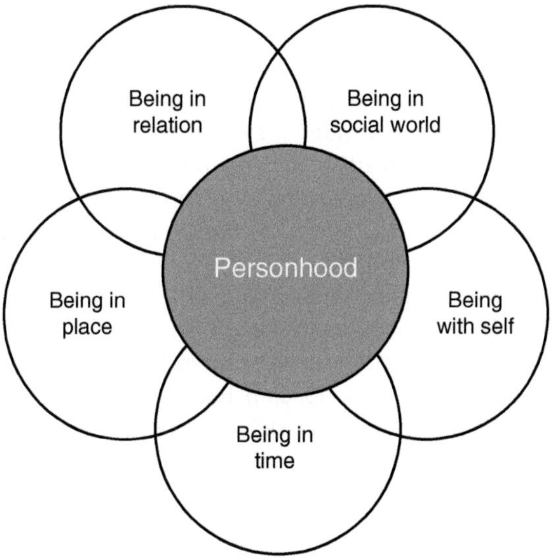

Sources: Dewing, J. (2007); McCormack 2004.

Working with the challenges of knowing and becoming

A community
A place of honesty; safe
Open yet contained

Stepping back; listening
There is sharing; creating
Learning gathered; held

I learn and absorb
My perspectives now shifting
Openness and trust

Person-centred ways of being are embedded in engaging in an authentic interconnected way with our fellow learners/colleagues to give us an opportunity to explore and question our responses to an experience. Working through a practice-based issue and consciously considering the alternative perspectives of peers, colleagues or mentors provides a clearer perspective of the world we operate in. This could be seen as the beginnings of a community of practice, with each person contributing to and engaging in learning – learning as belonging and becoming (Wenger 2018).

The experience of sharing our reflections requires living with some uncertainty; for example, we might feel insecure, worried about how others see us or struggle with self-doubt. Resulting behaviours might include defensiveness or using self-protective reasoning (Bolton 2014), which will hamper efforts in knowing and becoming a reflective person. Knowing and becoming involves balancing opening ourselves to new perspectives, through critical reflection, and making choices in how we will respond, rather than being driven by habitual reactions (Burch 2008; Mezirow 2012).

Linking knowing and becoming to experiences from practice

Habitual reactions are not unique to people who work in healthcare settings. We are frequently challenged by the person, as patient/client, who responds to their illness in ways that are opposed to our beliefs and values. For example, a person with chronic pain may habitually respond with learned helpless behaviours (Seligman 1972). Having repeatedly experienced pain, which they consider they cannot escape from, increases stress in the person experiencing pain (Müller 2011), making them reluctant or possibly resistant to trying new ways of increasing their physical activity. This challenges many of those providing healthcare who, through their frustration, may respond by avoiding the person they should care for. Those person-centred people who *know self* can be more sympathetically present with the person they are caring for and working with. With an increased sense of self-awareness and self-understanding, people providing healthcare can put aside their assumptions and begin to work with a sympathetic understanding of the person's motivations and limitations, developing a therapeutic relationship that focuses on the person's needs and life perspectives (*care processes*; see Chapter 3). This helps us realise that the person has a story, a history, and is seen with the layers of influence surrounding them (McCance and McCormack 2017).

Creating the conditions for knowing and becoming

It can be seen that taking steps to knowing and becoming reflective person-centred practitioners are challenging. However, it is important not to assume that reflection is just a fault-finding exercise; rather, the focus should be on what went well and why (Coward 2018). To create positive learning environments, it is crucial to establish the boundaries for supportive, non-judgemental reflection (see Chapter 4). This should be about creating openings for critical discourse and mutual learning opportunities, and at the same time acknowledging the need for the learner (and group of learners) to take ownership and responsibility and connect authentically (Mezirow 1994; McCance and McCormack 2017). Conducive learning environments need to take account of the reality of confidentiality and respect, acknowledging each person's beliefs and values in the context of practice (McCance and McCormack 2017). Mezirow (2000) suggests that the ideal conditions for transformative learning include being free from coercion or self-distorting deception, being able to assess arguments objectively, being open to alternative points of view and caring about the ways others think and feel. Agreeing clear ways of working is a must for those engaging in supporting others to achieve insight into their practice.

This is about 'becoming' and as we transition from one role to another, e.g. student to registered practitioner, how we view our professional identity can change (Illeris 2013). The transitions we experience in our careers can open us up to many experiences and opportunities, and also countless moments of disorientation along the way. Seedhouse (2017) refers to this as having an 'anti-delusion toolkit' in place to avoid complacency as we move on to new responsibilities and build new relationships. Drawing on all we have addressed so far in this chapter, consider working through the next activity to develop your knowing and becoming.

Activity

Looking back on the situation you were working on in the first activity, were you able to work through the discomfort and uncertainty? If so, what was your learning and understanding of this, your sense of knowing?

This question asks you to consider both your own and other people's perspectives and perhaps recognise that others have shared the same experiences as you (recognition of the connection). Often in clinical practice common issues arise that are relational to others. This can occur across different healthcare professions and services. Explore these perspectives through the different aspects of the Person-centred Practice Framework. Do you realise something different if you use the lens of person-centred processes than you do if you explore the issues in the care environment? Are they linked to prerequisites? How do they link with other colleagues' views? It is only by sharing experiences, in a safe environment, that we can learn and understand the situation, focus and transform our behaviours and reactions (see Chapter 4).

Take a sheet of paper and coloured pens and create a picture that represents a map of your learning from this chapter, including obstacles and a course of action. Where are you going?

> You have arrived at a point where you need to consider your new learning and plan to put into practice what you have learnt about the context or environment that you work in and what you now believe (prerequisites). Are you clear about the implications of potential changes you will make for either yourself or others (explorations of options for new roles/planning a course of action)?

How can you take this learning with you and connect it to new experiences you will encounter – and to theories, concepts and models of reflection – building on your sense of becoming?

> The final stage of transformation is realised through merging our old and new learning and reformed beliefs. This should be evidenced through our intention to find opportunities to use our new knowledge in practice and share it with others. It is also portrayed through our ability to logically apply our newly acquired knowledge and ways of thinking to meet future challenges. The reflective practitioner has 'become' (Wilcock 1998).

Activity

Having worked your way through this chapter, you are invited to take three minutes and use free writing to look at an aspect of your practice and unpick the issues it reveals. You are encouraged to consider thinking about the connections to the personal and the professional you. Perhaps they are different. Working through this process, have you noticed anything new about yourself or your practice? What would you change to be more person-centred in the future?

Conclusion

In this chapter we have reflected on the importance of knowing and becoming and considered how this may impact on therapeutic relationships and the way we engage with people in our practice. One strategy for doing this is reflective learning, telling (and questioning) stories of practice experiences, making connections and being open to other viewpoints – a sense of knowing. This can support and challenge our beliefs and values, and the decisions we make as we move onto new roles, new responsibilities and build new relationships – a sense of becoming.

Summary

- People who provide healthcare need to have an awareness of who they are and the ways in which they are connected with their world of practice, to become authentic persons who act in knowledge-informed person-centred ways.

- It is essential to be a reflective practitioner, embracing the change in our learning and thinking as we connect to 'others' to develop person-centredness in our own practice.
- People who work in healthcare require a strategy to support how they respond and learn from experience, cognitively and emotionally, which includes being self-aware, curious and questioning our assumptions and biases.

References

Bolton, G. (2014). *Reflective Practice: Writing and Professional Development*, 4e. London: Sage.

Burch, V. (2008). *Living Well with Pain and Illness: The Mindful Way to Free Yourself from Suffering*. London: Piatkus.

Clandinin, J.D. (2013). *Engaging in Narrative Inquiry*. New York: Routledge.

Coward, M. (2018). Reflection and professional learning. *Nursing Management* 25 (3): 38–41.

Denzin, N.K. (2014). *Interpretive Autoethnography*. Los Angeles, CA: Sage.

Dewing, J. (2007). Participatory research: a method for process consent with persons who have dementia. *Dementia* 6 (1): 11–25. https://doi.org/10.1177/1471301207075625 [Accessed 19/10/19].

Habermas, J. (1987). *The Theory of Communicative Action. Vol II: Lifeworld and System: A Critique of Functionalist Reason* (trans. T. McCarthy). Boston; MA: Beacon Press.

Illeris, K. (2013). *Transformative Learning and Identity*. London: Routledge.

McCance, T. and McCormack, B. (2017). The person-centred practice framework. In: *Person-Centred Practice in Nursing and Healthcare: Theory and Practice*, 2e (eds. B. McCormack and T. McCance), 13–68. Chichester: Wiley Blackwell.

McCormack, B. (2004). Person-centredness in gerontological nursing: an overview of the literature. *International Journal of Older People Nursing* 13 (3a): 31–38.

Merriam, S.B. and Bierema, L.L. (2014). *Adult Learning: Linking Theory to Practice*. San Francisco, CA: Jossey-Bass.

Mezirow, J. (1994). Understanding transformation theory. *Adult Education Quarterly* 44 (4): 222–232.

Mezirow, J. (2000). Learning to think like an adult. In: *Learning as a Transformation: Critical Perspectives on a Theory in Progress* (eds. J. Mezirow and Associates), 3–35. San Francisco, CA: Jossey-Bass.

Mezirow, J. (2012). Learning to think like an adult. In: *The Handbook of Transformative Learning: Theory, Research and Practice* (eds. E.W. Taylor and P. Cranton), 73–98. San Francisco, CA: Jossey-Bass.

Müller, M.J. (2011). Helplessness and perceived pain intensity: relations to cortisol concentrations after electrocutaneous stimulation in healthy young men. *Biopsychosocial Medicine* 5: 8.

Rolfe, G., Jasper, M., and Freshwater, D. (2011). *Critical Reflection in Practice: Generating Knowledge for Care*, 2e. New York: Palgrave McMillan.

Seedhouse, D. (2017). *Thoughtful Health Care: Ethical Awareness and Reflective Practice*. London: Sage.

Seligman, M.E.P. (1972). Learned helplessness. *Annual Review of Medicine* 23 (1): 407–412.

Tyler, J.L. and Swartz, A.L. (2012). Storytelling and transformative learning. In: *The Handbook of Transformative Learning: Theory, Research and Practice* (eds. E.W. Taylor and P. Cranton), 455–470. San Francisco, CA: Jossey-Bass.

Wenger, E. (2018). A social theory of learning. In: *Contemporary Theories of Learning: Learning Theorists... in Their Own Words*, 2e (ed. K. Illeris), 219–228. Oxford: Routledge.

Wilcock, A. (1998). Reflections on doing, being and becoming. *Canadian Journal of Occupational Therapy* 65 (5): 248–256.

Further reading

Bassot, B. (2016). *The Reflective Practice Guide: An Interdisciplinary Approach to Critical Reflection*. New York: Routledge.

Schon, D. (1983). *The Reflective Practitioner: How Professionals Think in Action*. London: Ashgate.

30

Becoming a critical thinker

Neal F. Cook[1], Sonyia McFadden[1], and Lindsey Regan[2]

[1] *Ulster University, Northern Ireland, UK*
[2] *University of Central Lancashire, Preston, UK*

Contents

Fundamentals of Person-Centred Healthcare Practice, First Edition. Edited by Brendan McCormack, Tanya McCance, Cathy Bulley, Donna Brown, Ailsa McMillan and Suzanne Martin.

Learning outcomes

- Define critical thinking and its centrality within person-centred practice.
- Reflect the importance of understanding self, being reflexive and reflective in becoming and being a critical thinker.
- Identify strategies that enhance the ability to think critically in practice.
- Begin or continue your journey in becoming and being a critical thinker.

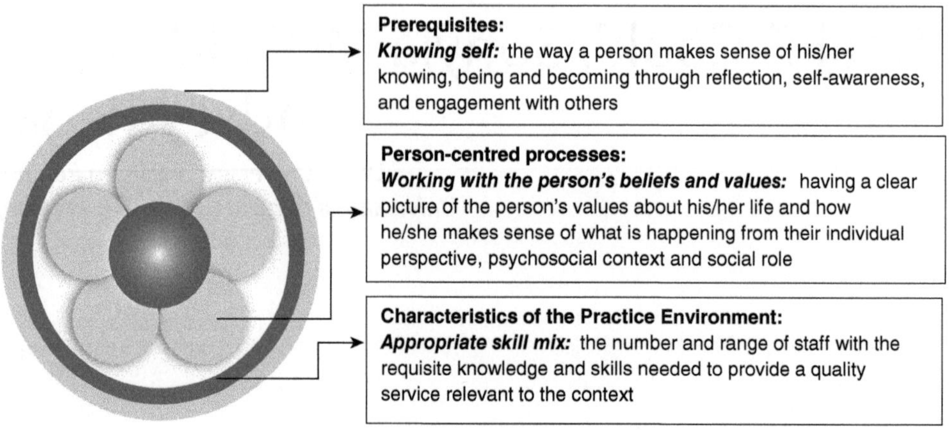
Prerequisites:
Knowing self: the way a person makes sense of his/her knowing, being and becoming through reflection, self-awareness, and engagement with others
Person-centred processes:
Working with the person's beliefs and values: having a clear picture of the person's values about his/her life and how he/she makes sense of what is happening from their individual perspective, psychosocial context and social role
Characteristics of the Practice Environment:
Appropriate skill mix: the number and range of staff with the requisite knowledge and skills needed to provide a quality service relevant to the context

Introduction

Within healthcare education and practice, reflective learning and critical thinking (see Chapters 28 and 29) are often discussed and expected of you as you develop your professionalism (see Chapter 7). The skill of being critical, however, can be difficult to acquire when you are immersed in complex care environments and team structures where the reality of practice can be stressful and turbulent, particularly when a novice within your profession. What can occur is an approach to learning and practice that becomes preoccupied with vocational and practical foci, i.e. a focus on doing. When a novice in practice, you can therefore find yourself focusing on competence, possibly to the neglect of considering what you are doing within a wider, more complex context. How you think and learn does not have to be, and should not be, distinct from how you practise. This chapter will take you through a journey of what critical thinking is and how to become a critical thinker, aligning it with living out the Person-centred Practice Framework (PcPF) (McCormack and McCance 2017).

What is critical thinking?

Critical thinking may conjure the image of something negative but it is actually positive, requiring people to be open-minded and committed to active, careful consideration of details. Active learning enables people to meaningfully talk and listen, to read, write and reflect on ideas and concerns of the topic under consideration (Zayapragassarazan and Zumar 2012). Underlying knowledge is essential to everyday professional practice. The ability to apply that knowledge to form a diagnosis and determine appropriate treatments in different situations is paramount. Critical thinking requires the use of the seven cognitive skills identified by Scheffer and Rubenfeld (2000): analysing, applying standards, discriminating, seeking information, logical reasoning, predicting, and transforming knowledge. These skills enable people to apply knowledge to adapt to situations and develop the ability to make judgements on their practice through informed decision making.

The importance of critical thinking in practice

The ability to apply critical thinking to practice is an essential skill across all health professions (Tanner 2006). It facilitates active learning through shaping knowledge development and the formation of informed professional judgement to enhance care. It also enables us to look for flaws in arguments and resist claims that have no supporting evidence. We can then generate possible explanations for findings, think of implications, and apply new knowledge to a broad range of social and personal problems. Scenario-based education promotes the use of critical thinking by engaging students with real-life scenarios, to formulate opinions and draw conclusions. This links directly with the 'shared decision-making systems' section of the PcPF and is of great importance as clinical decision making and planning interventions are complex processes. This is compounded by the fact that people present with a variety of symptoms, which are not classically 'textbook'.

A lack of critical thinking may lead to cognitive bias and error, increasing the risk for people in our care (Mezzio et al. 2018; Saposnik et al. 2016). Elliott et al. (2018) estimated that 237 million medication errors occur in England annually, costing £98.5 million for adverse drug reactions that could have been avoided. In this example, it is crucial to think critically about how medications may affect someone, rather than blindly administering medications because they are prescribed.

Activity

To improve your own critical thinking, try applying the points in Figure 30.1 to the scenarios below. This addresses the 'knowing self' element of the PcPF.

Scenario 30.1 Ava, 6 months old, is attending her physiotherapy appointment with her mother Megan (aged 16 years), for treatment of bilateral positional talipes. Megan says Ava fell out of her cot last night and is worried as she has been very drowsy for a couple of hours. On initial assessment both Megan and Ava look untidy and unkempt. A large bruise is visible on Ava's forehead.

Scenario 30.2 Steven is 45 years old and has been admitted to the emergency department at 3 a.m. He is alcohol-intoxicated, displaying behaviour that is challenging and reporting headache and dizziness. This is Steven's third admission to the emergency department in a month and he was intoxicated on each occasion. Previously, he was allowed to sleep and was discharged the following morning when sober. Currently, Steven is hypertensive and his speech is very slurred.

In Scenario 30.1, Megan presents with Ava who is drowsy. Immediately you consider Megan and Ava's ages and think about what questions to ask and what referrals, if any, to consider. How will you communicate with Megan, who is young and frightened, and Ava, who is drowsy and may have life-threatening injuries? Whilst a lot of this interaction is reflexive, you also need to think critically about what you are going to do. You need to rationalise what you believe is wrong with Ava and what the best course of action is for Megan and Ava. Does Megan's story

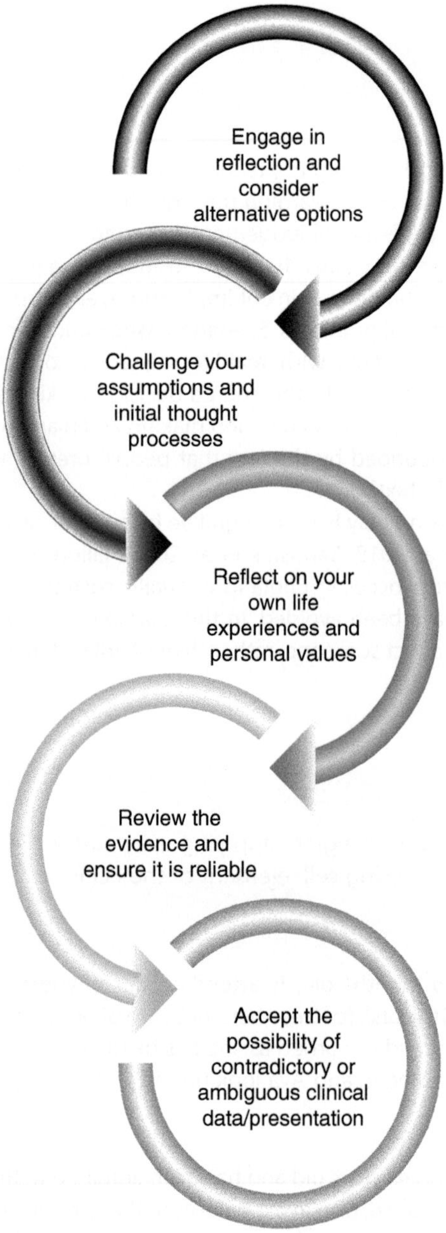

Figure 30.1 Tips for developing critical thinking skills.

of events seem plausible and does Ava need to go to radiology for imaging? Is there a possibility the child is at risk and if so, what other health professionals do you need to involve? What are your immediate priorities? Do you need to think of life-saving interventions first? Do you or others have the necessary skills to meet the most urgent presenting needs of both? This is where appropriate skill mix and effective staff relationships across the multidisciplinary team are essential to meet the needs of people.

In Scenario 30.2, Steven's admission to the emergency department may provoke a reflexive response to try to calm him and your initial impression may be that he needs paracetamol and a few hours of sleep. On reflection, you might consider that he has slurred speech and is very hypertensive. Is it safe to assume this is due to alcohol or, indeed, that he is intoxicated on this admission? Could Steven have fallen and hit his head? Should this be investigated immediately? In asking these questions, you are helping to eliminate the risk of diagnostic overshadowing.

Critical thinking is key to achieving the best possible solutions for people and adheres to the four concepts of the PcPF (McCormack and McCance 2017). Professional competence, as identified in the PcPF, and working within our code of practice will ensure welfare, health and safety are maintained. Engaging with our instinct, caring values and knowledge in a way that can often involve analysing complex scenarios leads to informed decisions that are in the best interests of the person in our care. Appropriate skill mix and effective staff relationships must be present alongside shared decision-making systems that work with the person's beliefs and values, to ensure they have a positive care experience. This is explicit in the care environment component of the PcPF. In both scenarios, the 'knowing self' component of the framework also comes into play. We must be aware of our own beliefs, values and prejudices in terms of how objective we are being in analysing a situation. For example, could Megan's socioeconomic background influence our views on how effective she is as a mother, or her age lead us to question her decision-making abilities or overlook her strengths? Are we more likely to focus on Ava's needs and forget that Megan may also have needs and be a vulnerable person too? Could possible prejudices impact on whether Steven's needs are met?

Activity

Reflect on a situation you have experienced either in the classroom or clinical environment where you have decided on an opinion quickly but could have used more critical thinking. Would this have changed the course of events? What would you do differently in the future?

Enablers and inhibitors of critical thinking

Storm and Patel (2014) identify that to be a critical thinker, you often need to have the ability to forget; critical thinking is not just about critically analysing and coming to conclusions, it is being able to see things from a new perspective. Preconceived views and experiences may lead to beliefs that a certain way of doing something is correct. By forgetting how we have always done something, we open our minds up to the possibility of alternatives. While critical thinking has an element of using our existing knowledge, experience and intuition to analyse a situation, we also need to forget, in order for new possibilities to emerge. Patterns and preferences from the past are sometimes inhibitors and forgetting, to some degree, enables all options to emerge equally without prejudice.

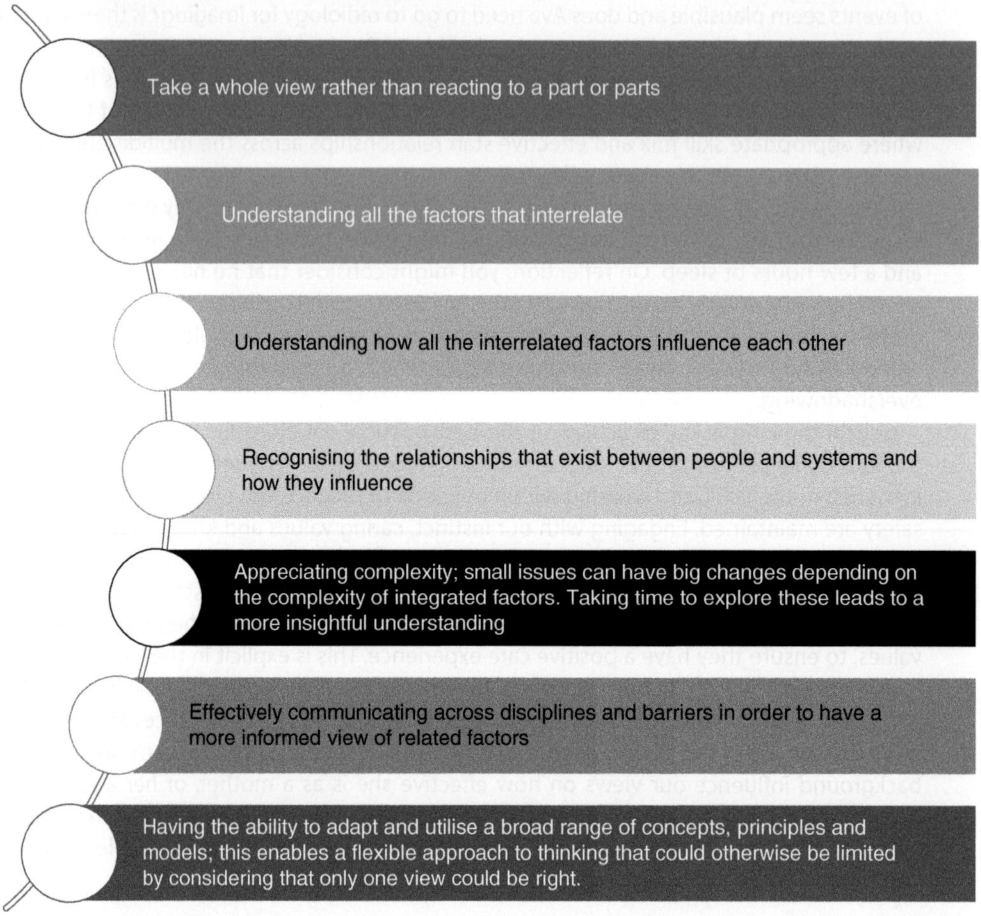
Take a whole view rather than reacting to a part or parts
Understanding all the factors that interrelate
Understanding how all the interrelated factors influence each other
Recognising the relationships that exist between people and systems and how they influence
Appreciating complexity; small issues can have big changes depending on the complexity of integrated factors. Taking time to explore these leads to a more insightful understanding
Effectively communicating across disciplines and barriers in order to have a more informed view of related factors
Having the ability to adapt and utilise a broad range of concepts, principles and models; this enables a flexible approach to thinking that could otherwise be limited by considering that only one view could be right.

Figure 30.2 Enablers of critical thinking through a systems approach.

A systems approach can be considered when identifying enablers of critical thinking. This means viewing a situation within the wider context of social, cultural and organisational factors. For example, you would not be fully considering why a person is malnourished if you did not look at various influences such as their ability to cook, whether they can afford healthy food, if they have the underpinning knowledge around nutrition, whether there is illness (physical or mental), whether global factors have influenced the price of food to make it affordable, or whether they have access to money following failure in a banking system. We do not exist in isolation and therefore taking a systems approach can be an enabler to viewing matters from a variety of contexts. Figure 30.2 identifies some of the enablers of critical thinking that a systems approach can bring (Valerdi and Rouse 2010), which are applicable in healthcare practice.

The ability to be reflective and reflexive is an essential co-enabler. Bringing these to practice requires the critical thinker to have the skill of high-level reasoning to assimilate and consider multiple perspectives simultaneously on a particular issue to make an informed analysis (Bonney and Sternberg 2017). High-level reasoning is a co-enabler, as is the ability to authentically engage with the perspective of others. In contrast, having a fixed, narrow focus and a tendency to focus only on your own views inhibits critical thinking. We must be prepared to learn and change based on authentic interactions. We therefore need genuine interest, motivation and passion. These enablers contrast with lack of interest and drive, overcoming inhibitors to critical thinking.

Another enabling factor is having cognitive 'space' to focus and reflect. While busy, noisy environments can cause sensory overload, inhibiting critical thinking, being able to focus the mind and filter out distractions can be enablers. You still need to be attuned to all the 'data' around you that inform your thinking, however, so this does not involve cutting yourself off from everything. Pausing where possible to reflect, rather than being reactionary, enables you to distinguish what is an accurate or inaccurate thought (or logical or unsound argument) (Bonney and Sternberg 2017). Filtering in this way will lead to more sound conclusions; we must be prepared to accept a sound conclusion from a sound analysis, even when it is contrary to what we expected. Therefore, being comfortable with discomfort is a further enabler, a central component of 'knowing self' in the PcPF.

The journey of becoming and being a critical thinker

Now that we have established what critical thinking involves, we turn our attention to the nature of the journey. In so doing, we present reflections on what has seemed significant to us, to provide you with some context and encouragement as you navigate your way through studies and practice.

Fundamentally, learning to think critically is a developmental process, taking us from a position of dependence to that of interdependence. In the early stages of our studies and practice, we tend to apply theory in concrete terms and from this novice position we are dependent on the skill and expertise of those more experienced than us as we look to them to highlight and explain the complexities of the 'real' world of healthcare. Having learned and applied the necessary theory, and trusting in the abilities of those around us, we feel safe to practise and we will do no harm to people in our care.

As we interact more with complexities in practice and explore and experiment with classroom theories, we begin to appreciate that healthcare does not operate in black or white, but rather in shades of grey. The acquisition of our growing knowledge base becomes the foundation on which our critical thinking processes are built and this enables us to make sound clinical decisions in practice (Brudvig et al. 2013). This process of independent thinking is perhaps the most anxiety provoking as we begin to 'forget' the truths we have accepted and accommodate new understandings, in what Mezirow (2003) calls the 'disorienting dilemma'.

The process of giving up our deeply held beliefs often compels us to hold on to *our* truths as we see them. On the other hand, we learn to appreciate that by actively seeking to understand others' experiences from *their* position, we access a wealth of resources to help us think more expansively and critically about ourselves, the care environment and the world around us. This is what Freire (1972) refers to as communing; when people come together to view the world around them from multiple perspectives in order to understand it and change it. In practice, acceptance of our interdependence helps us to work more adeptly with the values and beliefs of others in our efforts to work in person-centred ways. The world of healthcare no longer operates in shades of grey, but rather with the vibrancy of colour reflected in the human experience.

Understanding self in becoming and being a critical thinker

Fundamentally, it is the habitual act of being *present* and *actively* engaging with the 'self', others and the world which transforms the person who *thinks critically* into the *critical thinker*. Critical thinking is as much about the commitment of our will as it is the skilful application of our mind. Being able to identify and address barriers to knowing and understanding our 'self' is an important prerequisite in the development of the person-centred practitioner (McCormack and McCance 2017).

Amongst other influences, our ethnicity, cultural heritage, family background, social class, gender, religious/political persuasion and age provide context for our existence. We carry with us our values and beliefs, shaped by our worldview and a lifetime of experiences. Influenced by our perceptions of the world and interactions with it, we tend to think primarily from our own experiences, filtering information through our own lenses, which, when left unacknowledged, can diminish our objectivity. These cognitive biases may result in flawed decision making which can ultimately be harmful to others. In Scenario 30.1, for example, flawed decision making could result in Ava being subjected to unnecessary hospital treatment, or indeed failing to receive the required treatment, resulting in avoidable pain and distress. A lack of reflexivity diminishes our ability to recognise our own stance and understand its relationship to the way we think and interact with practice. Recognising that we are susceptible to cognitive biases is an important step in providing safe and effective person-centred care.

Critical thinking can be an uncomfortable process because of the interactions between the cognitions and emotions, particularly if new information is perceived as a threat. In the presence of strong emotions, the mind has a tendency towards subjectivity, which is the very antithesis of critical thinking because it diminishes rationality. You only have to look at what happens when people fall in love to understand the interplay between emotions and rational thought!

Returning to our case scenarios, imagine how an angry response to Steven's predicament may differ in outcome from that of a curious stance. Knowing and understanding the types of situations and circumstances in which strong emotions are triggered, and appreciating how these are likely to affect our ability to think critically, is crucial if we are to adopt the habits of the critical thinker. Our emotions can help indicate where we might be resistant to approaching or engaging in critical thought, by shining a light on our misgivings and motivations.

Knowing 'self' can be as confronting as it is empowering, and it is important to ensure you have access to a supportive environment where you feel accepted and validated (see Chapters 4 and 29). Action learning sets, critical companionship and conversational spaces can be helpful (McCormack and McCance 2017). Arguably, the most useful tool to understanding self is being open to new experiences and people. People who are very different from us often have the most to teach us about ourselves, akin to observing ourselves afresh in a mirror. Simply put, in order to better understand our self we must be committed to understanding the other.

Conclusion

This chapter has highlighted how critical thinking is central to safe, person-centred, effective, professional practice. Being a healthcare professional does not mean, however, that you passively inherit the ability to think critically. It is a conscious journey that you must go on to transition from what may be a monochrome view of practice to recognising the interplay and intricacy of a spectrum of factors that are brought together, analysed and translated to informed ways of working. Knowing self is central to being reflexive and reflective, whereby you can determine how your critical analysis of the world around you is influenced, sometimes negatively, by pre-existing views and experiences. Conversely, your historicity and life experiences also bring a richness and experience to your thinking that can enhance your ability to analyse complex situations by 'seeing' more influencing factors to which inexperience can cause blindness. What is clear is that we have to be comfortable with the uncomfortable and let our professional values, and those shared with others, guide us in being that person-centred, critical thinking practitioner.

References

Bonney, C.N.R. and Sternberg, R.R.J. (2017). Learning to think critically. In: *Handbook of Research on Learning and Instruction*, 2e (eds. R.E. Mayer and P.A. Alexander), 175–206. New York: Routledge.

Brudvig, T., Dirkes, A., Dutta, P., and Rane, K. (2013). Critical thinking skills in healthcare professional students: a systematic review. *Journal of Physical Therapy Education* 27 (3): 12–23.

Elliott, R.A., Camacho, E., Campbell, F. et al. (2018). *Prevalence and economic burden of medication errors in the NHS in England: Policy Research Unit in Economic Evaluation of Health & Care Interventions (EEPRU).* www.eepru.org.uk/prevalence-and-economic-burden-of-medication-errors-in-the-nhs-in-england-2/

Freire, P. (1972). *Pedagogy of the Oppressed.* New York: Herder and Herder.

McCormack, B. and McCance, T.V. (2017). *Person-Centred Practice in Nursing and Healthcare: Theory and Practice*, 2e. Chichester: Wiley Blackwell.

Mezirow, J. (2003). Transformative learning as discourse. *Journal of Transformative Education* 1 (1): 58–63.

Mezzio, D.J., Nguyen, V.B., Kiselica, A., and O'Day, K. (2018). Evaluating the presence of cognitive biases in health care decision making: a survey of U.S. formulary decision makers. *Journal of Managed Care & Specialty Pharmacy* 24 (11): 1173–1183.

Saposnik, G., Redelmeier, D., Ruff, C.C., and Tobler, P.N. (2016). Cognitive biases associated with medical decisions: a systematic review. *BMC Medical Informatics and Decision Making* 16: 138.

Scheffer, B.K. and Rubenfeld, M.G. (2000). A consensus statement on critical thinking. *Journal of Nursing Education* 39: 352–359.

Storm, B.C. and Patel, T.N. (2014). Forgetting as a consequence and enabler of creative thinking. *Journal of Experimental Psychology: Learning, Memory, and Cognition* 40 (6): 1594–1609.

Tanner, C.A. (2006). Thinking like a nurse: a research-based model of clinical judgment in nursing. *Journal of Nursing Education* 45 (6): 204–211.

Valerdi, R. and Rouse, W. B. (2010). *When systems thinking is not a natural act.* Presented at the 2010 IEEE International Systems Conference, pp. 184–189.

Zayapragassarazan, Z. and Zumar, S. (2012). Active learning methods. *NTTC Bulletin* 19 (1): 3–5.

Further reading

Carter, A.G., Creedy, D.K., and Sidebotham, M. (2017). Critical thinking skills in midwifery practice: development of a self-assessment tool for students. *Midwifery* 50: 184–192.

Cottrell, S. (2017). *Critical Thinking Skills: Effective Analysis, Argument and Reflection*, 3e. London: Palgrave Macmillan.

Price, B. (2015). Applying critical thinking to nursing. *Nursing Standard* 29 (51): 49–58.

Ruggiero, V.R. (2014). *Becoming a Critical Thinker.* Stamford: Nelson Education.

Sharples, J.M., Oxman, A.D., Mahtani, K.R. et al. (2017). Critical thinking in healthcare and education. *BMJ* 357: j2234.

Skills You Need (2019). Critical Thinking Skills. www.skillsyouneed.com/learn/critical-thinking.html

31

Developing and supporting practice educators

Fiona Stuart[1], Lucia Ramsey[2], and Jacinta Lynch[3]

[1] University of the West of Scotland, Paisley, Scotland, UK
[2] Ulster University, Northern Ireland, UK
[3] Milesian Manor Lifestyle Care Home, Magherafelt, Northern Ireland, UK

Contents

Fundamentals of Person-Centred Healthcare Practice, First Edition. Edited by Brendan McCormack, Tanya McCance, Cathy Bulley, Donna Brown, Ailsa McMillan and Suzanne Martin.

Learning outcomes

- Develop, support and promote a person-centred learning culture.
- Identify and apply the prerequisites of person-centredness that underpin the learning process.
- Identify and apply key evaluation processes to support the ongoing development of person-centred learning and practice.

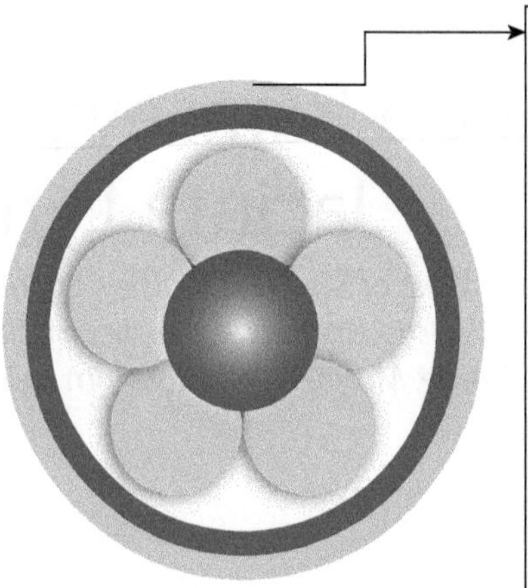

Prerequisites
Professionally competent: the knowledge, skills and attitudes of the person to negotiate care options, and effectively provide holistic care

Developed interpersonal skills: the ability of the person to communicate at a variety of levels with others, using effective verbal and non-verbal interactions that show personal concern for their situation and a commitment to finding mutual solutions

Knowing self: the way a person makes sense of his/her knowing, being and becoming through reflection, self-awareness, and engagement with others

Clarity of beliefs and values: awareness of the impact of beliefs and values on the healthcare experience and the commitment to reconciling beliefs and values in ways that facilitate person-centredness.

Commitment to the job: demonstrated commitment of persons through intentional engagement that focuses on achieving the best possible outcomes.

Introduction

The development of person-centred learning environments will enable all people to experience, internalise and enact person-centred values and skills. Whether you are a practice supervisor, assessor, mentor or educator responsible for providing learners with effective learning experiences, or a practice assessor responsible for conducting assessments to confirm learner proficiency (Health and Care Professions Council 2017; NMC 2018), this chapter will offer support to your role and enable you to promote a person-centred learning culture. Focusing upon the prerequisites of the Person-centred Practice Framework (professionally competent, developed interpersonal skills, knowing self, clarity of beliefs and values, commitment to the job), this chapter will guide you through a process of reflection and self-evaluation to enable you to develop in your role as an educator.

Person-centred learning cultures

The impact of organisational culture on the learning capacity of care environments cannot be overestimated (Chapter 3). Within large institutions, there is the potential for cultures to become deeply rooted. Unchallenged behaviours and accepted norms can negatively affect every person who engages with the organisation. In order to develop person-centred learning and practice that is sustainable, it is essential that the organisational culture is also person-centred (Carlström and Ekman 2012; McCormack and McCance 2017). A person-centred learning culture enables the competencies of individuals to be recognised, allows creative connections to be made and maximises the potential for personal and professional growth (Chapter 5) (McCormack and Titchen 2014). In order to maximise your potential to promote a person-centred learning culture, it is important that you recognise the difference between the concept of person-centred care and the broader concept of person-centredness.

The concept of person-centred care has been open to critique and has evolved over the course of time. Whilst retaining the key values of mutually beneficial, healthful relationships where compassion and shared decision making are key, the broader notion of person-centredness (or person-centred culture) takes account of all persons, including yourself as an educator, involved in care interactions. Within a person-centred learning culture, you will feel recognised and valued as a person and have a sense of belonging and feel integrated within the team. You will be offered or will create opportunities to share your ideas and insights and your own strengths and capacities will be recognised. You will also feel a sense of autonomy and be involved in decision-making processes. Overall, you will have opportunities to flourish within your role (McCormack et al. 2009; McCormack and Titchen 2014; Fagan 2017; O'Donnell et al. 2017; Slater et al. 2017).

Activity

Think about the culture where you work. Take some time to sit back and notice how people interact with each other. How do you demonstrate to colleagues and learners that they are valued? How do you support colleagues and learners to share their ideas and insights? How do you identify and celebrate the strengths and capacities of colleagues and learners? Is the culture person-centred? Perhaps you could have a conversation with your colleagues about this and reflect on your observations.

Professionally competent

You have a responsibility to maintain your professional competence, both in terms of your position as registered professional and also in your role as an educator (NMC 2018). This aligns with the promotion of a person-centred learning culture where a focus upon lifelong learning is key (Chapter 33). Within a person-centred learning culture, there is an individual, team and organisational commitment towards continual development. As an educator, you will engage, alongside colleagues and learners, in active learning processes including critical reflection and critical dialogue. You will examine events or established practices to develop new insights and the learning achieved will support the ongoing development of a person-centred learning environment (Manley et al. 2011; O'Donnell et al. 2017) (see Chapter 28). The open and constructive communication required to engage in this reflective process can only be achieved in the presence of effective staff relationships. This is also identified as a key component of the Person-centred Practice Framework. Overall, a person-centred learning culture promotes and values learning and innovation, adequately resources staff development, creates and nurtures opportunities for critical reflection and reflexivity and supports you as an educator to enable learners to be active in their learning journey (Manley et al. 2011).

Beliefs and values

Clarity of beliefs and values is also highlighted as a prerequisite within the Person-centred Practice Framework. Some of the key values of a person-centred learning culture include a commitment to fostering relationships characterised by dignity, respect and trust, where individuals feel valued and where their expertise and capacities are recognised and celebrated. Open communication within a context of high challenge and high support is the norm and is underpinned by care and compassion. Creativity and innovation are encouraged alongside a commitment to self-reflection and evaluation (McCormack et al. 2009; Manley et al. 2011; O'Donnell et al. 2017). As an educator, your own beliefs and values are likely to shape learners' experiences so it is essential that you have insight into how your beliefs and values are (or are not) enacted in your role with learners (Hegenbarth et al. 2015; O'Donnell et al. 2017).

Activity

Take some time to consider your beliefs and values about learning and your role in this. What helps you to enact your beliefs and values within your educator role? How might you enable learners to enact their beliefs and values in the practice environment? What could you do to overcome any barriers to the enactment of your beliefs and values?

By engaging learners in active learning processes within the work environment, you will enable them to emotionally connect with their practice. In so doing, they will have the opportunity to deepen their self-awareness and develop a clearer insight into their own beliefs and values (see Chapter 28).

Learning processes

Successful, person-centred learning experiences are more likely to occur in safe but challenging learning cultures and within a partnership model (O'Donnell et al. 2017). Introduction to the theoretical background to person-centred care prior to practice learning can begin the process of embedding the foundation and understanding for developing practice in a person-centred manner. Consistent exposure to and use of the concepts within the framework ensure that a common language and understanding of the breadth of constructs which are involved in person-centred practice are explored and developed. As a facilitator of learning, you should explore the extent and depth of understanding of person-centred practice with learners and identify any gaps in knowledge appropriate with stage of learning. Examples of theoretical issues which influence understanding of person-centred practice include health literacy, social determinants of health, carer awareness, person-centred outcomes and statutory and mandatory regulation and governance.

Chapter 1 illustrates that our insight into how we function as a person is vital to becoming effective in enabling others. This is the foundation on which person-centred practice grows and requires the ability to reflect on developing skills and practice. Appreciating the impact of teaching and learning styles and how these influence learners is key to creating the conditions to facilitate development as a person-centred practitioner.

Placement offers a learning environment that allows learners to experience, reflect and act on an extensive range of live situations within care environments. It offers them the opportunity to engage emotionally with these experiences, which then challenges the behavioural, perceptual, cognitive and affective learning dimensions which are necessary for effective, and potentially transformative, learning (Kolb and Kolb 2005) (see Chapter 28). Learning flexibility is described as engagement with the full breadth of learning styles in response to the learner's context (Peterson et al. 2015). A learning environment such as placement offers abundant opportunities for learners to engage with all learning styles. Learners may prefer certain learning styles to others, for example, sense or cognitive modalities; they may also have instructional preferences, such as learning in groups or alone. Peterson et al. (2015), however, challenge educators to offer a breadth of learning experiences in order to maximise learning flexibility within a person-centred culture. Chapter 28 shares the principles of active learning and demonstrates how you can align this with the prerequisites illustrated above.

In order to highlight how the Person-centred Practice Framework can be used to structure learning processes, the following section outlines two prerequisite attributes from the framework and suggests how you can engage learners to help them develop these in a person-centred manner.

Developed interpersonal skills

Fagan (2017) has outlined practical methods for developing and ensuring you are using person-centred interpersonal skills. These include the use of techniques such as active listening and open, focused questioning, clarification of what has been said and being aware of the environment. Exploring, discussing and using these strategies during practice learning will help foster effective person-centred interpersonal skills in learners.

A visible example of encouraging the development of interpersonal skills can be familiarising learners with the 'Hello my name is' campaign (Hello My Name Is 2019). A warm welcome into each practice learning environment will allow learners to more easily integrate into the team and create a sense of belonging. This will give them concrete experience of how they can reflect this behaviour within their own practice to ensure they are starting each care experience on a positive and welcoming note. Using kind and positive words can let the learner know you understand or are trying to understand how it is for them emotionally. Key guiding principles for mastering this complex skill include acknowledging and accepting the learner's perspective, avoiding judgemental behaviours, recognising emotion and communicating what you notice. Observation, modelling and reflection are encouraged to build the fundamental interpersonal skills that are essential within a person-centred learning culture. Learners should be encouraged to engage their primary senses (seeing, noticing, observing) during interactions and to reflect upon past and present experiences so that they develop a fuller insight into themselves, others and the situation at hand (see Chapter 28).

Activity

Explore the creative engagement programme outlined in McCormack et al. (2014). Consider whether you could adopt or adapt some of the creative learning sessions to explore interpersonal skills with learners, such as use of creative, interactive role-play exercises to provide insight into how others experience your communication methods. Discussion of and reflection on thoughts, feelings and experiences following these exercises can highlight the impact of how and where you communicate on the person with whom you are working. McCormack et al. (2014) suggest 'Games such as "Swords" which is focused on targeted and specific interactions that provoke differing responses'.

Knowing self

As discussed in Chapter 1, having insight into how you function as a person is a key determinant of how you develop as a person-centred practitioner. Each person brings a personal history influenced by, for example, their sociocultural background and experiences which shapes their unique view of the world. Taking time to help learners reflect on their personal 'story', thoughts and actions, and observe and reflect on the actions of others, creates opportunities to analyse and alter their experiences and subsequently impact positively on their behaviours. You can help learners in this process by asking them to keep a reflective diary, encouraging them to discuss their thoughts and experiences with peers and listening to and acting upon feedback from people who have used healthcare services. Creating the opportunity to discuss how you use reflection, self-awareness and engagement within your interactions with others will help people contextualise their learning (Peterson et al. 2015). The ability to self-assess is key to making sense of knowing, being and becoming a healthcare practitioner. You can encourage learners to take responsibility for evaluating their own person-centred evolution by providing early and frequent opportunities for self-assessment during both formal and informal supervision sessions.

Activity

Digital storytelling

Invite a learner to create a two-minute digital story of their personal experience in a healthcare environment. This could be a reflection on an appointment with a GP or their first experience of visiting a relative or friend in hospital. Create your own digital story of a similar experience. You can capture this on your phone or tablet device. Share your digital stories during a supervision session. Take some time to discuss similarities and differences in your experiences and how these have shaped your understanding of self on the journey to becoming a healthcare professional and educator.

Evaluation processes

To support the ongoing person-centred learning experience, as an educator you will be inviting the learner to engage in various evaluation methods. Learner feedback is key to developing your role as practice educator and to enhancing the overall practice learning environment. The process for evaluation enables feedback to be obtained, facilitates analysis of comments, and can lead to discussions which may result in changes being implemented (Kinnel and Hughes 2010).

The various evaluation processes include informal and formal methods. Gopee (2015) and Royal College of Nursing (RCN 2017) advocate both methods as being a fundamental requirement. Learners can provide you with verbal feedback during their practice learning experience and when they leave the learning environment. This feedback may be at the end of a working day or after you facilitate a formative or summative assessment. Some practice environments request learners to complete an in-house questionnaire in order to evaluate their experience, as this can provide more immediate feedback. Similarly, when the learner returns to their academic education institution, they are normally required to engage in a formal online evaluation process for the purpose of quality assurance. This may involve answering key questions that evaluate the learning environment in relation to the support and guidance offered by the educator. O'Donnell et al. (2017) stress the view that monitoring of the quality of learning experiences should be achieved through partnership, feedback and educational audit processes.

Evaluating your role and responsibility

To remain on a professional register, most of us are required to critically reflect on the feedback provided and evaluate our competence. You can use the prerequisites as a guide; several are discussed below to illustrate.

Professionally competent and commitment to the job

In Chapter 3 you explored the seven characteristics of the practice environment within the PcPF, exploring how person-centred practices can be established. You need to be professionally competent as an educator and committed to the role (Gopee 2015; RCN 2017). You must ensure the environment is conducive to learning and that everyone who contributes to the learning culture feels valued and respected (Manley et al. 2011; Carlström and Ekman 2012; O'Donnell et al. 2017).

To foster healthful relationships in the learning environment, it is essential that you encourage all staff to demonstrate excellent communication skills (Gopee 2015; RCN 2017). During their experience, learners may feel stressed or anxious so you should offer pastoral support as a key element in building confidence and trust. This will also enable you to keep abreast of their expectations and encourage learners to become active and motivated, facilitating ongoing development.

It is essential that in this ever-changing healthcare environment, you continually demonstrate commitment to your role. You need to ensure you are up to date in education and training requirements and have developed well-established networks with relevant universities. Bennett and McGowan (2014) claim that lack of preparation is having an impact on educators' confidence in fulfilling role requirements, especially the critical factor of assessment and determining competence (Bennett and McGowan 2014). Taking opportunities to participate in the review and development of programmes or professional standards are some examples of how you can stay current in your knowledge and understanding.

If you recognise that a learner is not performing to the expected standards, you must take appropriate action, such as devising tailored development plans that meet the learner's needs and exploring learning expectations. Feedback to the learner must be timely, constructive, meaningful and honest. Supporting a learner who is underperforming can be challenging and it is essential to seek the support and guidance of the educational link person.

Developing interpersonal skills and knowing self

As an educator, you need to continually evaluate how you develop your interpersonal skills and knowing self to role model person-centredness. You are required to welcome and integrate the learner into the team. Gopee (2015) advocates that the learner can only achieve a sense of 'belonging' if a relationship of respect is established. It is essential that you reflect on how you continually advocate for the learner to optimise learning opportunities. It is important that you continually assess your own performance in teaching the learner when exploring their learning needs and experimenting with different learning styles. Furthermore, sharing experiences with fellow educators and celebrating the positive rewards of the role of the educator can lead to personal development and flourishing.

Similarly, you need to be receptive to learner feedback and devise strategies that will address issues that emerge from practice learning. It is also important to have an awareness of knowing self and adhere to concepts previously outlined in Chapter 4. One example you may consider is how you foster critical thinking and reflective practice in your day-to-day care delivery. It is important to acknowledge, as an educator, that learners can influence and change practice, so encourage them to speak up and make their voice heard.

Taking guidance from this chapter, you as an educator should now be able to foster learning environments where you can observe, experience, internalise and enact person-centred values, skills and capacities to support person-centred learning. Engaging in evaluation processes will assist with the creation of practice environments that are conducive to learning as well as furthering your personal and professional development.

Ultimately, the goal of the educator is to encourage ongoing commitment to the development of a person-centred learning culture in which they can maximise the potential of learners to flourish as person-centred practitioners.

Summary

- Developing, supporting and promoting person-centred cultures can positively influence learning.
- The prerequisites of the Person-centred Practice Framework can be used to develop self and others as learners in practice.
- Identifying and applying key evaluation processes can support the ongoing development of person-centred learning and practice.

References

Bennett, M. and McGowan, B. (2014). Assessment matters – mentors need support in the role. *British Journal of Nursing* 23 (9): 454–457.

Carlström, E.D. and Ekman, I. (2012). Organisational culture and change: implementing person-centred care. *Journal of Health Organization and Management* 26 (2): 175–191.

Fagan, P. (2017). Person-Centred Approaches: Empowering People in Their Lives and Communities to Enable an Upgrade in Prevention, Wellbeing, Health, Care and Support. www.scie.org.uk/prevention/research-practice/getdetailedresultbyid?id=a110f00000NeJXwAAN

Gopee, N. (2015). *Mentoring and Supervision in Healthcare*, 3e. London: Sage.

Health and Care Professions Council (2017). *Standards of Education and Training*. London: HCPC. www.hcpc-uk.org/globalassets/resources/standards/standards-of-education-and-training.pdf.

Hegenbarth, M., Rawe, S., Murray, L. et al. (2015). Establishing and maintaining the clinical learning environment for nursing students: a qualitative study. *Nurse Education Today* 35: 304–309.

Hello My Name Is (2019). A Campaign for More Compassionate Care. www.hellomynameis.org.uk

Kinnel, D. and Hughes, P. (2010). *Mentoring Nursing and Healthcare Students*. London: Sage.

Kolb, A.Y. and Kolb, D.A. (2005). Learning styles and learning spaces: enhancing experiential learning in higher education. *Academy of Management Learning & Education* 4: 193–212.

Manley, K., Sanders, K., Cardiff, S., and Webster, J. (2011). Effective workplace culture: the attributes, enabling factors and consequences of a new concept. *International Practice Development Journal* 1 (2): 1–29.

McCormack, B. and McCance, T. (2017). *Person-Centred Practice in Nursing and Health Care: Theory and Practice*. Chichester: Wiley Blackwell.

McCormack, B. and Titchen, A. (2014). No beginning, no end: an ecology of human flourishing. *International Practice Development Journal* 4 (2): 1–21.

McCormack, B., Henderson, E., Wilson, V., and Wright, J. (2009). Making practice visible: the Workplace Culture Critical Analysis Tool (WCCAT). *Practice Development in Health Care* 8 (1): 28–43.

McCormack, B., McGowan, B., McGonigle, M. et al. (2014). Exploring 'self' as a person-centred academic, through critical creativity. *International Practice Development Journal* 4 (2): 1–16.

Nursing Midwifery Council (2018). *Realising professionalism: standards for education and training. Part 2: Standards for student supervision and assessment.* www.nmc.org.uk/globalassets/sitedocuments/education-standards/student-supervision-assessment.pdf

O'Donnell, D., Cook, N., and Black, P. (2017). Person-centred nursing education. In: *Person-Centred Practice in Nursing and Health Care: Theory and Practice*. Chichester: Wiley Blackwell.

Peterson, K., DeCato, L., and Kolb, D.A. (2015). Moving and learning: expanding style and increasing flexibility. *Journal of Experimental Education* 38 (3): 228–244.

Royal College of Nursing (2017). *Helping Students Get the Best from Their Practice Placements: A Royal College of Nursing Toolkit*. London: RCN.

Slater, P., McCance, T., and McCormack, B. (2017). The development and testing of the Person-Centred Practice Inventory- Staff (PCPI-S). *International Journal for Quality in Health Care* 29 (4): 541–547.

Further reading

Kreindler, S. (2013). The politics of patient-centred care. *Health Expectations* 18: 1139–1150.

McCance, J., Gribben, B., McCormack, B., and Laird, E. (2013). Promoting person-centred practice within acute care: the impact of culture and context on a facilitated practice development programme. *International Practice Development Journal* 3 (1): 1–17.

McCormack, B., Dickson, C., Smith, T. et al. (2018). "It's a nice place, a nice place to be." The story of a practice development programme to further develop person-centred cultures in palliative and end-of-life care. *International Practice Development Journal* 8 (1): 1–23.

McCormack, B., Borg, M., Cardiff, S. et al. (2015). Person-centredness: the state of the art. *International Practice Development Journal* 5 (1): 1–15.

NHS Leadership Academy (2013). *Health Care Leadership Module: The nine dimensions of leadership behaviour*. www.leadershipacademy.nhs.uk/resources/healthcare-leadership-model

32

Being curious through research and knowledge exchange

Cathy Bulley[1], Margaret Smith[1], and Alison Williams[1,2]

[1] *Queen Margaret University, Edinburgh, Scotland, UK*
[2] *Parkinson's UK*

Contents

Fundamentals of Person-Centred Healthcare Practice, First Edition. Edited by Brendan McCormack, Tanya McCance, Cathy Bulley, Donna Brown, Ailsa McMillan and Suzanne Martin.

Learning outcomes

- Engage in conversations that lead to collaborative identification of meaningful research or knowledge exchange questions or topics.
- Work with others to apply person-centred principles and values in designing a project.
- Plan further conversations with all persons engaged in implementing a project, leading towards co-production of findings and exploring ways to achieve broader impact.

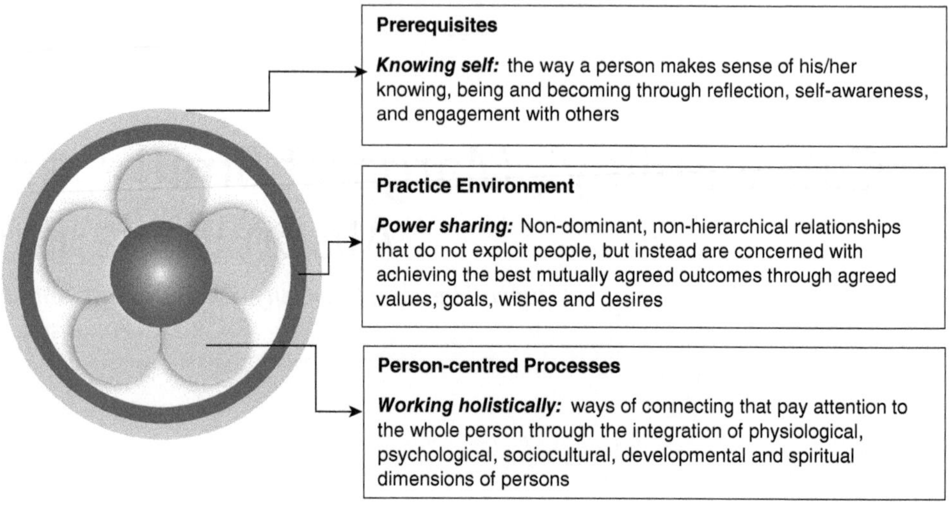
Prerequisites
Knowing self: the way a person makes sense of his/her knowing, being and becoming through reflection, self-awareness, and engagement with others
Practice Environment
Power sharing: Non-dominant, non-hierarchical relationships that do not exploit people, but instead are concerned with achieving the best mutually agreed outcomes through agreed values, goals, wishes and desires
Person-centred Processes
Working holistically: ways of connecting that pay attention to the whole person through the integration of physiological, psychological, sociocultural, developmental and spiritual dimensions of persons

Introduction

> What is wanted is not the will to believe, but the wish to find out, which is its exact opposite. Source: Bertrand Russell (1922).

Openness to experience and questioning can be seen in the curiosity of an enquiring mind and is integral to person-centredness (McCormack et al. 2017). Conversations between curious people can lead us to enquire together – we may want to find out something specific, explore better ways of doing things, or develop greater understanding. These conversations can trigger careful planning of activities such as research and knowledge exchange (KE).

Research is 'the systematic investigation into and study of materials and sources in order to establish new facts and reach new conclusions' (https://en.oxforddictionaries.com/definition/rese). This requires methods that aim to be trustworthy, transparent and credible to those making use of the results and outcomes. The term 'knowledge exchange' relates to exchange of knowledge between different people or groups to enable new developments, for example, development of better equipment or enhancement of service delivery.

A person-centred practitioner will use and generate new knowledge and ensure that this is used in practice (Dewing et al. 2017). This chapter aims to help you think through how you can use person-centred principles to explore your ideas and work out how to move them forward. This relates to much of the Person-centred Practice Framework, as illustrated in the image above.

Person-centred values and principles in research and knowledge exchange

According to Dewing et al. (2017), in order to undertake person-centred research, each researcher must develop clarity about their framework of thinking (paradigm). In simple terms, this should include:

- what they think it means to be a person
- their views on what is 'real', and what exists in the world (ontology)
- what they think knowledge is and how they 'create' it (epistemology).

The reading and thinking involved in developing your framework is a lifelong pursuit, and *Person-Centred Healthcare Research* by McCormack et al. (2017) will help you develop foundations for this. Many people studying and working in healthcare environments have started on this journey. We also frequently work in teams, where we may need to agree to use the same framework of thinking when making collaborative decisions. It can be valuable to use an existing framework, such as the Person-centred Practice Framework. Reading Chapters 1–3 of this book can help you reach early conclusions about whether you 'own' the values described in the Person-centred Practice Framework. Key assumptions of person-centredness for the researcher are respect, self-determination, reciprocity and mutuality (McCormack and McCance 2010). In this chapter we focus on 'application of person-centred values and principles' in research and KE, rather than 'doing person-centred research'. This makes use of person-centred processes from the Person-centred Practice Framework, such as taking a holistic view; practice environments that support the processes that are needed, such as power sharing; and prerequisites, such as knowing self (McCormack and McCance 2017) (see Chapter 4).

Starting off: developing ideas for research and knowledge exchange through conversation

The starting point is to decide on a focus for research or KE. Key person-centred values and principles in this decision are:

- working with the person's beliefs and values
- shared decision making
- authentic engagement and power sharing.

People bring different forms of knowledge and expertise; Tritter and McCallum (2006) explain that people who use services are experts in their own experience, and the different perspectives they bring are assets. They may ask new questions and challenge assumptions. Instead of seeing professional knowledge as more valuable or important than lay knowledge, the two can complement each other (Tritter and McCallum 2006). If we can put aside preconceptions and invite people with different 'forms of knowing' into discussions, we create a safe space for conversation and mutual learning. Good conversations can lead to meaningful questions and well-planned research that can have impact. This is well illustrated in an article written by three people living with Parkinson's disease who aim to work collaboratively with health professionals in both clinical and research settings (Williams et al. 2017).

We decided to illustrate this journey by engaging in a real conversation within the writing team with the intention of planning a research or KE project. We interrupt the 'story' of these conversations with activities to engage you in the reflection and planning journey. Initially, it would be useful to introduce ourselves briefly.

- AW: As a person with Parkinson's (PwP), an artist, an academic focusing on creativity and physical space, and a passionate enquirer into how people – including myself – take responsibility for our own well-being and wellness, I relish wide-ranging conversations.
- MS: As a nurse, researcher and educator, I currently lead a project exploring person-centred care in older persons at high risk of fracture due to osteoporosis. I am committed to genuinely person-centred practices in health and social care and in higher education.
- CB: I teach and research in physiotherapy at QMU and am fascinated by the different ways we all experience health, wellness and different services and interventions.

Margaret and Cathy started this conversation by asking Alison – 'What is the best question to start the conversation?'

Alison: 'A good question is: What is meaningful to you?'

Margaret and Cathy: 'What is meaningful to you right now?'

Alison: 'The Quality of Life Group (QoL Group: part of the Edinburgh Branch of Parkinson's UK) has been having vibrant discussions about the "nocebo effect".' (She explained that this term describes non-specific, harmful effects of intervention (Hauser et al. 2012; Williams et al. 2017).) 'The QoL Group has been discussing our experiences of health professionals unconsciously sending negative messages through their words and body language.'

Margaret and Cathy: 'What sort of messages, and how?'

Alison: 'For example, one healthcare professional told me: "Well, you're doing really well, we'll just plod on." And in an interaction with a different healthcare professional I said: "I don't need occupational therapy yet", and received the emphatic response: "'Yet' is a word we *never* use".'

Alison expanded further, that instead of exploring positive aspects of well-being: 'Even the questionnaires used by health professionals often focus on death, doom and disaster! Members of the QoL Group are considering ways of recognising when a "nocebo effect" may be coming, and batting it out of the way! We want to take control of our own wellness and go beyond an approach that focuses on a "restitution narrative" – the focus of health professionals on trying to "fix" things. This is unhelpful when people are living with a long-term condition (see Chapter 26). The QoL Group has been discussing the need for a "quest narrative" – focusing on the journey and living well. We really need to focus on wellness of spirit as well as body; on wellness of heart as well as mind.'

Continuing the conversation, we all felt this approach could be strengthened in the education and training of health professionals and wondered about how we might be able to work together to develop a project from this conversation. As we ended this conversation, we all expressed feelings of anticipation and excitement about what we could do. . .

Activity

We want you to engage in this thinking. Having read the overview of this conversation, how do you think the first healthcare professional could have rephrased their comment to Alison? From our conversation so far, what ideas do you have for possible research questions or knowledge exchange topics? We come back to this in the next section but if you wish to explore this further, please read Hauser et al. (2012), Williams et al. (2017), Williams (2019).

Continuing: developing ways of addressing research questions and knowledge exchange topics

This section focuses on making collaborative choices when planning research and knowledge exchange projects. We believe that keeping person-centred values and principles central cultivates a healthful research and KE culture. Jacobs et al. (2017, p. 51) describe specific principles for 'doing research in a person-centred way'. These relate to the values of respect for each other, reciprocity (exchanging with the other for mutual benefit) and self-determination (McCormack and McCance 2010). Considering 'connectivity' is important – instead of 'doing research about others', we research 'with' other persons (Jacobs et al. 2017). We must consider the following principles.

- 'Attentiveness and dialogue': we are aware, express mutuality, enter into dialogue and celebrate difference.
- 'Empowerment and participation': we use facilitation skills in individual and group settings, practise self-awareness, consider self-esteem, work non-hierarchically and build capacity for collective action.
- 'Critical reflexivity': we reflect on possible power imbalances between the researcher and others and consider social inclusivity, equality and diversity to ensure new insights reflect the range of views and ways of being and doing (Jacobs et al. 2017).

We need to think about how to apply these values and principles in different types of research. Returning to the first activity, our conversations could take us in different directions, for example exploring how people with Parkinson's take control of their own wellness or investigating how many health professionals are aware of the term 'nocebo effect'. The type of question asked will influence the type of research approach, such as qualitative, quantitative, mixed or multiple methods, action research or participatory research. Many possible resources are available to support you in understanding the advantages and disadvantages of specific study designs and how to make sure your study is trustworthy, for example Reason and Bradbury (2008), Polit and Beck (2017).

Some approaches have person-centred principles embedded within them, such as Participatory Action Research. Study designs like a randomised controlled trial (RCT) are rooted in a different framework of thinking about what knowledge is (Titchen et al. 2017) and strategies to increase their trustworthiness may seem less consistent with person-centred values. The assumption is that by randomly allocating people into intervention or control groups, it is possible to be sure that any changes in your measurements are due to the intervention (Polit and Beck 2017). This does reduce participant choice, but if we have decided collaboratively that an RCT is the best way to robustly address an unanswered question that is meaningful to people, we may still uphold person-centred principles, such as those suggested by Badian et al. (2017).

Table 32.1 Person-centred principles and values applied to different broad study approaches

Principles and values[a]	Quantitative study approach	Qualitative study approach	Participatory study approach
Healthful relationships with mutual respect and dialogue	Co-design of study question, approach, materials and methods with careful consideration of inclusivity and diversity. Involvement of people in ongoing decision making, e.g. project steering group		
	Co-design is predominantly within the design and planning stage, with less flexibility later. Consultation with steering group at key stages	Methods can be more fixed or fluid depending on the approach. More potential for dialogue throughout, and a sympathetic presence	Values are reflected throughout the journey, including co-design of methods and collaborative analysis leading to the study results
Reciprocity and mutuality	Promote understanding, interest and impact of the project by discussing motivations, decisions and outcomes with people who may be interested in participating or using results		
	Approachable updates for participants and stakeholders at key points	More potential to respond to queries and concerns that come up during interviews or focus groups, e.g. signposting to useful information	Project develops in a way that reflects the needs of everyone involved, through negotiating what each person needs and wants from the work
Self-determination and autonomy	Provision of full and clear information to inform potential participants about the study and their rights – ideally information is pre-reviewed by people who could be participants		
	Generally addressed through ethical principles of informed consent	Participants may have more ability to influence the topics and themes as the study progresses	Participants have far greater autonomy as they co-design processes and findings
Empowerment and participation	Integrate conversations throughout the journey about how people would like to receive project outcomes and how they would like these to be used – locally, nationally and internationally		

[a] McCormack et al. (2017).

In Table 32.1 we summarise suggestions of how they may be reflected within different broad study approaches, to help you think through ways of applying person-centred principles and values within your specific research or KE project.

We will summarise our next conversation to help you reflect on how these person-centred principles and values might be applied.

We discussed what might influence the 'nocebo effect', such as a negative state of mind due to tiredness or stress, lack of self-awareness, clumsiness or labelling of 'others'. We theorised about whether we could explore with people how their communication was experienced, possibly through a simulation activity in an educational setting or in a practical activity with a person from the QoL Group. We started to refine this into a research/KE topic, discussing ideas such as 'exploring people's experiences of conscious and unconscious communication during healthcare interactions' and 'strategies for becoming more person-centred in our communication'. The next step was to use the person-centred principles and values that we introduced earlier to help us plan a possible project and we would like you to do some of this thinking.

Activity

Pick one of the suggested topics (or your own): would this benefit from research or KE? How would you start to plan forward? Who would you involve and how?

If you are planning research, which approach might work best? How would you use the suggestions in Table 32.1 when planning study design, methods and materials?

Moving forward: ensuring that our work has positive impacts on people

It is important to ensure mutuality and reciprocity by making sure research and KE outputs are used, ensuring that everyone benefits (Jacobs et al. 2017). Dissemination of the knowledge and insights gained may involve presenting at conferences and submitting articles for publication in journals. Increasingly, social media are used to make new knowledge more approachable and accessible to people. The further step of implementation describes the application of new insights within everyday practice to increase the likelihood of positive change (impact) for the people who need this most.

Using our hypothetical project to illustrate, we would talk together about who could use our outcomes to make sure they benefit the QoL Group, other people living with Parkinson's and potentially people living with other conditions. Short updates, approachable explanations at meetings, blogs and micro-blogs such as tweets, mixed media including images or videos, and conversations with people and organisations with decision-making powers can all increase the likelihood of our work leading to impact.

Activity

It is important that you apply learning from this chapter to your own situation. Are you at the point of designing a project? Are you involved in or joining an existing project? The amount of influence you have over the design of a project varies depending on your answers to these questions. You can ask yourself the following questions.

- What decisions have already been taken? What influenced these decisions and how might I do things in future situations?
- What are the next steps? How can I use the learning from this chapter to involve people in collaboration from this point onwards?
- Using Table 32.1, how can I reflect person-centred values and principles in different aspects of my study or project?
- How can I increase the likelihood that insights from my/our work will be used by (and for) the people they relate to?

Conclusion

We believe that person-centred values and principles can – and should – be applied across all types of research and knowledge exchange to ensure ethical and healthful practices. Person-centred conversations can ensure meaningful projects and outcomes that have impact. While we do not always have 'control' over the process of developing ideas for research and knowledge exchange, for example through being allocated a dissertation topic or joining an existing team, we can seek to influence the journey. This can be challenging but incredibly fulfilling.

Summary

- Research and knowledge exchange should start with conversations with the people most affected, to ensure questions/topics are meaningful to all involved.
- Different types of questions and research designs may be chosen, and person-centred values and principles can be applied to all through insight into the Person-centred Practice Framework and careful thought.
- It is important to consider the use and potential impacts of project outcomes, and make sure conversations take place throughout the journey with people and organisations who can make good use of the results.

References

Badian, R., McCormack, B., and Sundling, V. (2017). Person-centred research: a novel approach to randomized controlled trials. *European Journal for Person Centred Healthcare* 6: 209–218.

Dewing, J., Eide, T., and McCormack, B. (2017). Philosophical perspectives on person-centredness for healthcare research. In: *Person-Centred Healthcare Research* (eds. B. McCormack, S. van Dulmen, H. Eide, et al.), 20–29. Chichester: Wiley.

Hauser, W., Hansen, E., and Enck, P. (2012). Nocebo phenomena in medicine: their relevance in everyday clinical practice. *Deutsches Ärzteblatt International* 109 (26): 459–465.

Jacobs, G., van Lieshout, F., Borg, M., and Ness, O. (2017). Being a person-centred researcher: principles and methods for doing research in a person-centred way. In: *Person-Centred Healthcare Research* (eds. B. McCormack, S. van Dulmen, H. Eide, et al.), 51–60. Chichester: Wiley.

McCormack, B. and McCance, T. (eds.) (2010). *Person-Centred Practice in Nursing and Health Care: Theory and Practice*. Chichester: Wiley.

McCormack, B. and McCance, T. (eds.) (2017). *Person-Centred Practice in Nursing and Health Care: Theory and Practice*, 2e. Chichester: Wiley.

McCormack, B., van Dulmen, S., Eide, H. et al. (2017). *Person-Centred Healthcare Research*. Chichester: Wiley.

Polit, D.F. and Beck, C.T. (2017). *Nursing Research. Generating and Assessing Evidence for Nursing Practice*, 10e. Philadelphia: Wolters Kluwer.

Reason, P. and Bradbury, H. (2008). *The Sage Handbook of Action Research. Participative Inquiry and Practice*, 2e. London: Sage.

Russell, B. (1922). *Free Thought and Official Propaganda*. www.gutenberg.org/files/44932/44932-h/44932-h.htm

Titchen, A., Cardiff, S., and Biong, S. (2017). The knowing and being of person-centred research practice across worldviews: an epistemological and ontological framework. In: *Person-Centred Healthcare Research* (eds. B. McCormack, S. van Dulmen, H. Eide, et al.), 31–50. Chichester: Wiley.

Tritter, J.Q. and McCallum, A. (2006). The snakes and ladders of user involvement: moving beyond Arnstein. *Health Policy* 76: 156–168.

Williams, A. (2019). Exploring the impact that quality of life assessments can have on Parkinson's patients, the values informing those measurements, the words that are used, and how those words can invoke the 'nocebo effect' – what one colleague calls 'the evil twin of the placebo effect'. https://measuringhumanity.org/words-cast-spells-and-why-this-matters-in-parkinsons

Williams, A., Bowler, K., and Wright, B. (2017). Adventures with Parkinson's: empowering Parkinson's patients to become active partners in research and treatment. *Regenerative Medicine* 12 (7): 737–742.

Further reading

Harding, E., Wait, S., and Scrutton, J. (2015). *The State of Play in Person-Centred Care: A Pragmatic Review of how Person-Centred Care Is Defined, Applied and Measured, Featuring Selected Key Contributors and Case Studies across the Field*. London: Health Policy Partnership.

Sandvik, B.M. and McCormack, B. (2018). Being person-centred in qualitative interviews: reflections on a process. *International Practice Development Journal* 8 (2): 8.

33

Being a lifelong learner

Lindesay Irvine[1], Patricia Gillen[2], and Owen Barr[3]

[1] Queen Margaret University, Edinburgh, Scotland, UK
[2] Southern Health and Social Care Trust and Ulster University, Northern Ireland, UK
[3] Ulster University, Northern Ireland, UK

Contents

Fundamentals of Person-Centred Healthcare Practice, First Edition. Edited by Brendan McCormack, Tanya McCance, Cathy Bulley, Donna Brown, Ailsa McMillan and Suzanne Martin.

Learning outcomes

- Debate the relationship between lifelong learning, person-centredness and practice learning.
- Identify and explore ways of understanding learning and its role in self-development.
- Apply strategies of learning to own role and development as a person-centred healthcare worker.

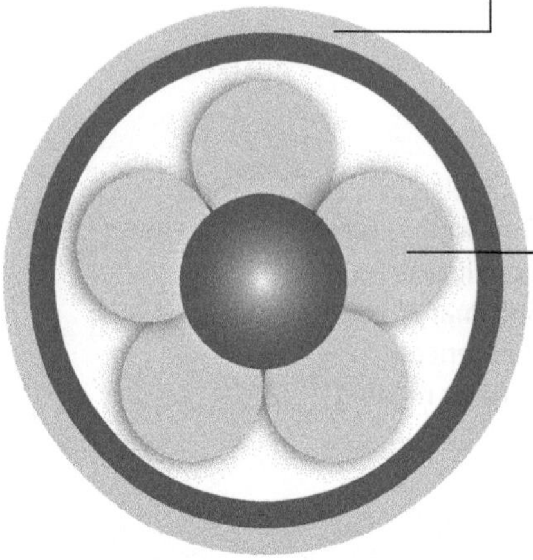

Prerequisites

Professionally competent: the knowledge, skills and attitudes of the person to negotiate care options, and effectively provide holistic care

Knowing self: the way a person makes sense of his/her knowing, being and becoming as a person-centred practitioner through reflection, self-awareness, and engagement with others

Person-centred Processes

Working with the person's beliefs and values: having a clear picture of the person's values about his/her life and how he/she makes sense of what is happening from their individual perspective, psychosocial context and social role

Engaging authentically: the connectedness between people, determined by knowledge of the person, clarity of beliefs and values, knowledge of self and professional expertise

Being sympathetically present: an engagement that recognises the uniqueness and value of the person, by appropriately responding to cues that maximise coping resources through the recognition of important agendas in their life

Introduction

In this chapter, we will discuss person-centred learning as a lifelong process and its role in assisting our development as healthcare practitioners, thus reflecting the philosophy of learning as being both about 'being' and 'becoming'. To this end, the nature and relevance of lifelong learning and how it is situated within the development of person-centredness will be reviewed. Approaches to learning that allow us to know 'self' as a learner and understand our self-identity through transformative learning are considered along with ways to reduce the challenges this may present during practice learning. Finally, the art of reflexivity and how we can learn from things that go well or not so well is addressed. We will focus on the prerequisites of the Person-centred Practice Framework – knowing 'self' and being professionally competent – along with three aspects of the person-centred processes – working with the person's beliefs and values, engaging authentically and being sympathetically present.

Lifelong learning and its relationship to person-centredness

Lifelong learning starts when we start – so depending on your view, this is either at our conception or birth, with the need to learn being fundamental to our humanity; it is by living that we learn and through our learning that we make sense of life and how we live. We are not always aware of the learning we are experiencing but often are aware of the outcome of learning. For example, we might recognise a cake is being baked by the smell emitted from the oven but we have not consciously learnt that the smell means a cake is baking.

However, in relation to adults as learners, we need to understand some brain development to better understand ourselves. The frontal cortex of the brain controls executive functions such as thinking, creativity and setting goals. In younger people (up to about age 26), the cortex has not finished developing so they rely more on teachers and facilitators to offer direction and control of learning. As you progress in your career, you will find that lifelong learning becomes more relevant as you feel the need to know the 'who, what, why and how' of the learning journey (Knowles et al. 2015).

Learning normally occurs because we wish to grow and develop ourselves. However, Dweck (2012) suggested that there are two different mindsets (Figure 33.1) for learning linked to our most basic beliefs: fixed mindset versus growth mindset; here we can see a link to the Person-centred Practice Framework. Our beliefs and values, whether conscious or unconscious, affect what we want as learners and how we achieve that. Thus, our mindset can either promote or prevent us from fulfilling our potential. Our view of ourselves which we have developed over time, often based on our previous experiences and the nature of feedback from others, can determine everything. If you believe that your qualities are unchangeable (a fixed mindset), you will want to prove yourself correct over and over again rather than learning from your mistakes. This is normal in a culture that values intelligence, personality and character such as Western cultures. However, a growth mindset, where you situate yourself as the starting point for development and learning, is based on your belief that your basic qualities are things you can cultivate and nurture through your own efforts in order to flourish. The growth mindset creates a powerful passion for learning and changing our beliefs can have a significant impact on how we think, feel and practise.

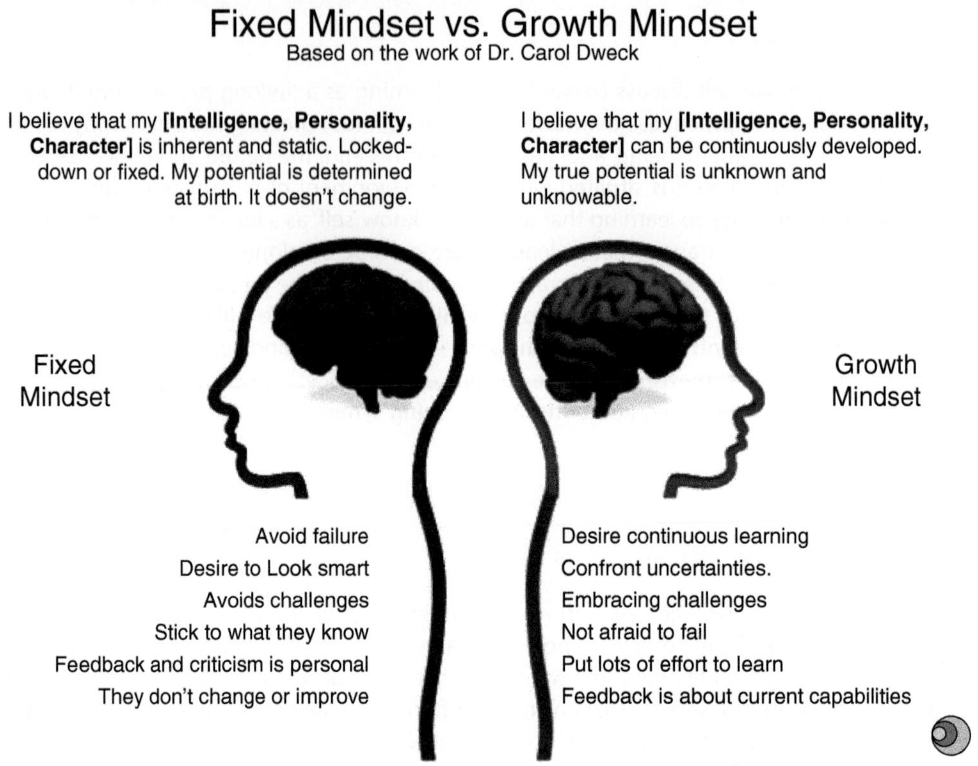
Fixed Mindset vs. Growth Mindset
Based on the work of Dr. Carol Dweck
I believe that my [Intelligence, Personality, Character] is inherent and static. Locked-down or fixed. My potential is determined at birth. It doesn't change.
I believe that my [Intelligence, Personality, Character] can be continuously developed. My true potential is unknown and unknowable.
Fixed Mindset
Growth Mindset
Avoid failure
Desire to Look smart
Avoids challenges
Stick to what they know
Feedback and criticism is personal
They don't change or improve
Desire continuous learning
Confront uncertainties.
Embracing challenges
Not afraid to fail
Put lots of effort to learn
Feedback is about current capabilities

Figure 33.1 Fixed mindset versus growth mindset. Source: From Fixed Mindset vs Growth Mindset, Rio District Blog.

Activity

Linda, a pre-registration student, is persistently 10 minutes late for the start of her physiology lectures regardless of the time they are starting. This disrupts the session for the other learners and is causing tension in the lecture room. The lecturer asks Linda's personal academic tutor to have a meeting with her to discuss this to try to find out what the issue might be.

Thinking points and discussion

- From your understanding of lifelong learning what might be the cause of this behaviour? Write down your ideas.

Through their facilitated discussion, it seems that Linda cannot see why she needs to know all this physiology because, as she says, 'she just wants to look after people and help them recover'.

- How might Linda gain an understanding of the effects of her late arrival in class? Give some reasons for your answer.
- Which part of the prerequisites domain of the Person-centred Practice Framework can be used to explore this situation?

In your thinking and discussion, you may have considered the relationship between Linda's learning and practice and her understanding of self in terms of the impact of behaviour.

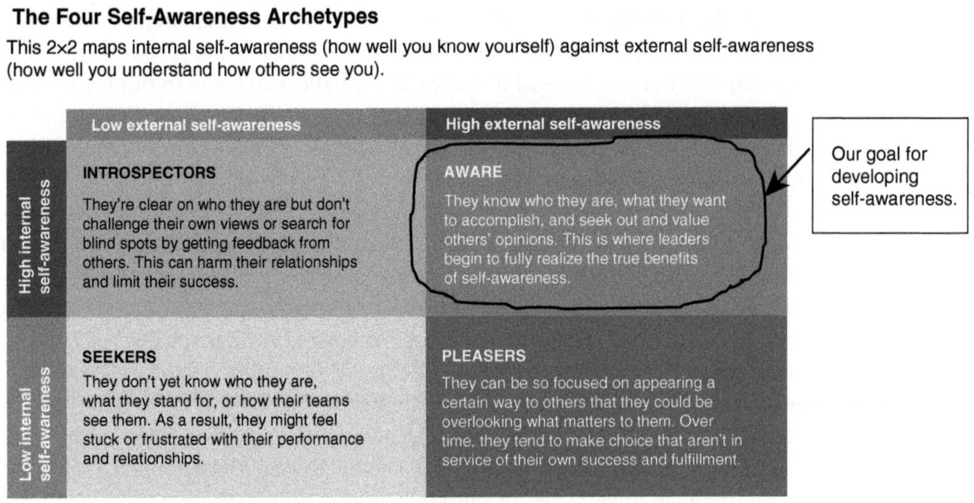

Figure 33.2 Map of internal/external awareness. Source: From What Self-Awareness Really Is (and How to Cultivate It) by Tasha Eurich, Harvard Business Review 2018 © Harvard Business School.

A crucial aspect of lifelong learning is the idea of continual growth and development through self-awareness, authenticity of actions and axiological values and beliefs that map with three aspects of the Person-centred Practice Framework. Axiology is a branch of philosophy that studies judgements about the value of things and, in the context of practice learning, engages us in assessing our own values in all stages of the learning process. Self-awareness is vital, as knowledge of self helps us to respond positively to the challenges inherent in lifelong learning through the processes of transformative learning. Figure 33.2 illustrates the importance of self-awareness generally.

Taylor and Cranton (2012) suggested an important facet for transformative learning is that the educator (and arguably the adult learner also) has a strong sense of self-awareness. Transformative learning is supported by a well-developed self-awareness that enables a person to reflect upon, illuminate and question previously held assumptions that underpin their worldview (Mezirow 2000). It is through such processes of thinking and reflecting that a person can revise their assumptions and their wider perspectives which influence their approaches to learning. These processes can be particularly effective when working together in groups in which people feel safe to express their views and question their ideas. Illeris (2014) argues that transformative learning has been developed in relation to adult learners, as in order for transformation to occur there must be a base from which to transform. This base comes from our socialisation in childhood and youth where our understanding has not been founded on independent considerations and thus as adults, we should have reason and need to revise our perspectives (Mezirow 2000). An interesting perspective of this in relation to lifelong learning is by Kathryn Schulz in her TED talk which you can find at: www.ted.com/talks/kathryn_schulz_on_being_wrong?referrer=playlist-the_love_of_lifelong_learning.

Activity

You might wish to try this self-awareness questionnaire as a starting point to consider where you locate yourself at present:

www.higherawareness.com/awareness-level-test.php

There is no doubt that if we do not know where we are starting from, it is hard to move forward in developing ourselves.

In terms of learning and education, authenticity of self and in relationships is essential, particularly in the practice setting. This requires us to be open-minded and receptive to new ways of thinking that expand our minds, lead to opportunities and add value to our lives, reflecting the growth mindset identified earlier (Lynch and McCance 2018). The following broadcast by Melvin Bragg's *In Our Time* series discusses what being oneself means in today's world: www.bbc.co.uk/programmes/m00035z4.

An authentic relationship is particularly important between learners and educators as it is a trusting relationship that is decisive in transformative learning. Both the educator and the learner need to be 'present' and open to learning. Social presence is an important aspect of learning and often a key ingredient of successful online courses and communities of practice, whether in educational institutions or practice learning settings (Wenger 1998; Garrison 2011). This meaning of being 'present' is about nurturing a social connection with another person, being focused on them and your interaction, which is much more than being physically in the room. The need for presence is core to the Person-centred Practice Framework in the context of 'engaging authentically' and 'being sympathetically present', particularly within the healthcare practice setting. It has been argued that there are three circles of presence (Rodenburg 2009; hear more about this by watching Patsy Rodenburg talk about it at www.ted.com/speakers/patsy_rodenburg) which roughly correspond to Illeris's (2014) three layers of identity as illustrated in Figure 33.3.

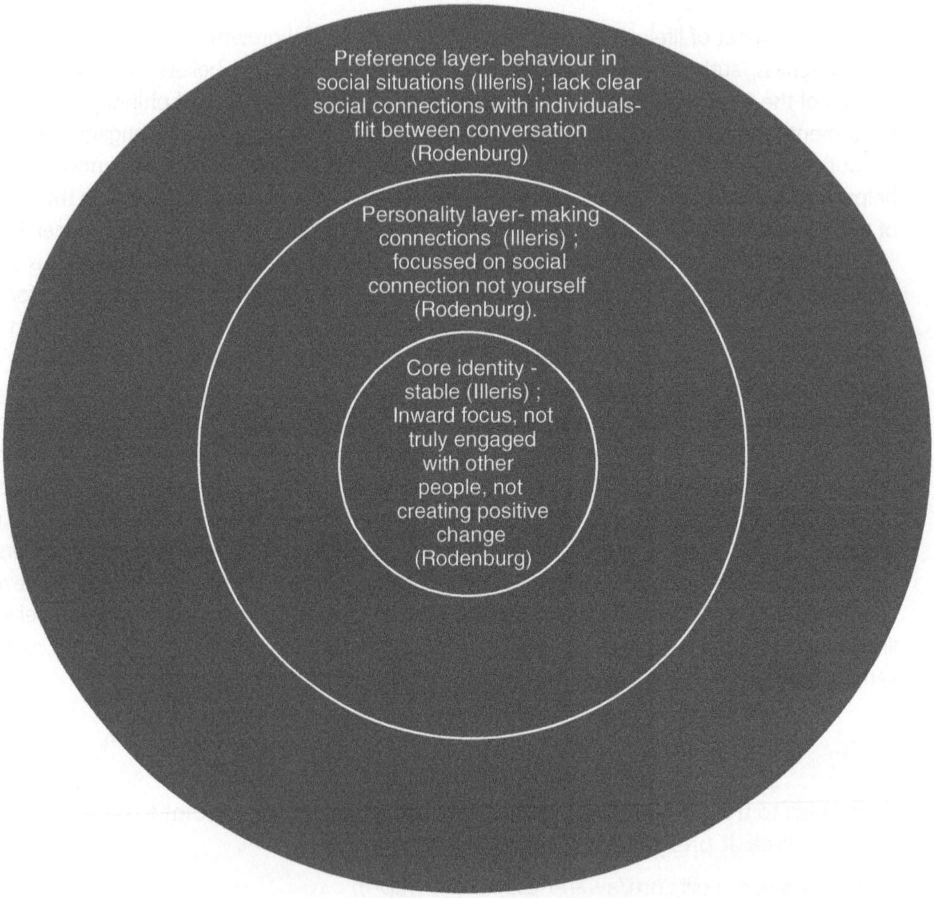

Figure 33.3 Comparison of Rodenburg's and Illeris's notions of identity and presence. Source: Modified from ILLERIS, K. 2014.

Engaged social connections between learners and educators is as important as between healthcare workers and service users (second circle of presence) in assisting in the development of emotional confidence. A learner-centred approach where the educators take the role of initiator and facilitator rather than teacher is important in enabling the transformation of the learning experience. Both educator and learner need to come to each interaction with an openness to learning, willingness to change and the security and freedom to recognise their own failings. This can be particularly challenging when we have spent a lot of time and energy investing in our self-identity as a competent skilled professional. However, accepting our fallibility provides opportunities to become more creative and learn new approaches (see the Kathryn Schulz TED talk mentioned above). Indeed, the professional duty of candour requires honesty and openness to recognise our potential for fallibility and to use this to provide safer and more person-centred practice (www.nmc.org.uk/globalassets/sitedocuments/nmc-publications/openness-and-honesty-professional-duty-of-candour.pdf).

If we understand ourselves through our mindset for learning and the role of authenticity, how then do we engage in effective and active learning? A crucial aspect of knowing ourselves is understanding how we prefer to learn as this also affects how we can facilitate others to learn. The next section of this chapter will address this and how our learning can become transformative. How the fundamental attributes of lifelong learning relate to the Person-centred Practice Framework is shown in Figure 33.4.

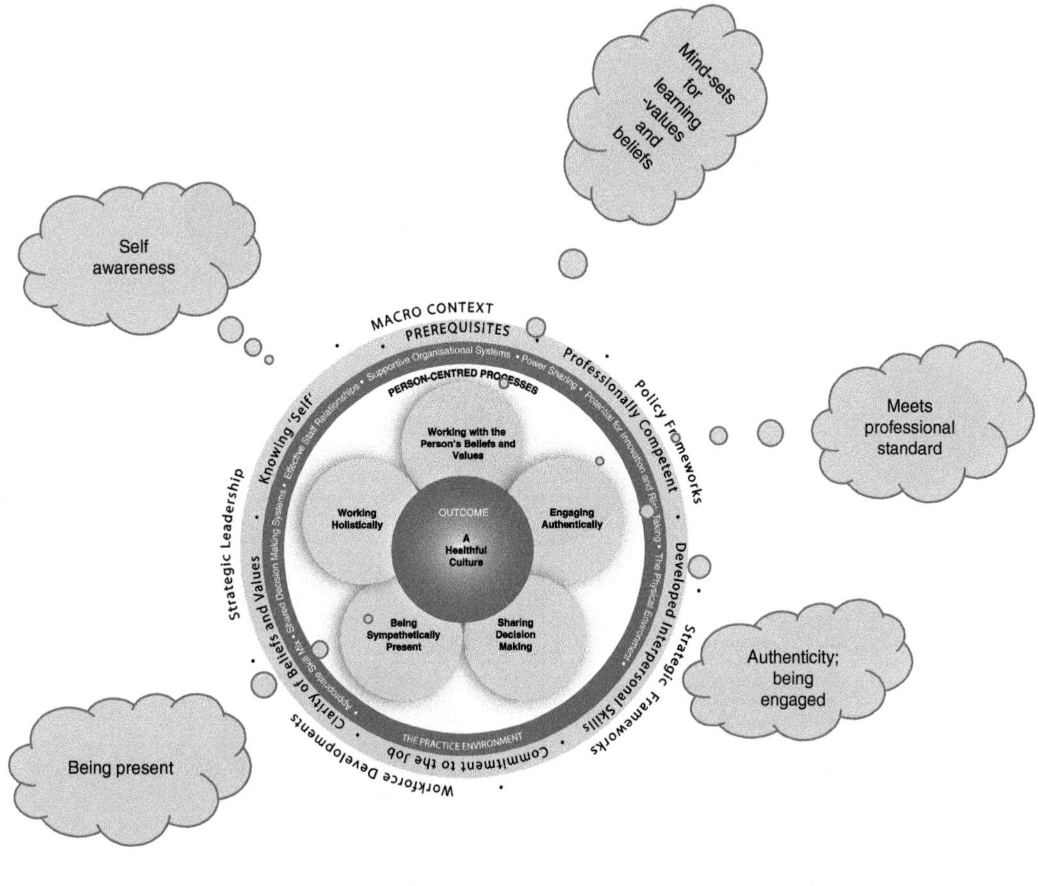

Figure 33.4 Lifelong learning attributes mapped to the Person-centred Practice Framework.

Practice learning as adult learners

Much has been written about the characteristics of successful adult learning (*andragogy*) (Knowles et al. 2015). Knowles' approach to supporting adult learning is built on five assumptions and underpinned by four principles (Figure 33.5).

Assumptions underpinning adult learning theory

These assumptions from the theories available suggest that adult learners:

- have moved from a dependent learning approach, being directed by other people, to a self-directed approach to learning
- have previously accumulated experience that is an important resource for future learning
- increasingly orientate their readiness to learn to the developmental tasks of their social roles
- have an orientation towards problem solving and problem-based learning and application to practice as opposed to a subject knowledge-based approach
- have developed an internal motivation to learn (as opposed to being directed to learn by others).

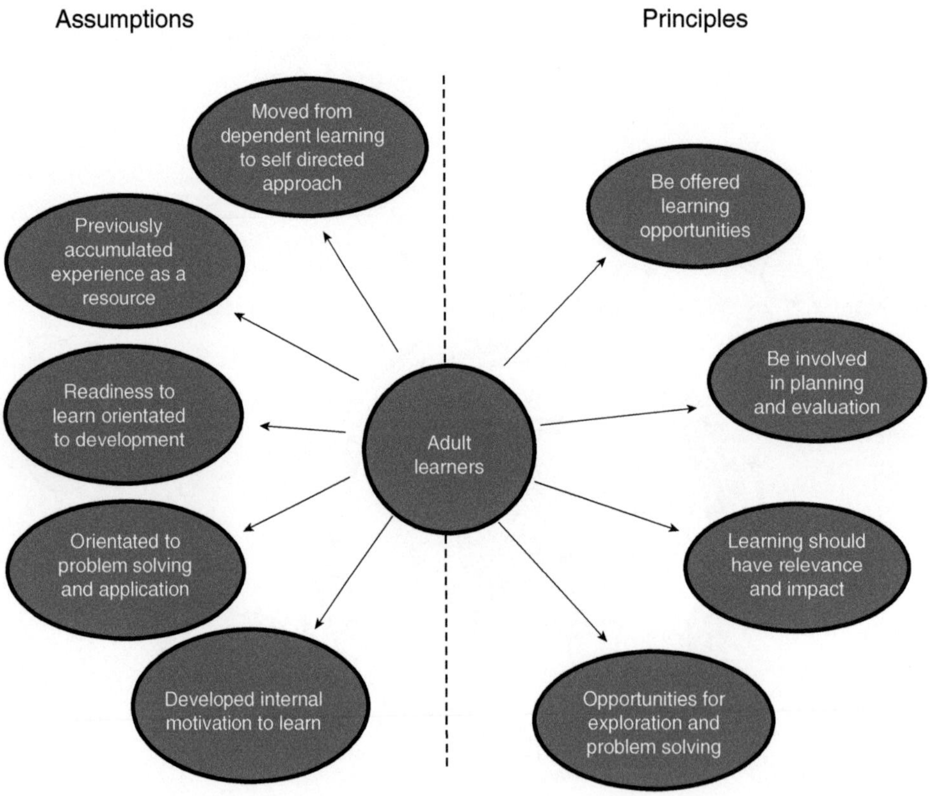

Figure 33.5 Assumptions and principles underpinning adult learning.

Principles that underpin adult learning

Adult learners should:

- be involved in the planning and evaluation of their instruction
- be offered opportunities to gain experience (including mistakes) which will provide the basis for the learning activities
- understand that experience and learning should have a clear relevance to and impact on their current or future role
- have opportunities to explore and solve problems, as opposed to being provided with answers.

Building on andragogy, with its emphasis on self-directed learning, *heutagogy* moves this further by focusing on a student-centred learning strategy that emphasises the development of autonomy, capacity and capability. It emphasises the need for learners to be facilitated to move beyond being self-directed and embrace self-determination in relation to their learning. The role of the learner is therefore to take responsibility for developing their own learning pathway, including creating learning goals and deciding upon the most appropriate methods for them to achieve their learning. In this approach, the educator facilitates learning through offering opportunity and space to learn, and the student takes responsibility for their learning. Key concepts in heutagogy include double-loop learning and self-reflection (see Chapter 29) where learners question and test their personal values and assumptions as being central to their learning (Blaschke 2012).

Activity

Hassan is a pre-registration learner who has a first degree in biology. He is undertaking a second degree in a healthcare subject at an Egyptian university and is currently in a practice learning environment. His personal academic tutor is concerned as his practice educator has contacted her to suggest Hassan is failing on practice learning. The practice educator indicates that he thinks Hassan is too confident as he keeps questioning the approach being used by qualified staff in their care roles. Hassan also is asking to attend various activities that he feels will assist him in his learning whereas the practice educator feels he should be on the unit at all times, working with his practice educator.

Based on your understanding of person-centred learning, what issues can you identify in this scenario that may be causing the problem for Hassan? Suggest how Hassan, the educator and the practice educator could work to resolve these issues.

In your discussions, you might have considered the practice educator's understanding of adult learning and heutagogy, Hassan's own stage of learning and the cultural context of the practice learning setting.

How we learn, and its effect on practice learning

As noted earlier in this chapter, as we evolve into adult learners we have opportunities to make decisions about our mindset (fixed or growth), and we need to develop an increased self-awareness about how we best learn. Unfortunately, formal learning opportunities (including practice) may be constrained in some of the approaches they adopt. This may be due to the need to try and meet the learning approaches of the largest number of people in a group, time and environment constraints or the limited range of approaches used by educators.

Reflecting on the Person-centred Practice Framework in the context of adult learning, and noting the importance of being present, we need to think about our values and beliefs about learning and be actively and authentically engaged in making informed decisions about what we are willing to do to grow and flourish as a person and professional. This requires us as adult learners to think about how we learn most effectively and to seek out these opportunities. We should reflect on our previous and current learning to explore why it is or isn't being successful. Often a defence is offered that the learning approaches used do not really 'suit me'. Reasons used to justify this may be that it is 'too academic', 'not relevant', 'not applicable to our specialist level of practice' or other comments to defend our lack of engagement to change the opportunities or consider how we can benefit most from them. Jack (1995) argued that one of the greatest factors that prevented new learning and creative approaches to change was what he named the DATA effect. This stands for our ability to defend our self-esteem and self-identity when faced with new ideas that may challenge our practice or thinking, and to claim there is little learning in these ideas for us because we are 'Doing All That Already'. As human beings, we are prone to staying in our 'comfort zones' so even when we are not embracing the new challenges presented, we may draw tentative similarities and comparisons to make it appear that we are doing this work and do not need to change.

From research on learning, we know that learners learn most when they feel valued – by themselves, those they are learning alongside and whoever is facilitating their learning. Thus, there needs to be a climate of mutual respect in these situations and learning will flourish in an environment of acceptance, empathy and trust (Taylor and Cranton 2012; Illeris 2014; Knowles et al. 2015). Mezirow (2000) suggested that for transformational learning to occur, learners, co-learners and educators should engage in a process of reflective discussion where 'taken for granted' assumptions are challenged and explored (see Chapter 29).

Developing reflexivity in learning

One of the most challenging aspects of becoming truly person-centred in all aspects of our life is developing the skills of reflexivity, as opposed to reflection. Reflection is a good starting point for 'knowing self' (Johns 2004); however, the disadvantage of imposing an external framework (such as a model or tool) for reflection is that it leaves little scope for us to draw on our own intuitions, values and priorities. Thus, reflexivity is an opportunity to help us push deeper into a situation to understand and grow from it, thus engaging in transformative learning.

Strategies for students to foster transformative learning

- Consider your mindset – fixed or growth; what factors may be impacting on this for you and how do you challenge these?
- Engage in developing self-awareness.
- Develop learning plans with clear outcomes to be achieved.
- Set goals/targets for yourself about what knowledge and skills you want to develop and why this is important to you.
- Engage with educators as a peer, in a person-centred, self-aware manner and be clear about how your learning can be supported.
- Through a process of discussion with educators, agree goals and learning contracts; these have two aspects – what you will do and what you need from them to succeed.

Strategies for educators to foster transformative learning

- Create a climate that supports transformative learning – immediate and helpful feedback that provides support for future learning, promote learner autonomy, participation and co-creation, engage in problem solving and critical reflection.
- Know yourself and the learners – what types of learning activities will appeal; ask the learners.
- Develop and use learning activities that expose and explore different points of view and different learning preferences.
- Provide adequate support, time, resources, opportunities and tools for reflection.
- Be self-aware and critically evaluate your own responses to practice learning situations. (This last strategy is a requirement for many professionals as part of their revalidation process.)

As reflection and reflexivity can potentially be stressful and ethically challenging, it is important to have plenty of time and to be well supported when engaging in reflection. We need to feel safe and to have access to others who are effective at reflecting and on whom we can model (see Chapter 29). Often learners value the opportunity to undertake solitary reflection *in private*. This is especially important when we reflect on situations that revealed ourselves in a less positive light and when there are issues of confidentiality to consider. These opportunities for reflection can be particularly meaningful and enduring. However, by working through discussion with peers and educators, we will also hear alternative perspectives and views that support development of our reflective adult learning.

Conclusion

Person-centred facilitated learning has the potential to encourage a growth mindset that fosters compassion and reflects the philosophy of learning as being about both 'being' and 'becoming'. To this end, the nature and relevance of lifelong learning and how it is situated within the development of person-centredness have been explored. Approaches to learning that allow us to know 'self' as a learner and understand our self-identity through transformative learning and critical reflectivity have been considered, with examples and ideas offered on how to continue developing as a person. Finally, the role of reflection and reflexivity in developing person-centred approaches to learning is discussed. Contrary to the belief that Darwin's theory is about survival of the fittest – meaning the strongest and most ruthless – it is 'survival of the kindest and most co-operative' that will ensure survival of our societies in the long term (Doty 2017).

Summary

- Understanding self and how we can use that to continue our learning throughout life is crucial in person-centred learning.
- Having a growth mindset will assist in facilitating our own and others' learning.
- Developing and continuing to use reflexivity in our practice will foster transformative learning.

References

Blaschke, L.M. (2012). Heutagogy and lifelong learning: a review of heutagogical practice and self-determined learning. *International Review of Research in Open and Distributed Learning* 13 (1): 56–71.

Doty, J.R. (2017). *Into the Magic Shop: A Neurosurgeon's Quest to Discover the Mysteries of the Brain and the Secrets of the Heart*. New York: Penguin.

Dweck, C. (2012). *Mindset: How You Can Fulfil your Potential*. New York: Random House.

Garrison, D.R. (2011). *E-Learning in the 21st Century: A Framework for Research and Practice*, 2e. New York: Routledge.

Illeris, K. (2014). *Transformative Learning and Identity*. Oxford: Routledge.

Jack, R. (1995). *Empowerment in Community Care*. New York: Springer.

Johns, C. (2004). *Becoming a Reflective Practitioner*, 2e. Oxford: Blackwell.

Knowles, M., Holton, E.F. III, and Swanson, R.A. (2015). *The Adult Learner*. Oxford: Routledge.

Lynch, B. and McCance, T. (2018). The development of the person-centred situational leadership framework: revealing the being of person-centredness in nursing homes. *Journal of Clinical Nursing* 27: 427–440.

McCance, T. and McCormack, B. (eds.) (2017). *Person-Centred Practice in Nursing and Health Care: Theory and Practice*. Oxford: Wiley Blackwell.

Mezirow, J. (2000). *Learning as Transformation: Critical Perspectives on a Theory in Progress*. San Francisco: Jossey-Bass.

Rodenburg, P. (2009). *Presence: How to Use Positive Energy for Success in Every Situation*. London: Penguin.

Taylor, E.W. and Cranton, P. (eds.) (2012). *The Handbook of Transformative Learning. Theory Research and Practice*. San Fransisco: Jossey-Bass.

Wenger, E. (1998). *Communities of Practice: Learning, Meaning, and Identity*. Cambridge: Cambridge University Press.

Further reading

Finlay, L. (2008). *Reflecting on 'Reflective practice'*. Practice Based Professional Learning Paper 52. Practice based Professional Learning Centre for Education Teaching and Learning, Open University. oro.open.ac.uk/68945/1/Findlay-(2008)-Reflecting-on-reflective-practice-PBPL-paper-52.pdf

Illeris, K. (ed.) (2018). *Contemporary Theories of Learning: Learning Theorists in Their Own Words*, 2e. London: Routledge.

O'Donnell, D., Cook, N., and Black, P. (2017). Person-centred nursing education. In: *Person-Centred Practice in Nursing and Health Care: Theory and Practice*, 2e (eds. B. McCormack and T. McCance), 99–117. Oxford: Wiley Blackwell.

Taylor, E.W. (2017). Critical reflection and transformative learning: a critical review. *PAACE Journal of Lifelong Learning* 26: 77–95.

34

The future of person-centred practice – a call to action!

Brendan McCormack[1], Tanya McCance[2], Donna Brown[2], Cathy Bulley[1], Ailsa McMillan[1], and Suzanne Martin[2]

[1] *Queen Margaret University, Edinburgh, Scotland, UK*
[2] *Ulster University, Northern Ireland, UK*

Contents

Fundamentals of Person-Centred Healthcare Practice, First Edition. Edited by Brendan McCormack, Tanya McCance, Cathy Bulley, Donna Brown, Ailsa McMillan and Suzanne Martin.

In this final chapter, we reflect on the work presented in this book and what it means for person-centredness and person-centred practice in the context of health and social care. We are conscious that you have been introduced to a variety of perspectives about person-centredness and a range of approaches to the practice of person-centred healthcare in a range of contexts. To the casual reader, this can feel a bit overwhelming and maybe even 'overkill' in paying attention to issues that for some people are routine everyday practices. It is precisely that tension that challenges all of us in the development of person-centred healthcare, in learning about person-centredness and in embodying it in everyday work. 'We do it but we don't call it that' is a retort that is familiar to all of us and it challenges us to language person-centred practice in a way that demonstrates its uniqueness, worthwhileness and transferability across contexts.

So in this the final chapter, we want to reflect on 'where we are at' and challenge all of us to be clear about our intentions and meanings as we take forward the future development of person-centred healthcare services. We will focus on two key discussion points that, for us, transcend the chapters of this book – (i) the need for conceptual and theoretical clarity and (ii) the KISS Principle!

The need for conceptual and theoretical clarity

It is still common for practitioners, academics and researchers to express the view that person-centredness is difficult to develop, implement or teach because we don't *really* know what it means and there are multiple definitions of the concept. In reality, there is little evidence to support such assertions as few definitions of person-centredness and person-centred practice have actually been published and those that have lack conceptual clarity, use patient and person-centredness interchangeably and mainly focus on care delivery (e.g. Slater 2006; Edvardsson 2015; The Health Foundation 2016; Suhonen et al. 2018) as opposed to a holistic view of the concept. The use of the term 'person-centred' and its derivations without any definition of terms being offered is prolific in published research and this does little to help practitioners develop a clear understanding of person-centredness and the elements they need to focus on. There is also a tendency to focus on the patient at the centre of care and decision making. Whilst nobody could object to such an important focus, it is only part of the story. Throughout this book, you will have seen that whilst we focus on professional practice for care delivery, we balance this focus with that of the practitioner and their needs. For an organisation to expect high-quality evidence-informed person-centred care to be provided to service users without an equal focus on the personhood of staff and their well-being is immoral. Thus, McCormack and McCance (2017) defined person-centredness as:

> . . .an approach to practice established through the formation and fostering of healthful relationships between all care providers, service users and others significant to them in their lives. It is underpinned by values of respect for persons (personhood), individual right to self-determination, mutual respect and understanding. It is enabled by cultures of empowerment that foster continuous approaches to practice development. (p. 3)

Whilst this definition resonates with the other definitions, through its focus on providing care that is consistent with persons' beliefs and values and how these are realised in different contexts, it differs significantly through its emphasis on a central outcome of 'healthful cultures' of practice. In working with that focus, we have challenged the dominance of focusing on person-centred care provided to, with and for patients at the expense of staff well-being. While none of us would challenge the centrality of the patient experience in determining outcomes from person-centred practice, we cannot overestimate the significance and importance of healthful cultures in enabling such care to be realised.

Healthfulness is not a concept that is generally used in the narrative of healthcare and in general terms is used to mean 'promoting good health'. This idea of promoting good health is a necessary but insufficient condition for person-centred practice. In this book, we have argued that healthfulness is *the* outcome arising from the development of person-centred cultures. Yes, it means promoting good health but in addition, it means ensuring that the environment in which healthcare is experienced has the individual health and well-being of all persons at the core of our concerns. It embraces outcomes of good care experiences, feeling of well-being and involvement in care arising from person-centred practice, previously articulated by McCormack and McCance (2017). For such outcomes to be achieved, all persons need to be energised by the context in which they work and for that energy to connect with the personhood of all persons. This perspective on well-being ensures that person-centredness is not a unidirectional activity focusing on ensuring that service users have a good care experience at the expense of staff well-being. Indeed, without a focus on staff well-being, we contend that person-centred care is an impossible and idealistic goal.

This is not a new argument and indeed, it is one that has been made by some of us for many years. However, it remains the case that the person-centredness of care providers is placed on a lower level of importance and significance to that of service users. Previously, McCormack and McCance (2010) argued that this is a morally inconsistent position for organisations to adopt, as without the same person-centred values being applied to *all persons*, person-centred care can never be fully realised and normalised in practice. We view this challenge as a conceptual one – a challenge whereby thought leaders, strategic planners, managers and decision makers stop using the 'it's too difficult to define' argument to defend organisational cultures that are non-conducive to the achievement of person-centred care for service users but instead, strive to make sense of what person-centredness could look like for all persons in an organisation.

In Chapters 1 and 2 we present conceptual and theoretical perspectives of person-centredness that can be applied in any (healthcare) organisation, any setting and with any team. The perspectives offered ground what might seem like complex concepts in the everyday realities of practice. We would argue that this application needs to go beyond student learning and individual staff responsibility to become a systems-wide responsibility for adoption. It is inappropriate for organisations to espouse the values of person-centredness and person-centred practice without doing the work needed to achieve conceptual clarity. For too many organisations, an obsession with 'quick-fix' solutions means that the time needed to achieve such clarity is sacrificed at the altar of expediency. Person-centred practice needs to be understood as a concept that is embedded in every strategy and policy that shapes healthcare planning and delivery. It needs to be based on conceptual frameworks that are inclusive of all persons and that clearly articulate how these concepts are to be embedded in everyday practices at macro, mezzo and micro levels of practice.

Lewin and Cartwright (1951) famously stated 'There is nothing so practical as a good theory' and this is an assertion that we would support. Conceptual clarity about person-centredness is critical as a basis for building shared understanding, shared meaning and a common language for practice. However, locating those concepts in a theory that explains how these concepts operate, as well as the relationships between concepts, is essential for ensuring consistency of practice, developing knowledge about practice and evaluating effectiveness. In Chapter 3 we identified the key components of a mid-range theory and the importance of these theories to the abstraction of key concepts and principles for practice. We discussed how a mid-range theory explains how we operationalise concepts such as health, environment and care and locate these in the context of perspectives of persons. Person-centred theory connects key concepts through the lens of personhood and whilst there are diverse philosophical perspectives on personhood (see Chapter 2), what is common is a shared understanding of the importance of recognising that persons are complex beings, shaped by embodied ways of being that in turn inform how we shape our actions.

This is an important consideration when reflecting on the practices you have read about in this book. In each chapter, the authors identified key activities to enhance your learning about person-centred practice in different contexts. Without locating these activities in theoretical perspectives, they are merely reflective activities about practice. But considering them through a theoretical lens means we can determine the relationships between these everyday practices and how they connect to build a person-centred culture. We would contend that if we are to advance person-centred practice, then we need facilitators, educators and leaders who are able to do this as an integral part of their engagement with others.

The Person-centred Practice Framework through which the theoretical lens of this book is framed has been developed through 23 years of research and scholarship by McCormack and McCance. They have critiqued concepts, tested relationships between concepts and explored different theoretical perspectives in order to create a framework that informs person-centredness at the level of systems. The development of this framework has been important in challenging the often dominant discourse of person-centred practice being the responsibility of individual practitioners, without systems-level engagement in providing the necessary infrastructure support to enable it to happen. In a review of person-centredness in healthcare (Harding et al. 2015), the Person-centred Practice Framework was recognised as one of the few that provided a systems lens on person-centred practice. The framework helps to bring alive the conceptual and theoretical perspectives that we contend are critical to having a deeper understanding of person-centredness, beyond those of choices and preferences, whilst we are realistic enough to understand that in busy and challenging practice environments, a theoretical framework of person-centredness is not the first 'tool' a healthcare worker will draw upon! Nor indeed is it likely that a single framework can cover everything we need to explain in order for person-centredness to become more of an everyday reality.

However, we would make the case for frameworks to be used by leaders and facilitators of culture change to help healthcare workers understand why person-centredness is important and, probably even more importantly, why it is difficult to achieve. As editors of this book, we have needed to engage with these difficult and challenging conversations too. We all feel passionately about the centrality of the person in healthcare and share values such as dignity, respect, compassion and social justice as central components of personhood, but how these values shape our lives and our engagements is different for all of us. These differences have the potential to divide us as a team, with each of us arguing for our particular view of the world shaped by our experience, or they can unite us around key concepts and life experiences that are embraced through our combined (but unique) narratives. In committing to a collaborative relationship, we each needed to embrace that which united us and learn to understand why we differed in other respects. These differences create points of contention and opportunities for transformation through learning from our unique narratives. The person-centred practice framework acted as a focus for these conversations – debating linkages with concepts, agreeing chapter titles, understanding why particular perspectives are located in certain chapters and even agreeing on writing teams for each chapter. Through the lens of the framework, we were able to listen and be listened to, connect and be connected, challenge and be challenged, and be present for each other as we engaged in complex concept clarification processes. Our process was no different from that of many healthcare workers lived out day after day.

So, if healthcare organisations are committed to developing person-centred cultures for all persons, we need decision makers to think about how they create opportunities for all persons to have spaces 'to be' with others and explore opportunities for increasing connections with personhood and for further developing person-centred practices. Developing complex systems is not the answer, but neither are simple quick fixes to complex problems.

The KISS Principle

In the 1960s, Kelly Johnson formulated the KISS (Keep It Simple Stupid) Principle. At the time, Johnson was working as an engineer in the development of aircraft. He coined this phrase to emphasise the importance of designing systems that were based on straightforward principles and that could be repaired by the 'average mechanic'. Johnson wasn't implying that mechanics who couldn't repair these systems were somehow 'stupid' – quite the opposite! Instead, he challenged the growing threat of systems becoming increasingly complex, to the point whereby the 'average mechanic' couldn't make sense of it without continuous development and training – so the system is stupid and not the person!

This principle resonates with us very strongly, as persons committed to advancing knowledge, skills and expertise in person-centredness and person-centred practices. Throughout this book, collaborating authors have worked with concepts, theories and frameworks to help make sense of what might seem like everyday practice in different contexts, with different client groups and articulating different knowledge and skills to bring to life person-centred practice in real-life situations. At the start of this chapter, we articulated the 'we do it anyway' principle that often dominates (and indeed kills!) conversations about person-centredness and person-centred practices. This is not the same as the KISS Principle. Indeed, it is clear to us that there is an increasing need for leaders and decision makers in organisations to engage in KISS Principle-based conversations in order to dig deeper into the landscape of person-centredness that might result in fundamental changes in how systems embrace and promote person-centred cultures. What do we mean by this?

Since person-centredness became a foundation principle underpinning healthcare strategy around the world, there has been a proliferation of initiatives to develop, implement and improve person-centred care in healthcare settings. A number of organisations have adopted a leading role in supporting person-centred care, especially through the use of quality improvement methods, including the World Health Organization (WHO 2015), the Institute of Health Improvement People and Family-centred Care Programme (http://www.ihi.org/Topics/PFCC/Pages/default.aspx) and The Health Foundation (2015). Some of these initiatives have become global foci for person-centredness, for example the 'What Matters to You' movement which focuses on changing the nature of conversations with service users from 'what's the matter with you?' to 'what matters to you', thus generating more personalised understanding of the needs of service users. Each year, June 6th is the designated 'what matters to you' day where healthcare organisations focus on these conversations as a means of promoting person-centred care (Healthcare Improvement Scotland 2019). Whilst these initiatives serve an important purpose in shining a light on the need for continuous and sustained efforts in developing person-centredness, the extent to which they create cultures of person-centredness that sustain practice over time needs to be questioned. Indeed, recent research into the long-term impact of 'Releasing Time to Care' (a global initiative to create more time in clinical teams for direct patient care) showed that six months after the end of formal projects, there was little evidence of the practices being sustained (Robert et al. 2020).

Many of the strategies used are 'simple' in that they are locally designed, informed by consensus and local information and make sense in the immediate context. However, the dominant focus is on the provision of person-centred care, without addressing the deep and complex factors that shape the workplace cultures where these initiatives are implemented. And as is the case with the 'Releasing Time to Care' research, simple solutions to freeing up time for practitioners to spend with patients require complex change processes to systems, processes, leadership, decision making and ways of working. Streamlining certain parts of a system to free up time will not on its own create a sustained change in how practitioners relate to service users. In the various chapters of this book that apply the concepts, philosophies and practices outlined in Section 1 in different contexts, we begin to understand that person-centred practice is not a 'one-off' event or a short-term project.

Instead, the authors outline the variety of key factors that need to be considered in order to bring about sustained culture change. We can also see that whilst the cultural and contextual nuances of the particular setting inform how these concepts, philosophies and practices are adopted, the concepts, philosophies and practices themselves are universal and apply to any setting or service user grouping. So the need for continuous reflection, reflexive practices and life-long facilitated learning is paramount. None of us can ever be assured of our person-centredness or judge the person-centredness of others. Instead, we need to be open to the everyday challenges that striving to be person-centred in our ways of being and doing present to us; to be able to work in a culture that enables reflection on our experiences and a system that supports facilitated engagement with reflexive learning throughout our careers. If organisations are to be taken seriously about their commitment to person-centred cultures, then these requirements are fundamental to our progress.

Resting place

So we have reached the end of this particular journey. However, the development of person-centred cultures is a never-ending process and one that needs tangible and real sustained commitment from healthcare organisations. For too long, providing person-centred care has been predominantly seen as an individual practitioner responsibility without the same degree of overt corporate responsibility from healthcare organisations. The sustainability of person-centred care is dependent on the existence of person-centred cultures and without this it remains an elusive ideal that is fragile and transient in nature. However, as the authors of the chapters of this book have demonstrated, if a whole-systems approach is adopted, then person-centredness can be a reality for all persons.

Person-centred healthcare
Alive
Living through our humanness

References

Edvardsson, E. (2015). Notes on person-centred care: what it is and what it is not. *Nordic Journal of Nursing Research* 35 (2): 65–66.

Harding, E., Wait, S., and Scrutton, J. (2015). *The State of Play in Person-Centred Care*. London: Health Foundation.

Health Foundation (2015). *Person-centred Care Resource Centre*. www.health.org.uk/publications/person-centred-care-made-simple

Healthcare Improvement Scotland (2019) 'What Matters to You?' Supporting More Meaningful Conversations in Day-to-Day Practice. A Multiple Case Study Evaluation. www.whatmatterstoyou.scot/wp-content/uploads/2019/09/wmty-evaluation-report-May2019.pdf

Lewin, K. and Cartwright, D. (eds.) (1951). *Field Theory in Social Science*. New York: Harper.

McCormack, B. and McCance, T. (2010). *Person-Centred Nursing: Theory, Models and Methods*. Oxford: Blackwell Publishing.

McCormack, B. and McCance, T. (2017). *Person-Centred Practice in Nursing and Healthcare: Theory and Practice*, 2e. Chichester: Wiley-Blackwell.

Robert, G., Sarre, S., Maben, J. et al. (2020). Exploring the sustainability of quality improvement interventions in healthcare organisations: a multiple methods study of the 10-year impact of the 'Productive Ward: releasing time to care' programme in English acute hospitals. *BMJ Quality and Safety* 29 (1): 31–40.

Slater, L. (2006). Person-centredness: a concept analysis. *Contemporary Nurse* 23 (1): 135–144.

Suhonen, R., Charalambous, A., Berg, A. et al. (2018). Hospitalised cancer patients' perceptions of individualised nursing care in four European countries. *European Journal of Cancer Care* 27: e12525.

The Health Foundation (2016). *Person-Centred Care Made Simple. What Everyone Should Know About Person-Centred Care*. London: The Health Foundation www.health.org.uk/sites/default/files/PersonCentredCareMadeSimple.pdf.

World Health Organization (2015). *WHO global strategy on people-centred and integrated health services. Interim Report*. https://apps.who.int/iris/bitstream/handle/10665/155002/WHO_HIS_SDS_2015.6_eng.pdf;jsessionid=86231CFDB4E5267E1B73A49EE634E1C6?sequence=1

Index

Page locators in **bold** indicate tables. Page locators in *italics* indicate figures. This index uses letter-by-letter alphabetization.

Fundamentals of Person-Centred Healthcare Practice, First Edition. Edited by Brendan McCormack, Tanya McCance, Cathy Bulley, Donna Brown, Ailsa McMillan and Suzanne Martin.